INVESTING IN THE HEALTH AND WELL-BEING OF YOUNG ADULTS

Committee on Improving the Health, Safety, and Well-Being of Young Adults

Board on Children, Youth, and Families

Richard J. Bonnie, Clare Stroud, and Heather Breiner, *Editors*

INSTITUTE OF MEDICINE *AND*
NATIONAL RESEARCH COUNCIL
OF THE NATIONAL ACADEMIES

THE NATIONAL ACADEMIES PRESS
Washington, D.C.
www.nap.edu

THE NATIONAL ACADEMIES PRESS 500 Fifth Street, NW Washington, DC 20001

NOTICE: The project that is the subject of this report was approved by the Governing Board of the National Research Council, whose members are drawn from the councils of the National Academy of Sciences, the National Academy of Engineering, and the Institute of Medicine. The members of the committee responsible for the report were chosen for their special competences and with regard for appropriate balance.

This study was supported by contracts and grants between the National Academy of Sciences and the Health Resources and Services Administration (HHSH25034014T), the Office of the Assistant Secretary for Planning and Evaluation (HHSP23337004), the Robert Wood Johnson Foundation, the Annie E. Casey Foundation, and the Department of Defense (HHSP23337009). Any opinions, findings, conclusions, or recommendations expressed in this publication are those of the author(s) and do not necessarily reflect the views of the organizations or agencies that provided support for the project.

International Standard Book Number-13: 978-0-309-30995-0
International Standard Book Number-10: 0-309-30995-6
Library of Congress Control Number: 2014959552

Additional copies of this report are available for sale from the National Academies Press, 500 Fifth Street, NW, Keck 360, Washington, DC 20001; (800) 624-6242 or (202) 334-3313; http://www.nap.edu.

For more information about the Institute of Medicine, visit the IOM home page at: **www.iom.edu.**

Printed in the United States of America

The serpent has been a symbol of long life, healing, and knowledge among almost all cultures and religions since the beginning of recorded history. The serpent adopted as a logotype by the Institute of Medicine is a relief carving from ancient Greece, now held by the Staatliche Museen in Berlin.

Suggested citation: IOM (Institute of Medicine) and NRC (National Research Council). 2014. *Investing in the health and well-being of young adults.* Washington, DC: The National Academies Press.

THE NATIONAL ACADEMIES

Advisers to the Nation on Science, Engineering, and Medicine

The **National Academy of Sciences** is a private, nonprofit, self-perpetuating society of distinguished scholars engaged in scientific and engineering research, dedicated to the furtherance of science and technology and to their use for the general welfare. Upon the authority of the charter granted to it by the Congress in 1863, the Academy has a mandate that requires it to advise the federal government on scientific and technical matters. Dr. Ralph J. Cicerone is president of the National Academy of Sciences.

The **National Academy of Engineering** was established in 1964, under the charter of the National Academy of Sciences, as a parallel organization of outstanding engineers. It is autonomous in its administration and in the selection of its members, sharing with the National Academy of Sciences the responsibility for advising the federal government. The National Academy of Engineering also sponsors engineering programs aimed at meeting national needs, encourages education and research, and recognizes the superior achievements of engineers. Dr. C. D. Mote, Jr., is president of the National Academy of Engineering.

The **Institute of Medicine** was established in 1970 by the National Academy of Sciences to secure the services of eminent members of appropriate professions in the examination of policy matters pertaining to the health of the public. The Institute acts under the responsibility given to the National Academy of Sciences by its congressional charter to be an adviser to the federal government and, upon its own initiative, to identify issues of medical care, research, and education. Dr. Victor J. Dzau is president of the Institute of Medicine.

The **National Research Council** was organized by the National Academy of Sciences in 1916 to associate the broad community of science and technology with the Academy's purposes of furthering knowledge and advising the federal government. Functioning in accordance with general policies determined by the Academy, the Council has become the principal operating agency of both the National Academy of Sciences and the National Academy of Engineering in providing services to the government, the public, and the scientific and engineering communities. The Council is administered jointly by both Academies and the Institute of Medicine. Dr. Ralph J. Cicerone and Dr. C. D. Mote, Jr., are chair and vice chair, respectively, of the National Research Council.

www.national-academies.org

COMMITTEE ON IMPROVING THE HEALTH, SAFETY, AND WELL-BEING OF YOUNG ADULTS

RICHARD BONNIE (*Chair*), Harrison Foundation Professor of Medicine and Law, University of Virginia School of Law
CLAIRE D. BRINDIS, Director, Philip R. Lee Institute for Health Policy Studies, University of California, San Francisco
GLADYS CARRIÓN, Commissioner, New York City Administration for Children's Services
MARK E. COURTNEY, Professor, School of Social Service Administration, University of Chicago, Illinois
ROBERT CROSNOE, The Elsie and Stanley E. (Skinny) Adams, Sr., Centennial Professor in Liberal Arts, Department of Sociology, The University of Texas, Austin
MARYANN DAVIS, Research Associate Professor, Systems and Psychosocial Advances Research Center, Department of Psychiatry, University of Massachusetts Medical School, Worcester
KATHLEEN MULLAN HARRIS, James E. Haar Distinguished Professor of Sociology, University of North Carolina at Chapel Hill
HARRY J. HOLZER, Professor, McCourt School of Public Policy, Georgetown University
CHARLES E. IRWIN, JR., Distinguished Professor of Pediatrics, UCSF Benioff Children's Hospital, University of California, San Francisco
BEATRIZ LUNA, Director, Laboratory of Neurocognitive Development, University of Pittsburgh, Pennsylvania
VELMA McBRIDE MURRY, Professor of Human Development and Lois Autrey Betts Chair, Department of Human and Organizational Development, Peabody College, Vanderbilt University, Nashville
ZIZI PAPACHARISSI, Professor and Head, Department of Communication, University of Illinois, Chicago
JOHN SCHULENBERG, Professor of Psychology and Research Professor, Institute for Social Research and Center for Human Growth and Development, University of Michigan, Ann Arbor
MARTIN SEPÚLVEDA, IBM Fellow & Vice President, IBM Research
KASISOMAYAJULA VISWANATH, Professor of Health Communications, Harvard School of Public Health
LESLIE R. WALKER, Professor and Chief, Adolescent Medicine Division, Seattle Children's Hospital and the University of Washington, Seattle

YOUNG ADULT ADVISORY GROUP

MARCUS BROWN, Chief Executive Officer, Adolesco Services
HERNAN CARVENTE, Research Assistant, Vera Institute of Justice
JENNIFER COLLINS, Student, University of Maryland
AMY DOHERTY, Board President, National Youth Leadership Network
SEMIRA ABDULMALIK KASSAHUN, Former Youth Advisor, Colorado Department of Public Health and Environment
JACKIE MALASKY, Public Health Professional, Baltimore, Maryland
PAUL RASTRELLI, Community Health Action Team Member, Kaiser Permanente
ANDREA VESSEL, Student, American University

Consultants

RONA BRIERE, Consultant Editor
VICTORIA FAUST, Doctoral Student, School of Ecology, University of Wisconsin–Madison
CONSTANCE FLANAGAN, Professor, School of Ecology, University of Wisconsin–Madison
RACHEL FAULKENBERRY McCLOUD, Doctoral Student, Harvard School of Public Health
LAUREN MIMS, Doctoral Student, University of Virginia
EVELYN STRAUSS, Consultant Writer
LAUREN TOBIAS, Principal, Maven Messaging and Communications
JOANNA WILLIAMS, Assistant Professor, University of Virginia

Project Staff

CLARE STROUD, Study Director
HEATHER BREINER, Associate Program Officer
DOUGLAS KANOVSKY, Senior Program Assistant
AMANDA PASCAVIS, Senior Program Assistant (July-August 2014)
FAYE HILLMAN, Financial Associate
PAMELLA ATAYI, Administrative Assistant
KIMBER BOGARD, Director, Board on Children, Youth, and Families

Reviewers

This report has been reviewed in draft form by individuals chosen for their diverse perspectives and technical expertise, in accordance with procedures approved by the National Research Council's Report Review Committee. The purpose of this independent review is to provide candid and critical comments that will assist the institution in making its published report as sound as possible and to ensure that the report meets institutional standards for objectivity, evidence, and responsiveness to the study charge. The review comments and draft manuscript remain confidential to protect the integrity of the deliberative process. We wish to thank the following individuals for their review of this report:

ANNE-MARIE BRAGA, Colorado Department of Public Health and Environment
ELLEN WRIGHT CLAYTON, Vanderbilt University
DONNA FUTTERMAN, Albert Einstein College of Medicine
ADRIANA GALVÁN, University of California, Los Angeles
RENÉE R. JENKINS, Howard University College of Medicine
MEREDITH KLEYKAMP, University of Maryland
ROBERT I. LERMAN, American University and Urban Institute
ELIZABETH LOWER-BASCH, Center for Law and Social Policy
MICHELLE R. MUNSON, New York University
ALICE SHOBE, Building Changes
PATRICK H. TOLAN, University of Virginia
PATIENCE WHITE, Got Transition

JOY JOHNSON WILSON, National Conference of State Legislatures
JONATHAN F. ZAFF, America's Promise Alliance

Although the reviewers listed above provided many constructive comments and suggestions, they were not asked to endorse the report's conclusions or recommendations, nor did they see the final draft of the report before its release. The review of this report was overseen by **ANTONIA M. VILLARRUEL,** University of Michigan School of Nursing, and **SARA ROSENBAUM,** The George Washington University School of Public Health and Health Services. Appointed by the National Research Council and the Institute of Medicine, they were responsible for making certain that an independent examination of this report was carried out in accordance with institutional procedures and that all review comments were carefully considered. Responsibility for the final content of this report rests entirely with the authoring committee and the institution.

Prologue[1]

Marcus Brown is working toward a business management degree at Davenport University in Grand Rapids, Michigan. He spent 5 years in the foster care system before being adopted into a family of 23 children.

Lack of contact with one's biological family raises significant questions that many people never encounter, Marcus said. "I have had experiences where I had to go to the hospital. They say, 'Tell me about your family.' I go, 'Your guess is as good as mine.'" Boys who grow up without a father can lack other basic information, too, and Marcus relied on social media to learn some basic life skills. "I did not know how to tie a tie, so I had to YouTube that," he said. "My other parent is the Internet."

Marcus offered ideas about ways to smooth and improve the transition from the foster care system into independent life. As adulthood looms and people are about to age out, "It is like, 'oh yeah, we want to talk to you about housing now.' I say, 'Should we not have talked about that a year ago so I could start saving for the deposit?'"

Hernan Carvente will soon graduate from the City University of New York with a bachelor's degree in criminal justice. He is a research assistant at the Vera Institute of Justice, where he works on projects related to juvenile justice and family engagement. Many of Hernan's insights and sug-

[1] The vignettes presented here are from eight young adults who served as a young adult advisory group to the committee that prepared this report. They provided written permission to include their stories, quotes, and names. Their stories are not intended to be representative of all young adult experiences and views. A description of the group and its work is in Chapter 1.

gestions are based on his experiences with various government institutions and programs. Beginning at age 15, he served 4 years at a secure juvenile detention facility. "My family was broken, so the gang became my family," he said. "The only system that could hold onto me was the criminal justice system, unfortunately."

Hernan highlighted the importance of problem-solving skills. "In public schools, I never experienced any structured lesson on how to deal with conflicts," he said. "With my troubled background, I had no ways to deal with issues impacting me at home, which led to issues with peers at school." He sees family-centered initiatives as a priority. Rather than telling parents that "you did no good," so "we are going to take care of your child," Hernan suggested that government programs "give the responsibility back to the people who brought that child into the world by offering them the appropriate resources." He also emphasized the value of communication among agencies. "When a young person goes into the foster care system and ends up in the criminal justice system, it is hell to get the data that was in the foster care system," said Hernan. Yet that information is essential to "understand what the young person went through" and provide the services he or she needs. "The systems fall apart when we don't have that collaboration."

Jennifer Collins entered foster care for the first time at age 7. As a teen, she struggled with mental health issues. Now pursuing a bachelor's degree in family science at the University of Maryland at College Park, she credits numerous "tireless advocates"—her social worker, foster mother, and adoptive mother—with helping her get the help she needed to persevere and succeed.

Jennifer spoke about the difficulties she faced while trying to navigate the Medicaid system, particularly when she was dealing with serious emotional challenges. "The most frustrating thing is just getting on the phone with someone," she said. "It usually took a drastic event, like me attempting to off myself, to access care. The only way you could get into the mental health system, as I recall, was the police had to take you there after you tried to take your own life." Jennifer raised other issues that are commonly misunderstood, such as abuse. "I don't think a lot of people realize that abuse may start at any point—and many people discount abuse of older kids," she said. "I was stuck in a situation for three years until I could get someone to listen. If I had been younger, someone would have done something sooner."

Jennifer pointed out that low Medicaid reimbursement rates lead to high turnover in the system and a lack of experienced professionals—a problem that has particularly grave ramifications in the area of mental health. When a person starts working with a new psychologist, "you are not starting where you dropped off before," she said. "You are starting all the way back at square one."

Amy Doherty graduated from Mount Holyoke College in South Hadley, Massachusetts, and conducts research in a vision rehabilitation lab. She was born legally blind and currently serves as board president for the National Youth Leadership Network, a group that works to break down isolation and build community among young people with disabilities.

Amy discussed the many challenges young adults face as they grow toward independence. "One of the things that I noticed in transitioning from high school to college was that you lose a lot of your support system," she said. The people who previously had played that role are no longer "right there with you." She talked about the importance of helping young adults access health care, which has been difficult for her, even with private insurance, and she also pointed out that young people typically do not learn financial management skills. That crucial topic "is missing from education," she said, "but it could be incorporated in lots of ways."

Semira AbdulMalik Kassahun came to the United States at age 3. Her English fluency grew, and she soon was translating for her parents at doctor appointments and teacher conferences to "make everything go smoothly . . . which is a typical scenario for U.S. immigrant families." Semira is the first person in her family to graduate college and is now pursuing a master's degree in public health, focusing on maternal and child health, at The George Washington University in Washington, DC.

"Growing up, you sometimes have to take charge," she said. "My parents always supported me by saying, 'Keep going,' but due to language and education barriers I needed to take the initiative of finding guidance and role models who I could ask about college and higher education." She now feels "proud and happy" to serve a similar role for young people in her community. In addition, she is reaching out to individuals beyond her cultural circle to raise awareness about issues that matter to her, such as religion. "I'm a Muslim and I follow Islam," she said. "There's a lot of work I've tried to do to fight misconceptions about Islam." Semira stressed the value of connections with older people to whom young adults can direct personal and professional questions. "Relationships are like fuel," she said, "helping young people move forward in their lives."

Jackie Malasky majored in public health and anthropology at New York University. She then earned a master's degree in education at The George Washington University, where she concentrated on maternal and child health. Jackie did her master's thesis on how men and women use the Internet differently to access sexual health resources online. She currently works as an HIV program evaluator.

Technology—especially social media—is changing how young adults mature and establish themselves in the world. "We are developing our self-identity by using two-way media," she said, but often "people post without really thinking about what it means or what it says about them." Jackie is especially interested in using entertainment to educate young adults. She also would like to see that they are trained to recognize and assist with mental health problems in their communities. "Our friends may be depressed," she said, but "we are not psychologists. How can I have the tools I need to really provide resources?"

Paul Rastrelli has always been interested in health, perhaps because both of his parents work in that field. In high school, he was already making significant contributions to his community's welfare. For instance, he spearheaded an antibullying campaign. Paul was a member of Kaiser's Community Health Action Team (CHAT), which is creating classroom resources that help students learn about comprehensive health. He commuted 2.5 hours to attend CHAT meetings, "but it was totally worth it," he said. He is now studying mechanical engineering at the University of Colorado Boulder.

Through his work with CHAT and other enterprises, Rastrelli encountered—and was captivated by—the concept of human-centered design. "When you are designing a product or an experience, you design around the eventual end user and really get their input," he said. He talked about the importance of following one's enthusiasm—and how social status can interfere with that endeavor. "Regardless of who you are, you contribute the most to the world when you feel you are doing something you are passionate about," he said.

Andrea Vessel grew up in a middle-class household with both of her parents. She often was racially isolated—the only black person in predominantly white communities—and felt pressured to "represent my culture," she said. As she advanced through school and noticed that fewer people "looked like me," she wanted "to prove myself." Because of her involvement in 4-H and Girl Scouts, she said, "I never thought, 'I couldn't do this' or 'people around me may not be doing this and I can't do it either.' I saw myself as being able to achieve." Now studying justice and law at American University in Washington, DC, she also serves as a youth trustee on the National 4-H Council Board of Trustees.

Andrea spoke about mistrust among young adults that can interfere with public health campaigns. "For example," she said, "when people say marijuana is bad, we think they are full of it. It's just some way to get us to not do drugs." Providing information about drugs rather than telling young adults what to think, Andrea suggested, might help empower them to make wise choices.

Preface

Young adulthood (spanning the ages of approximately 18-26) is a significant and pivotal time of life. During this time, young women and men typically complete their education, start working, develop relationships, and pursue other endeavors that help set them on the path to a healthy and productive adult life. Older adults, myself included, who have the opportunity to work on a daily basis with successive generations of young adults, often marvel at the energy, talent, creativity, and hopefulness they bring to their classrooms and workplaces and to their relationships with each other and their elders. Almost every new insight I have had in recent memory emerged from my interactions with the young adults I see every day. It is therefore all the more troubling that many young adults in our country are having difficulty accomplishing these transitions, particularly in the aftermath of the Great Recession and in the face of escalating costs of higher education. The dizzying pace of change in modern life also has confounded the traditional pathways to marriage, parenting, and other hallmarks of independent adulthood. Any conversation with today's young adults is likely to evoke observations about the stresses and uncertainties they confront.

The needs of young adults, and the challenges they face, do not receive a great deal of systematic attention in policy and research. Accordingly, the Health Resources and Services Administration asked the Institute of Medicine (IOM) to convene a committee to examine, analyze, and synthesize information and knowledge on the health, safety, and well-being of young adults. The IOM appointed a planning committee to design, organize, and conduct a workshop to review the current state of knowledge in this area.

The workshop was held on May 7-8, 2013, and a summary of the presentations was published in September 2013.[1] The Committee on Improving the Health, Safety, and Well-Being of Young Adults was then formed to conduct a consensus study and develop a set of recommendations for policies, programs, practices, systems development, service delivery, and research to address the needs of young adults and guide policy makers and other stakeholders in meeting those needs. (See Chapter 1 for the committee's full statement of task.) This report is the product of that study.

The central aim of this report is to draw attention to young adulthood as a distinct and important period in the life course of young people who are growing up in modern society. From a developmental standpoint, young adults are different, biologically and psychologically, from both adolescents and older adults in ways that affect their decision making, health, and behavior. From a social point of view, many of today's young adults confront major challenges in making a successful transition to adult roles in a rapidly changing and stressful world. Policy makers and service providers need to understand these differences in designing and implementing policies and programs to help young people accomplish these transitions successfully.

It is also important for public and private agencies monitoring the health, safety, and well-being of young adults to collect, classify, and maintain data in a way that permits researchers to analyze the status, behavior, and well-being of young adults, as well as their correlates and causes and the outcomes of interventions designed to improve them. Many of the report's recommendations focus on advancing understanding of young adulthood and the effects of policies and programs focused on this critical period of life. While the committee's recommendations include specific substantive changes in current policies and programs where the evidence is sufficiently compelling to warrant action, we were generally content to sketch our policy prescriptions with broad strokes, pointing the way for others to conduct more specialized investigations.

I would like to express my sincere appreciation to each member of the committee and the talented IOM staff for their extraordinary commitment to this important project. The health, safety, and well-being of young adults are of immense interest to us all as parents, colleagues, scientists, and members of the body politic. I am particularly grateful to our young adult advisory group for their uniquely insightful contributions to the committee's work.

Richard Bonnie, *Chair*
Committee on Improving the Health, Safety, and Well-Being of Young Adults

---

[1] The full text of the summary is available online via www.iom.edu/youngadults.

Acknowledgments

The committee would like to express its sincere gratitude to everyone who assisted in the development of this report. This work would not have been possible with the support of our sponsors—the Health Resources and Services Administration and the Office of the Assistant Secretary for Planning and Evaluation in the U.S. Department of Health and Human Services, the Robert Wood Johnson Foundation, the Annie E. Casey Foundation, and the U.S. Department of Defense. We thank them for generously providing information and responding to our questions.

Shortly after the study was initiated, a young adult advisory group was formed to give the committee opportunities for ongoing dialogue with young adults during the research phase of the study and the preparation of this report. We are grateful to the following individuals for their thoughtful comments throughout the study process: Marcus Brown, Hernan Carvente, Jennifer Collins, Amy Doherty, Semira AbdulMalik Kassahun, Jackie Malasky, Paul Rastrelli, and Andrea Vessel. Their efforts proved invaluable to the committee.

The committee would also like to acknowledge several consultants who contributed to this study: Constance Flanagan and Victoria Faust (University of Wisconsin–Madison) for their synthesis of research on civic engagement among young adults and service programs in which many young adults participate; Rachel Faulkenberry McCloud, a doctoral candidate in the Department of Social and Behavioral Sciences at the Harvard School of Public Health, for her assistance with the committee's review of the literature on public health interventions; Joanna Williams and Lauren Mims (University of Virginia) for their assistance in reviewing the literature on diversity; Sandra Graham at the University of California, Los Angeles, Graduate School of Education and Information Studies for her technical review; Evelyn Strauss for her assistance with writing and her advice on incorporating young adult voices throughout the report; and Lauren Tobias of Maven Messaging for her advice on presenting the evidence in a compelling manner. The committee is also grateful to Rona Briere and Alisa Decatur of Briere Associates, Inc., for their assistance in editing the report.

Many individuals volunteered significant time and effort to address and educate the committee during our information-gathering meetings (see Appendix A for the names of these speakers). In addition, Rebecca Gudeman of the National Center for Youth Law provided valuable information about confidentiality issues in young adult health. These contributions informed our deliberations and enhanced the quality of this report.

The committee also expresses its deep appreciation for the opportunity to work with the talented and dedicated members of the staff of the Institute of Medicine and the National Research Council on this important project. We are grateful for the ongoing contributions of Kimber Bogard, director of the Board on Children, Youth, and Families. The assistance of associate program officer Heather Breiner and senior program assistant Douglas Kanovsky were indispensable. Finally, special praise is due to study director Clare Stroud, whose impeccable planning, superb judgment, and faithful support made serving on (and especially chairing) this committee a genuine pleasure.

Contents

APPENDIXES

Summary[1]

Young adulthood—ages approximately 18 to 26—is a critical time in life. What happens during these years has profound and long-lasting implications for young adults' future employment and career paths and for their economic security, health, and well-being. Young adults are key contributors to the nation's workforce and military services and, since many are parents, to the healthy development and well-being of the next generation.

In recent decades, the world has changed in ways that place greater demands on young adults and provide less latitude for failure. The disruption and lengthening of established social and economic pathways into adulthood—graduating from high school, entering college or the workforce, taking on civic engagement and national service, leaving home, finding a spouse or partner, and starting a family—have presented more choices and opportunities for some young adults, and more barriers for others. And the transition to adulthood reflects the end of trial periods and the beginning of more consequential actions.

Providing educational, economic, social, and health supports will help young adults assume adult roles, develop marketable skills, and adopt healthy lifelong habits that will benefit them, their children, and the nation. Despite popular attention to some of the special circumstances of young adults, however, they are too rarely treated as a distinct population in policy, program design, and research. Instead, they are often grouped with adolescents or, more often, with all adults.

---

[1] This summary does not include references. Citations and detailed supporting evidence for the findings presented in the summary appear in the subsequent report chapters.

STUDY CHARGE

In light of these gaps in attention to the needs of young adults, the Health Resources and Services Administration (HRSA) and the Office of the Assistant Secretary for Planning and Evaluation in the U.S. Department of Health and Human Services, the Robert Wood Johnson Foundation, the Annie E. Casey Foundation, and the U.S. Department of Defense (DoD) commissioned the Institute of Medicine (IOM) and the National Research Council (NRC) to review and summarize what is known about the health, safety, and well-being of young adults and to offer recommendations for policy and research. The statement of task for this study is in Chapter 1. To respond to this charge, the IOM and the NRC convened a committee comprising experts in public health, the private sector, health care, behavioral health, social services, human development, psychology, neuroscience, demography, justice and law, sociology, economics, family studies, and media and communication. The committee prepared this report to assist federal, state, and local policy makers and program leaders, as well as employers, nonprofit organizations, and other community partners, in developing and enhancing policies and programs to improve young adults' health, safety, and well-being. The report also suggests priorities for research to inform policy and programs for young adults.

YOUNG ADULTS IN THE 21ST CENTURY: KEY FINDINGS

Young Adulthood Is a Critical Developmental Period

Young adulthood always has been a critical period of development, bridging adolescence and independent adulthood. It is a time when individuals face significant challenges and are expected to assume new responsibilities and obligations. Success or failure in navigating these paths can set young adults on a course that will strongly affect the trajectories of their adult lives. Earlier periods of the life course (e.g., early childhood) are widely viewed as critical windows of development and occasions for intervention, and young adulthood should also be seen in the same light.

The World Has Changed in Ways That Place Greater Demands on Young Adults

Although the normal course of physiological and biological development of young adults probably has not changed in many generations, the world in which they live has changed greatly. Today's young adults live in a more global and networked world, marked by increased knowledge and information transfer, heightened risks, fairly low social mobility, and greater economic inequality. Economic restructuring, advances in information and communication technologies, and changes in the labor market have radically altered the landscape of risk and opportunity in young adulthood. For example, earnings gaps between those with a BA and high school only have roughly doubled since 1980. The demands placed upon young adults are greater, and there is less latitude for failure.

Young Adults Today Follow Less Predictable Pathways Than Those in Previous Generations

Beginning in the 1970s, several well-established patterns of social and economic transition that once defined young adulthood have been altered. In previous generations, the path for most young adults was predictable: graduate from high school, enter college or the workforce, leave home, find a spouse, and start a family. While there were always exceptions, these established milestones provided structure and direction for young adults as they assumed adult responsibilities. Today, those pathways are considerably less predictable, often extended, and sometimes significantly more challenging, as the following examples illustrate:

- The cost of college has grown substantially, and many students have difficulty financing the investment or repaying the debt they incur, yet prospects for well-paying jobs for high school graduates without some postsecondary credential are slim. Although many young adults enter college, dropout rates are high, and degree programs take longer to complete.
- Even for young college graduates, well-compensated entry-level jobs are becoming more difficult to find, especially in the aftermath of the Great Recession that began in late 2007. Many companies do not provide health insurance or other nonsalary economic benefits. Low earnings plague many young workers because they lack skills needed for higher-paying knowledge-based jobs. Increasing numbers of the jobs available to them are part time.
- The estimate of a recent study is that 6.7 million youth and young adults aged 16-24—about 17 percent of the population in this age range—are neither in school nor working. The rates are highest among African Americans and those aged 20-24, almost all of whom have left high school.
- Partnership and parenting patterns have shifted substantially. Educated young adults often live together for many years before marrying and having children, while less-educated young adults often have children outside of marriage before gaining skills and income to support them. In addition, rapidly changing laws on same-sex

marriage are providing new opportunities for family formation among lesbian, gay, bisexual, and transgender young adults.
- The high cost of living independently has encouraged many young adults to move back into their parents' home.

Inequality Can Be Magnified During Young Adulthood

The disruption of these established social and economic pathways has presented more choice and opportunity for some young adults and more barriers for others. Marginalized[2] young adults—such as children of low-income immigrants, those aging out of foster care, those in the justice system, those with disabilities, those who dropped out of school, and those who bear responsibility for raising young children—are much less likely than other young adults to experience a successful transition to adulthood. Compared with their peers, for example, former foster youth are less likely to graduate from high school, have low rates of college attendance, suffer from more mental health problems and often experience poorer health, have a much higher rate of involvement with the criminal justice system, have a higher rate of dependence on public assistance, are more likely to be unemployed, and experience high levels of housing instability and homelessness. They also are less likely to marry or cohabit, but have higher rates of out-of-wedlock parenting and more children.

Despite extensive challenges, some of these young people ultimately fare very well as adults, and their hopes and aspirations are similar to those of young people who have not been marginalized. Meeting the needs of marginalized young adults not only improves their lives and can reduce persistent inequalities due to family background, but also has the potential to help them become fully contributing members of society. Absent deliberate action, however, this period of development is likely to magnify inequality, with lasting effects through adulthood.

Young Adults Are Surprisingly Unhealthy

Young adulthood is a critical period for protecting health, not just during the transitional years but over the life course. Despite some positives, however, the dominant pattern among young adults today is declining

[2] The committee's use of this term is informed by the concept of social exclusion, a concept denoting the economic, social, political, and cultural marginalization experienced by specific groups of people because of social forces such as poverty, discrimination, violence and trauma, disenfranchisement, and dislocation. Commitment to social inclusion is based on the belief that a democratic society benefits when all its members participate fully in community affairs. Viewing marginalized populations from this perspective helps shift the focus from individuals' difficulties or limitations to how society portrays and treats them.

health, seen most clearly in health behaviors and related health statuses such as the following:

- As adolescents age into their early and mid-20s, they are less likely to eat breakfast, exercise, and get regular physical and dental checkups, and more likely to east fast food, contract sexually transmitted diseases, smoke cigarettes, use marijuana and hard drugs, and binge drink.
- In many areas of risky behavior, young adults show a worse health profile than both adolescents and older adults. For example, compared with adolescents and adults aged 26-34, young adults aged 18-25 are more likely to be injured or die in motor vehicle crashes and to have related hospitalizations and emergency room visits. Thus, young adulthood is when many risky behaviors peak, but it is also the time when involvement in risky behaviors begins to decline.
- Young adulthood is a time of heightened psychological vulnerability and onset of serious mental health disorders, a problem compounded by failure to recognize illness or to seek treatment. Recent data show that almost one-fifth of young adults aged 18-25 had a mental illness in the past year, and 4 percent had a serious mental illness. Yet two-thirds of those with a mental illness and almost half of those with a serious mental illness did not receive treatment.
- The current generation of young adults appears to be at the forefront of the obesity epidemic and is more vulnerable than previous generations to obesity-related health consequences in later years. The National Longitudinal Study of Adolescent Health (Add Health) found that obesity rates more than tripled from adolescence (11 percent in 1995) to young adulthood (37 percent in 2008). More than one in four of those aged 24-32 had hypertension, 69 percent were prehypertensive, 7 percent had diabetes, and 27 percent were prediabetic.
- Prejudice and discrimination can negatively impact the health and well-being of young adults of color, but such factors as high racial/ethnic pride and exposure to both the familial and the dominant cultures can be protective.

The higher levels of poor health in young adulthood have important consequences for future health, educational attainment, and economic well-being. Rapid technological changes, economic challenges, and a prolonged transition to adulthood appear to be contributing to the health problems of young adults by increasing their stress and sedentary habits while making them less likely to participate in work and family roles that serve as strong social controls on risk taking. Therefore, these worrisome trends in young adult health can be expected to continue or worsen.

Supporting Young Adults Will Benefit Society

Much of the burden of the restructured economy has been borne by America's young adults. Young adults are resilient and adaptable, and many make remarkable accomplishments, demonstrating an extraordinary capacity for creative insight and innovation. At the same time, however, too many young adults are struggling to find a path to employment, economic security, and well-being. Healthy, productive, and skilled young adults are critical to the nation's workforce, global competitiveness, public safety, and national security. However, estimates indicate, for example, that 12 percent of all age-eligible men and 35 percent of all age-eligible women were unable to meet U.S. Army standards for weight-to-height ratio and percent body fat in 2007-2008. Furthermore, the DoD reported that between 2006 and 2011 62,000 individuals who arrived for military training failed their entrance physical because of their weight.

RECOMMENDATIONS FOR ACTION

Three common themes emerged from the committee's review of public and private policies and programs pertaining to young adults in the areas of education and employment, civic engagement and national service, public health, health care systems, and government programs for marginalized young adults. First, current policies and programs addressing this population too often are fragmented and uncoordinated. Second, these policies and programs often are inadequately focused on the specific developmental needs of this population. And third, the evidence base on interventions, policies, programs, and service designs that are effective for young adults is limited in most areas.

What is needed now is a coordinated effort by the public and private sectors to raise public awareness of the need to improve policies and programs that address the needs of young adults. To meet the unique needs of young adults will require heightened public understanding of the challenges they face and a robust public and private investment in their education and opportunities for employment. Investments in marginalized populations are particularly needed to reduce inequalities during the young adult years and increase the supply of skilled workers to serve the nation's future needs. Investing in public health and clinical preventive services will also be important because health underlies young adults' abilities to be successful in education, employment, and social relationships. Efforts to prevent and ameliorate the effects of behavioral health problems, including mood disorders, stress-related dysfunction, and substance use disorders, are critical as well.

Also key will be engaging young adults themselves—and not just high achievers—in the development of policies and programs that affect them. The powerful influence of young people who have lived in foster care in developing federal and state child welfare policy over the past two decades illustrates the potential of better engaging young adults in policy and program development.

While the need to invest in young adults is clear, the ideal nature of those investments is less so. As a result, the committee has generally avoided making recommendations for large-scale policy change. Instead, the current state of knowledge calls for coordination among federal, state, and local governments and philanthropies in engaging in experimentation to help identify the most effective approaches to improving the prospects of young adults. The most immediate tasks are to improve data and research and to make a concentrated effort to evaluate existing policies and programs at every level so as to achieve greater specificity and improve outcomes for young adults, while exploring new policies and programs. In the few contexts in which the evidence appears sufficient (e.g., education and employment), we have recommended some specific actions.

The committee first offers a cross-cutting recommendation that applies to all policies and programs addressing young adults, whether public or private, in all sectors of society. Subsequent recommendations focus on the key domains of education and employment, civic engagement and national service, public health, health care systems, and government investments in marginalized young adults.

Cross-Cutting Recommendation

Recommendation 9-1[3]: Federal, state, and local governments and nongovernmental entities that fund programs serving young adults or research affecting the health, safety, or well-being of this population should differentiate young adults from adolescents and older adults whenever permitted by law and programmatically appropriate.

To implement this recommendation, specific actions should be taken to

- modify reporting of data to identify young adults (aged 18-26) as a distinct age group in all reports, evaluations, and open data systems in which they are included;

[3] The committee's recommendations are numbered according to the chapter of the main text in which they appear.

- enhance new or existing surveys or experimental research focused on either adolescents or adults to advance knowledge regarding the health and well-being of young adults and healthy transitions into young adulthood;
- ensure that services provided to young adults are developmentally and culturally appropriate, recognizing that while adolescent or general adult services may sometimes be appropriate, modifications to existing services or entirely new approaches may be needed;
- engage diverse young adults in designing and implementing programs and services;
- support workforce training for health and human services providers to develop the skills and knowledge needed to work with young adults and their families;
- seek opportunities for coordinating services and, where possible, integrating them to achieve greater effectiveness and efficiency; and
- develop, implement, and evaluate systematic policy and program experiments to help identify the most effective approaches to improving the prospects of young adults.

It is important to note that this recommendation is not intended to imply the creation of an extensive set of new programs targeted only at young adults. Such an approach would have the potential to create new silos and similar concerns about discontinuities and lack of coordination as are found currently across programs for children/adolescents and adults. Rather, the intent is to increase focus on how policies and programs are currently working for young adults. We recommend the adaptation or creation of new policies, programs, and practices *only when the evidence indicates that young adults' specific needs are not being met*, with an emphasis on first attempting to modify existing efforts to better suit young adults. Further, we emphasize the importance of considering the transitions into and out of young adulthood to avoid inadvertently creating new discontinuities.

Relationships

Findings from recent two-generation programs, which invest simultaneously in young children and their parents, are promising and could be monitored closely, with successful programs being expanded to new sites. Such programs show potential for enhancing the outcomes experienced by young adults, and it is important that the programs value the parents as individuals in addition to the vital role they play in relation to the children.

Recommendation 3-1: In funding the implementation and evaluation of two-generation programs, philanthropic funders and federal government agencies should actively monitor the outcomes of the young parent participants in addition to early childhood outcomes. Doing so would be valuable for programs that target primarily health and well-being (such as home visiting programs), as well as those that target primarily human capital development.

Education and Employment

Enhancing the opportunities and the success of young adults will require (1) raising completion rates in high school and among those who enroll in postsecondary institutions, and (2) ensuring that the skills and credentials attained are ones the labor market actually rewards. To accomplish these goals will require better integrating institutions of secondary and higher education with workforce agencies and ensuring that both are more responsive to labor market needs than is the case today. In addition, more research is needed on what works for young adults who are neither working nor in education and those with disabilities and chronic health conditions.

Recommendation 4-1: State governments, with support from the U.S. Department of Education, should experiment with and evaluate a range of interventions designed to improve graduation rates at high schools and colleges, as well as the rates at which high school dropouts receive their General Educational Development (GED) credential and enroll in college or job training. These experiments should be primarily attempts to scale up interventions that have already been rigorously evaluated and generated positive impacts, such as (1) GED preparation or accelerated developmental education programs in college that integrate training (or at least labor market information) with remediation, (2) financial assistance that is more closely tied to individual performance as well as family income, (3) the provision of more information about college quality to high school students, and (4) mandated academic and career counseling for college students.

To encourage experimentation and evaluation of these interventions, the committee recommends the following specific actions:

- The U.S. Department of Education should continue to provide competitive grants for states that implement such interventions state- or county-wide and rigorously evaluate them, as it has done recently through its High School Graduation Initiative.

- The U.S. Department of Education should provide technical assistance for any states that undertake such interventions.
- State governments should encourage local school systems and the 2- and 4-year colleges in their state to implement such interventions, including by providing resources and assistance, and should rigorously evaluate them.
- State and local school systems should particularly experiment with and evaluate programs designed to reduce the enormous disparities in high school and college completion that now exist by race, family income, and geographic location (urban versus rural).
- State governments should promote the adoption by colleges of health and social supports that appear to encourage academic success among young adult enrollees.

Recommendation 4-2: State governments, with support from the U.S. Departments of Education and Labor, should implement and evaluate education and workforce development approaches that are more closely tied to high-demand economic sectors. These approaches should include sectoral models and partnerships (e.g., among employers, community colleges, and intermediaries), career pathways, high-quality career and technical education in high school, apprenticeships, and other forms of work-based learning.

To facilitate the implementation of these education and workforce development approaches, the committee recommends the following specific actions:

- The U.S. Departments of Education and Labor should provide competitive grants—perhaps modeled on the Race to the Top program for K-12 education, which had large impacts on state policy and practice—for states that implement such interventions at a medium or large scale and rigorously evaluate them.
- The U.S. Departments of Education and Labor should provide technical assistance for any states that undertake such interventions.
- State governments should encourage local colleges and workforce boards to implement such interventions, including by providing resources and assistance, and should rigorously evaluate them.

To improve the education and employment outcomes of young adults and also the efficiency of resources spent on higher education and workforce development, it will be necessary to improve both the information available to students and workers and the incentives for education institutions to improve the outcomes they generate.

Recommendation 4-3: State governments should experiment with and evaluate providing performance-based subsidies to their public colleges and universities, with performance being measured by credits earned, time to degree, and graduation rates. Weight also should be given to the subsequent labor market employment and earnings of graduates. States should ensure as well that college students have access to up-to-date labor market information and career counseling based on that information.

To facilitate state governments' implementation of these education and workforce development incentives, the committee recommends the following specific actions:

- The U.S. Departments of Education and Labor should provide competitive grants for states' use of performance-based subsidies for public colleges and universities. These grants should be targeted at states that implement such incentives state-wide and rigorously evaluate them.
- The U.S. Departments of Education and Labor should provide technical assistance for any states that undertake such incentives.
- States should give substantial weight to performance measures for specifically disadvantaged populations to help ensure that colleges meet performance requirements by applying improved practices to populations similar to those they have been serving, rather than by raising admission requirements to exclude more-disadvantaged students.

Civic Engagement and National Service

Civic engagement and national service, including military service, can contribute to optimal development during the transition to adulthood by providing new and alternative opportunities to contribute to society in meaningful ways, to form one's identity, and to explore the larger world. For some, national service is a logical next step after college; for those who do not go on to college, it can be a path to social incorporation and to skill and network building. If national service is to serve this function for marginalized young adults, however, it must provide at least some of the scaffolds (mentoring, counseling, education and training, guided practice in leadership and teamwork) that are built into curricular and co-curricular college life. To this end, sponsors of such programs need to focus on the development of the participants as well as community impact when evaluating program success. Unfortunately, the Corporation for National and Community Service recently shifted its evaluation priorities to focus primarily on community impact rather than on participants' development. This policy should be modified.

Recommendation 5-1: The Corporation for National and Community Service, the U.S. Department of Labor, and other entities that fund service programs should expand and improve opportunities for service for all young adults. They also should emphasize member development (in addition to community impact) in program evaluations, including the short- and long-term effects of service on participants' health and well-being.

Public Health

Because young adults confront more challenges to health and safety than is commonly assumed, and given the desirability of nurturing lifelong healthy habits, public health programs and clinical preventive services for young adults should be a high priority. Mobile digital media and social networking have the potential to play a pivotal role as vehicles for public health interventions, and research on the effectiveness of these technologies is a high priority.

Community interventions focused on binge drinking and alcohol-impaired driving, as well as tobacco control, demonstrate the effectiveness of multipronged and reinforcing community interventions that target and are tailored to individual behavior as well as the social environment and legal context. Such interventions require concerted and sustained implementation and a clear commitment to documenting outcomes for different groups of young adults (e.g., rural versus urban, by educational status). Very few state or local public health programs, however, have attempted to coordinate or integrate programs for young adults, although such initiatives have been undertaken in a handful of states. Several recent federal initiatives also represent a nascent effort to promote and support policies and practices reflecting an integrated understanding of young adulthood. Under the new Adolescent and Young Adult Health Program funded by HRSA, states and localities will be encouraged to expand services beyond adolescents.

Recommendation 6-1: State and local public health departments should establish an office to coordinate programs and services bearing on the health, safety, and well-being of young adults. If a separate office is not established for young adults, these responsibilities should be assigned to the adolescent health coordinator.

This initiative would promote the development of state- and community-level partnerships to advance coordination and integration through collaborative activities that promote the health, safety, and well-being of young adults.

In addition, to strengthen the collective ability to address the needs of young adults, the committee makes the following recommendation:

Recommendation 6-2: Each community should establish a multistakeholder private-public coalition on "Healthy Transitions to Adulthood," with the goal of promoting the education, health, safety, and well-being of all young adults. State or local public health agencies should take the lead in convening these coalitions. The coalitions should include young adults; colleges and universities; providers of career and technical education; employers; youth organizations; nonprofit organizations; medical specialties providing primary care to young adults; and other community organizations serving, supporting, or investing in young adults. These initiatives should mobilize public and private engagement and support; set priorities; formulate strategies for reaching all groups of young adults who need services and support; and design, implement, and evaluate prevention activities and programs. Initiatives should also incorporate the valuable input of young adults in shaping their scope and activities to ensure that there is traction among those initiatives aimed at improving their health, safety, and well-being.

Forty percent of the U.S. population is anticipated to be affected by the Centers for Disease Control and Prevention's Community Transformation Grant (CTG) program. The measurable performance goals of the CTG program are to reduce the following by 5 percent within 5 years: death and disability due to tobacco, the rate of obesity through nutrition and physical activity interventions, and death/disability due to heart disease and stroke. This program presents a good opportunity to address some of the issues that are important for young adults.

Recommendation 6-3: Recipients of Community Transformation Grants—including state and local government agencies, tribes and territories, and nonprofit organizations—should incorporate specific targets for young adults in their plans to reach the 5-year measurable performance goals in the areas of reducing death and disability due to tobacco use and reducing the rate of obesity through nutrition and physical activity interventions.

Health Care Systems

The majority of young adults' health problems are preventable. However, efforts to provide preventive care to young adults are complicated by

(1) the lack of a consolidated package of preventive medical, behavioral, and oral health guidelines focused specifically on the young adult population; (2) the fact that navigating the health care system during the transition from pediatric to adult providers is confusing and difficult, especially for those with behavioral health problems or a chronic condition; and (3) the limited availability of behavioral health interventions developed specifically for young adults, the early stages of development of those interventions for young adults that do exist, and the limited availability of interventions with demonstrated efficacy specifically in this population.

Recommendation 7-1: Health care delivery systems and provider organizations serving young adults (e.g., medical homes, accountable care organizations)—with input from the Agency for Healthcare Research and Quality (AHRQ) and the Centers for Medicare & Medicaid Services (CMS)—should improve the transition process for young adults moving from pediatric to adult medical and behavioral health care.

To implement this recommendation, the committee recommends the following specific actions:

- AHRQ should develop quality performance metrics on the transition-of-care process to ensure continuity of care for young adults making this transition.
- CMS should encourage greater attention to this transition within the innovation models that it solicits and funds, such as those from the Center for Medicare & Medicaid Innovation.
- Health care delivery systems and provider organizations serving young adults should develop a coordinated pediatric-to-adult transition-of-care process within their organizations.
- Pediatric-to-adult transition-of-care performance metrics should be incorporated into quality measurement and reporting frameworks by the National Committee for Quality Assurance, the National Quality Forum, and other quality measurement entities for all health care delivery models serving young adults, such as medical homes, accountable care organizations, and integrated delivery systems.
- The Office of the National Coordinator for Health Information Technology should ensure that meaningful use criteria enable the capture of relevant data elements for reporting on the pediatric-to-adult transition-of-care process.
- CMS, health insurers, and purchasing entities such as employer coalitions should incorporate young adult transition-of-care met-

rics into pay-for-performance initiatives, contracting, and other provider assessments.

- The Maternal and Child Health Bureau in the Health Resources and Services Administration should expand its work on transition-of-care metrics for youth with special health care needs to include all youth and young adults, incorporate such metrics in Title V program requirements, and support related capacity development and training in states.

Recommendation 7-2: The U.S. Preventive Services Task Force should develop a consolidated set of standardized evidence-based recommendations for clinical preventive services such as screenings, counseling services, and preventive medications specifically for young adults aged 18-26. Behavioral and oral health should be included in these recommendations.

Federal, state, and local government entities that fund or provide physical or behavioral health services—including the U.S. Department of Health and Human Services (through the Substance Abuse and Mental Health Services Administration, HRSA, AHRQ, CMS, and the Indian Health Service), DoD, the U.S. Department of Veterans Affairs, and corresponding state and local agencies, in partnership with commercial insurers and employer-sponsored health plans, should be involved in improving preventive care for young adults.

Recommendation 7-3: Federal, state, and local governments, commercial insurers, employer-sponsored health plans, and medical and behavioral health systems should adopt the clinical preventive services recommended by the U.S. Preventive Services Task Force, include the delivery of those services in quality performance metrics used for pay-for-performance and other health care provider assessments, and require public reporting of compliance.

Recommendation 7-4: The National Institutes of Health should support research aimed at developing a set of evidence-based practices for medical and behavioral health care, including prevention, for young adults. This research should build on the existing and established evidence-based practices (EBPs) for populations that are older (i.e., adults in general) or younger (i.e., adolescents) to

- **identify those EBPs that hold promise for being effective in this age group and test them for efficacy;**

- **identify EBPs that are likely to be effective with modification for this age group and test the efficacy of the modified versions; and**
- **identify behavioral and medical health care needs that are unlikely to be addressed by existing or modified EBPs and conduct research to develop and establish new EBPs for young adults in these areas.**

In developing methodologies for implementing this recommendation, it will be important to take into account socioeconomic position and racial, ethnic, and geographic disparities and differences, as well as differences according to immigrant and refugee status, across the full spectrum of the social, behavioral, and health indicators under discussion.

Government Investments in Marginalized Populations

Although young adults from marginalized populations are a heterogeneous group, they share a number of characteristics and experiences, such as living in poverty and behavioral health problems. Similarly, there is considerable overlap in the populations reached by the many programs that serve marginalized young adults. However, the lack of a comprehensive view of these populations limits the development of policies and programs intended to reduce their marginalization.

Recommendation 8-1: Federal and state government agencies—including the U.S. Departments of Health and Human Services, Labor, Justice, Housing and Urban Development, and Education and the corresponding state agencies—should incorporate a greater focus on marginalized young adults in ongoing and new population-based cross-sectional and longitudinal studies of young adults.

To implement this recommendation, the committee recommends the following specific actions:

- In conducting ongoing studies and developing new studies, agencies should actively involve planning and advisory groups comprising researchers and program managers familiar with the various marginalized populations, as well as representatives from these populations who have experienced such life events. Doing so would help ensure that study designs, including sampling and recruitment strategies and survey items, will better capture the experiences of these populations.
- Agencies should consider oversampling of marginalized populations to better distinguish their experiences from those of other young adults.

Recommendation 8-2: Federal and state governments should continue encouraging programs that serve marginalized populations to make better use of administrative data for describing the overlap of populations across service systems and young adults' trajectories into and out of these systems, and for evaluating policies and programs affecting young adults.

To implement this recommendation, the committee recommends the following specific actions:

- Federal agencies operating programs that affect young adults should aggressively implement the recent Office of Management and Budget "Guidance for Providing and Using Administrative Data for Statistical Purposes."
- Federal agencies serving young adults—including the U.S. Departments of Health and Human Services, Labor, Justice, Housing and Urban Development, and Education—and philanthropic funders should fund demonstration projects at the state level to support states in integrating program administrative data to better understand marginalized young adults and evaluate programs serving them.
- State government agencies serving marginalized young adults should expand on existing state and local efforts to integrate and use administrative data to better understand and serve these young adults.

Fragmented programs have narrow and idiosyncratic eligibility criteria that hinder young adults from obtaining the help they need, often create lapses in help when it is provided, and too often are stigmatizing. Major entitlement programs intended to help marginalized populations provide limited support for young adults, and discretionary programs targeting these populations often fall far short of meeting demonstrable needs. Collective accountability for improving the overall health and well-being of marginalized young adults is hampered by the multiple distinct, and often fragmented and uncoordinated, outputs and outcomes associated with the plethora of programs.

Recommendation 8-3: Congress and the Executive Branch should amend federal laws and regulations to allow for more flexible and efficient eligibility determination and service provision across marginalized young adult populations.

Recommendation 8-4: Congress and the Executive Branch at the federal level and state legislatures and governors at the state level should amend laws and regulations to create accountability for achieving improvement on a limited set of key outcomes for marginalized young adults (e.g., employment, education, housing stability, safety, health, connections to responsible adults, and effective parenting).

Recommendation 8-5: In funding evaluations of programs for marginalized young adults, the federal government and philanthropic funders should emphasize evaluation of programs aimed at improving outcomes across multiple marginalized populations while remaining sensitive to differences across subpopulations.

CONCLUSION

Focusing on the health and well-being of the current cohort of young adults (those becoming adults in the first third of the 21st century) is especially important because of the powerful (and perhaps transformative) economic and social forces now at work—the restructuring of the economy, widening inequality, a rapidly increasing "elder dependency ratio" (i.e., the ratio of the population aged 65 and older to the working-age population), a substantial increase in immigration, and the increasing diversity of the U.S. population. The future well-being of the nation rests on the investments made in *all* young adults today—particularly those whose background and characteristics put them at risk of experiencing the greatest struggles. Providing more of the educational, economic, social, and health supports they need will help ensure equal opportunity, erase disparities, and enable more young adults to successfully embrace adult roles as healthy workers, parents, and citizens.

1

Introduction

Young adulthood, spanning approximately ages 18 to 26,[1] is a transitional period during the life course when young people are traditionally expected to become financially independent, to establish romantic relationships and become parents, and to assume responsible roles as productive and engaged members of the community. From a developmental point of view, young adulthood is characterized by a period of normal and predictable biological and psychological maturation, but the specific social roles and tasks expected of each cohort of young adults are determined by the characteristics of the particular society at a particular time in history. In contemporary American society, young adulthood is marked by great heterogeneity of transitional experiences, with considerable variability in the timing, sequencing, and content of social roles and tasks.

The social expectations associated with young adulthood in the United States have changed markedly in recent decades. Many people do not view or treat young people aged 18-26 as adults, perhaps because their life experiences do not match traditional views of adulthood as a time of being both independent and responsible for others (Settersten and Ray, 2010). Indeed, national surveys reveal that only a bare majority of Americans label people in their early 20s as adults, even though large majorities did so in the past (Taylor et al., 2012). As they move from adolescence into adulthood, therefore, young adults do not seem to be either adolescents or adults, but

[1] The ages of 18 and 26 are arbitrary markers of the boundaries of both the developmental process and the social transitions that define young adulthood. Moving the markers to 16 and 30 would encompass a wider range of individual variation.

a little of both. The uncertainty of this "in-between" period and the ways in which it flows out of early life trajectories and shapes future life trajectories make it a time of both individual risk and opportunity, and a time when societal inequalities may be reproduced or reduced. As a result, social and institutional supports that may help young people navigate these uncertain years toward more certain futures assume particular importance (Arnett, 2004; Furstenberg, 2010; Roisman et al., 2004).

A systematic approach to understanding and responding to the unique circumstances and needs of today's young adults can help pave the way to a more productive and equitable tomorrow for young adults in particular and U.S. society at large. Unfortunately, despite popular attention to the special circumstances of young adults,[2] they are rarely treated as a distinct subpopulation in research and policy. Instead, they are often grouped with adolescents or, more often, with all adults. As the "in-between" subpopulation, they are getting lost in the shuffle.

STUDY CHARGE

Recognizing this paucity of attention to young adulthood as a distinct period of life in policy and research, the Health Resources and Services Administration and the Office of the Assistant Secretary for Planning and Evaluation in the U.S. Department of Health and Human Services, the Robert Wood Johnson Foundation, the Annie E. Casey Foundation, and the U.S. Department of Defense commissioned the Institute of Medicine (IOM) and the National Research Council (NRC) to review and summarize what is known about the health, safety, and well-being of young adults and to offer recommendations for policy and research. To respond to this charge, the IOM and the NRC appointed the Committee on Improving the Health, Safety, and Well-Being of Young Adults, drawn from both the public and private sectors, with expertise in public health, health care, behavioral health, social services, human development, psychology, neuroscience, demography, justice and law, sociology, economics, family studies, and media and communication. The committee's full statement of task is in Box 1-1, and biosketches of the committee members are in Appendix D.

CONTEXT FOR THIS STUDY

The committee's work is well situated in a rich intellectual and scientific tradition focused on understanding and studying the development of trajectories over the life course, as described below. In addition, several recent federal initiatives reflect a nascent effort to focus research and policy

---

[2] See the 2010 *New York Times Magazine* cover asking, "What Is It About Twentysomethings?"

BOX 1-1
Statement of Task

An ad hoc committee will conduct a study and prepare a report on the state of the science and policies pertinent to the life course of young adults (approximately 18-26 years old), as well as their transitions from adolescence (starting at about age 16) and to full adulthood (up to about age 30). The study will constitute Phase 2 of a three-part effort, following the completion in Phase 1 of the workshop titled "Improving the Health, Safety, and Well-Being of Young Adults, a Hidden Population." The study committee will review the available literature on young adults in the context of their health and development, building on the workshop as appropriate; the committee will also consider systems and institutions that provide pathways from adolescence into adulthood; and policies that impact young adult health and well-being. The following topics are of interest:

- The demographic profile of young adults today and historical shifts over time
- Neurobiological development of young adults
- Health behaviors, including substance abuse, and relationship to later outcomes
- Health and well-being of vulnerable populations
- Health and well-being of first-, second-, and third-generation immigrants
- Well-being of young adults in public systems and institutions (e.g., military, justice, welfare, college/university)
- Application of public health practices, and access to and use of health services
- Shifting roles and responsibilities within the family unit
- Labor force, economic, and civic engagement
- Policies that foster young adult health and well-being
- How young adults receive information and make decisions

Based on currently available evidence, the report will include—but will not necessarily be limited to—consideration of the above topics. Among these topics, the report may provide particular attention to policy and program areas that have the greatest potential for impacting young adults' lives. The report will provide recommendations for policies, programs, research, systems development, and service delivery that can facilitate the health, safety, and well-being of all young adults and inform policy makers and other stakeholders. The report will also inform institutions serving young adults. Recommendations will be primarily geared toward federal departments and their agencies (e.g., U.S. Department of Health and Human Services and such agencies as the Health Resources and Services Administration/Maternal and Child Health Bureau; National Institutes of Health; Centers for Disease Control and Prevention; Agency for Healthcare Research and Quality; Substance Abuse and Mental Health Services Administration; U.S. Department of Defense; U.S. Department of Labor; U.S. Department of Justice) as well as state agencies. As appropriate, the report may also provide recommendations aimed at legislatures, local governments, and nongovernmental entities. The report will also identify areas for further research to answer questions raised during the study process. Phase 3 will be planned to cover the dissemination/communication of the reports resulting from Phases 1 and 2.

BOX 1-2
Selected Federal Initiatives on Young Adults

My Brother's Keeper. This initiative of President Obama is intended to address persistent employment and education gaps for boys and young men of color, which continue throughout their lives, and to encourage action and partnerships to this end across multiple sectors, including government, business, nonprofit, philanthropic, faith, and community partners (My Brother's Keeper Task Force, 2014; Obama, 2014).

Young Adult Indicator Data. The Federal Interagency Forum on Child and Family Statistics released a special issue report on young adult data indicators in July 2014. This report provides data from nationally representative, federally sponsored surveys on young adults aged 18-24 in the following key areas: education; economic circumstances; family formation; civic, social, and personal behavior; and health and safety (Federal Interagency Forum on Child and Family Statistics, 2014).

Healthy People 2020 Adolescent and Young Adult Indicators. Healthy People establishes health goals and objectives, which are revised every 10 years to reflect changes in the health challenges facing the nation. *Healthy People 2020* addresses adolescents and young adults in greater depth than in previous decades by identifying 41 indicators for adolescent and young adult health (HHS, 2012). These include outcome and system-level indicators in seven areas: health care, healthy development, injury and violence prevention, mental health, substance abuse, sexual health, and prevention of chronic diseases of adulthood.

The Substance Abuse and Mental Health Services Administration's (SAMHSA's) Grants to Improve Mental Health Services for Young People. In September 2014, the U.S. Department of Health and Human Services announced $99 million in grants for an expanded set of mental health initiatives, with a particular focus on children and young people (HHS, 2014a). This effort is a component of President Obama's *Now Is the Time* plan, which is focused on reducing gun violence (The White House, 2013). The fiscal year 2015 budget provides SAMHSA with $130 million to use for mental health treatment for students, which is estimated to impact 750,000 young people (HHS, 2014b). Two of these SAMHSA initiatives are particularly relevant to young adults. First, working with the Health Resources and Services Administration, SAMHSA will provide $35 million toward training mental health professionals to serve students and young adults. Second, SAMHSA will award $20 million in grants in the Healthy Transitions program, which will support young adults aged 16-25—and their families—at high risk for mental illness, substance abuse, and suicide (SAMHSA, 2014).

The above are examples of initiatives that include a major focus on young adults. Other government initiatives focus on preparing adolescents for the transition to adulthood. An example of such an initiative is Promoting Readiness of Minors in Supplemental Security Income (PROMISE), a major interagency initiative to help youth with disabilities transition successfully to adult self-sufficiency (U.S. Department of Education, 2014).

development on the distinct capacities, vulnerabilities, and needs of young adults (see Box 1-2). This report is intended to build on these efforts, with a particular focus on the health and well-being of young adults.

The Intellectual and Scientific Context

This report builds on the work of an influential sequence of research networks funded by the John D. and Catherine T. MacArthur Foundation over several decades, including initiatives on successful aging, midlife, and adolescent development. The Network on Transitions to Adulthood brought together a diverse group of scholars from 2000 to 2009 to examine the changing nature of early adulthood (MacArthur, 2014). Major program areas were education, labor economics, marriage and relationships, changing attitudes and norms, and various populations of young adults. This fruitful initiative resulted in many books, briefs, and articles (e.g., Carr and Kefalas, 2009; Danziger and Rouse, 2007; Osgood et al., 2005; Settersten and Ray, 2010; Settersten et al., 2005; Waters et al., 2011). The present report extends the MacArthur network's extensive body of work by incorporating a focus on health and well-being, connecting the study of young adulthood to recent advances in developmental neuroscience, incorporating research published since the network finished its work, and offering concrete policy and program recommendations.

The Policy Context

The importance of focusing policy attention on young adults has become increasingly evident. An aim of this report is to consolidate information on these efforts and encourage similar initiatives by other federal agencies.

METHODS

This report represents the second phase of a three-phase project. The first phase was a large public workshop held in May 2013 to highlight research on the development, health, safety, and well-being of young adults. A published summary of the workshop presentations and discussions is available (IOM and NRC, 2013). The second phase was the consensus study that produced this report and is described in more detail below. The third phase will be extensive communication and dissemination activities.

The committee's work on this report was accomplished over a 12-month period that started in October 2013. The committee held four meetings between December 2013 and June 2014 that included both closed-session deliberations and open-session information-gathering dialogues with subject matter experts and stakeholders. During the first meeting, the committee received its charge from sponsors and held an information-gathering session to gain an overview of selected federal policies and programs relevant to the health, safety, and well-being of young adults. The second meeting included a 1-day workshop focused primarily on state policies and programs that impact young adults' health, safety, and well-being. That workshop also included a session on social media and information technology. The third meeting included a brief information-gathering session that explored the experience of young adults in the justice system. The agendas for these public sessions are available in Appendix A. The May 2013 workshop and its published summary, mentioned above, also were an important source of information for the committee (IOM and NRC, 2013).

In addition to the above information-gathering sessions, the committee examined the relevant peer-reviewed literature and available information on state and federal policies and programs; gathered information through personal contacts; and commissioned a paper on civic engagement, volunteerism, and national service programs and their impact on young adults' well-being. This paper provided extensive material for Chapter 5 of this report and is included in full on the project website.[3]

A young adult advisory group also informed the committee's work. This group of eight young adults met with the committee twice in person and several times by conference call to provide input and feedback on the topics the committee was examining. A brief vignette about each member appears in the prologue to this report, and the members are quoted throughout the report. The group's members were identified through organizations that work with young adults and through individual recommendations, and several had spoken at the May 2013 public workshop. Collectively, they brought diverse perspectives and experiences to this study, but their stories and views are not intended to be representative of all young adults. The group's members provided written permission to include their stories, quotes, and names.

STUDY APPROACH

This section explains the use of key terms in this report and provides some brief comments about how the committee approached its task. Chapter 2 offers a broader introduction to the report, including background information and key findings and their implications for policy and programs.

[3] See http://www.iom.edu/youngadults.

Key Terms and Definitions

Young Adults

This report defines *young adults* as individuals aged approximately 18-26 and focuses primarily on this age range. Recognizing the continuity of human development and the fact that some individuals will take on typical "young adult" tasks at slightly younger and slightly older ages, the report also considers the transitions from adolescence (starting at about age 16) into full adulthood (up to about age 30). There are no definitive reasons to select these specific cut-off points, and it will sometimes make sense to adjust the age period to take account of unique considerations in a particular policy context. However, in an effort to promote consistency in data analysis across domains of research and policy, the committee arrived at the age range 18-26 after considerable deliberation. The choice of 18 as the lower bound of young adulthood is conventional from a societal point of view—it is the "age of majority," the point at which individuals are legally considered adults not only in this country but in many other countries around the world as well. The choice of 26 as the upper bound is less clear. From biological and societal perspectives, no compelling evidence supports 26 versus 24, 25, 27, or 28. The committee's selection of 26 rests primarily on societal considerations. Based on the evidence reviewed in Chapter 2, 26 (up to the 27th birthday) denotes a point at which a large portion of young adults have completed some of the transitions typically associated with adulthood and are settling into adult status in society. Many current data sources use 24 as the upper bound,[4] which appears to underestimate the duration of this transitional period for most young adults. Further, it is noteworthy that the 26th birthday is the age used in the Patient Protection and Affordable Care Act to mark the point at which young adults are no longer covered under a parent's health insurance policy—the most prominent policy to date to recognize the special needs of young adults during this transitional period.

To refer to the age group immediately younger than young adults, the committee uses the terms *adolescents* and *youth* in the disciplinary contexts in which these terms are typically used. For example, *adolescent* is more common in health fields, while *youth* is commonly used in economics and can sometimes encompass both older adolescents and young adults (e.g., ages 16-24). Just as we have described for young adults, a variety of different age ranges also are used for adolescents (for an overview, see NRC and IOM [2009]). To differentiate adolescents from young adults for the

---

[4] For example, the data sources used in the *Healthy People 2020* core indicators for adolescent and young adult health use the following age ranges for young adults: 18-24, 18-21, 22-24, 20-24, and 21-24 (HHS, 2012).

purposes of this report, we consider age 17 to be the upper boundary of adolescence. We use the term *children* to refer to the youngest individuals.

Health and Well-Being

The report takes a broad view of the health and well-being of young adults, applying the World Health Organization's definition of health as a resource for active living encompassing social, physical, and mental well-being (WHO, 2006). Being healthy in this sense requires access to comprehensive, quality, and affordable medical care. But it also necessitates the use of system-level approaches to create and sustain the conditions needed for health and well-being, including strong families, supportive social networks, educational attainment, and productive employment.

Health Care

The term *health care* is used broadly in this report to include both physical and behavioral health. *Physical health* is a general term encompassing the human body's capacity to meet life's demands. It includes the promotion of overall physical fitness and the prevention and treatment of diseases and medical conditions that impair the normal functions of the body, including dental, medical, and developmental functions. The term *behavioral health* is a general term encompassing the promotion of emotional health; the prevention of mental and substance use disorders; and treatments and services for substance abuse, addiction, and mental and substance use disorders (SAMHSA, 2011). When one of these two areas of health care is specifically being discussed, the particular term is used; otherwise the term *health care* applies to both physical and behavioral health.

Young Adults Who Are Marginalized, Disadvantaged, and Disconnected

Studies and official policy documents pertaining to young adults use different terms to refer to those who face the most challenging obstacles in making a successful transition to independent adulthood. The committee has chosen to use *marginalized young adults* as the primary term in referring to this population, while reserving two other terms for contexts in which their use is standard in the pertinent discipline.

Marginalized young adults are young adults who exhibit characteristics that put them at risk for poor outcomes during young adulthood. Examples of young adults who may be marginalized are those living in poverty, children of low-income immigrants, those aging out of foster care, those in the justice system, those with disabilities, those who have dropped out of school, and those who bear responsibility for raising young children. Our use of this term is informed by the concept of social exclusion, a concept denoting the economic, social, political, and cultural marginalization experienced by specific groups of people because of social forces such as poverty, discrimination, violence and trauma, disenfranchisement, and dislocation (Daly and Silver, 2008; Mathiesen et al., 2008; Sen, 2000). Commitment to social inclusion is based on the belief that a democratic society benefits when all its members participate fully in community affairs. Viewing marginalized populations from this perspective helps shift the focus from individuals' difficulties or limitations to how society portrays and treats them. An emphasis on social inclusion calls for the identification of policies that exclude certain groups from full participation in society and the development of policies that enhance opportunities for full participation. We believe social exclusion is a useful lens through which to view how policies contribute to or ameliorate the relatively poor outcomes experienced by the groups of young people on which we focus here.

While *marginalized young adults* is the primary term used in this report, two other terms with related but distinct meanings are used in the context of young adults' educational attainment and employment. *Disadvantaged young adults* refers to young adults who come from families with lower incomes and/or educational attainment, while *young adults who are disconnected* are those without parental responsibilities who are neither enrolled in education nor employed.[5]

A Lens on Young Adults

The primary lens of this report is on young adults themselves, and of course this is an important focus, particularly in areas in which morbidity, mortality, and well-being indicators show worse outcomes for this age group relative to younger and older groups or long-term impacts throughout adulthood. However, the research presented in the report also makes clear that young adults' well-being has a critical impact on society at large, in both the short and long terms. Since many young adults are parents of young children, the report also highlights that investing in young adults has potential benefits for their young children, and therefore can complement existing efforts to support the health, safety, and well-being of the youngest members of society.

[5] A report by Belfield and colleagues (2012) coined the term *opportunity youth* to describe young people, disconnected from all major institutions, who present an opportunity for society to devise new ways to reengage them. Although this term conveys an important point about the promise associated with better supporting these young adults, we have elected to use *marginalized* to emphasize society's role in the circumstances of these young adults, as described above in the Key Terms and Definitions section.

Program Selection and Data Limitations

A challenge entailed in preparing this report was the overwhelming number and range of state and federal policies and programs that are potentially relevant to young adults and, at the same time, a paucity of data specific to young adults within these programs.

Young adults are eligible for inclusion in a majority of federal programs aimed at adults in such domains as labor, education, justice, health, and social services, with the exception of programs that target solely adults of retirement age and older. Young adults, particularly those aged 18 to 21, also are included in many programs and systems for children and adolescents. Only a couple of federal programs exclusively target young adults. Therefore, the committee had to consider both youth- and adult-targeted programs, as well as transitions between the two, which occur at different ages depending on the system and state. There are also a large number of specialty programs that target specific populations and outcomes, as illustrated particularly in Chapter 8, which examines government programs for marginalized young adults. In selecting programs for particular attention within the report, the committee focused primarily on those that serve a large number of young adults and those that are most relevant to the critical tasks of young adulthood, such as completing education, finding and keeping a job, obtaining health care coverage, and learning to navigate the adult health system.

Despite the abundance of programs that potentially impact young adults, specific information on young adults is frequently missing because they often are combined with adolescents in youth-focused programs and with older adults in adult-focused programs. In many cases, it was difficult to ascertain the number of young adults within the population served, and evaluation efforts typically did not assess effectiveness specifically for young adults. As described further in Chapter 2, there are developmental reasons why programs that show effectiveness across adults generally may not necessarily be effective for young adults, and vice versa.

Scope and Focus of the Report

The committee faced several challenges in determining how to carry out a charge that was so broad in scope (see Box 1-1). First, the charge called for reviewing the "the state of the science . . . pertinent to the life course of young adults." A wide-angle lens was required to synthesize knowledge and draw general conclusions about the health and well-being of the whole population of young adults. We have attempted to accomplish this in Chapter 2, which provides a broad overview of the complex transition from adolescence to young adulthood. At the same time, the charge invited specific recommendations for action in those "policy and program areas with the greatest potential" to affect the lives of young adults. To this end, we exercised our collective judgment in selecting several areas to explore in depth in the remainder of the report.

Topics Explored in Depth

The committee chose to concentrate on five policy-relevant domains. The programs and policies most central to the study charge are those relating to health (Chapters 6 and 7) and education and employment (Chapter 4). In addition, we chose to focus on policies and programs designed to serve populations of young adults perceived to be in need of help beyond what is available from their families and communities (Chapter 8). We also examined the relationships that are created during young adulthood, as well as the continuing relationships with parents, and considered policy and program implications of findings in this domain (Chapter 3). Finally, we chose to focus on civic engagement and national service because of the many government programs in this area and the salience of these activities to young adulthood (Chapter 5).

Many other policy areas also merit attention, including parental support obligations, correctional programs for young adult offenders, and services and supports available to unauthorized immigrants. While these topics are mentioned in the report, the committee was not well constituted to delve deeply into family policy, criminal justice administration, or immigration policy. Another area we chose not to address in depth is the highly specialized body of law, policies, and programs pertaining to young adults with severe developmental disabilities. While these individuals and their families confront transitions related to legal classifications and services during the age period of interest (18-26), those transitions differ substantially, in developmental and social terms, from those that lie at the center of this report for young adults who have opportunities for a successful transition to independent adulthood.

Heterogeneity

Another challenge the committee faced was finding the right approach for conveying, in a single, integrated report, the diverse experiences, pathways, and trajectories of the heterogeneous population of young adults. The same challenge would confront a committee charged with characterizing the "current status" of "children" or "adolescents" in the United States. Any such developmentally oriented inquiry will reveal wide differences in health and well-being among the individuals in the focal population, divergent trajectories as they age, and variations in the need for interventions to improve and shift these trajectories. In such a mixed picture, how does the observer develop an integrative narrative? Does one focus on vulnerabilities and risks or on strengths and resilience?

Choice of tone and emphasis was a constant theme in the committee's deliberations from the outset of the study. Inevitably, a policy-oriented discussion of the health, safety, and well-being of any population will tend to focus on the left end of the distribution (on young adults with greater needs) and on the potential value of interventions, rather than on those who are more successful and who do not require interventions to keep them on track. However, this tendency to focus on the negative was frequently counteracted by reminders that the period of young adulthood is also a time when even the most disadvantaged young people demonstrate resilience and when many young people make remarkable accomplishments, demonstrating an extraordinary capacity for creative insight and innovation. That being said, this report does tend to focus on those areas in which opportunities for healthy productive futures are now being squandered and in which support and protection are most needed to help young adults live healthy and productive lives and contribute to the well-being of their families and communities.

Haves and Have-Nots

Chapter 2 provides a broad overview of the diverse pathways into adulthood taken by recent cohorts of young adults, ranging from those who progress through these transition years with strong financial and emotional support from parents to those who have no connections with parents and little financial support for education, workforce entry, and the creation of strong social relationships. One of the committee's concerns is that the demands of education, workforce entry, and parenting faced by young adults today tend to magnify the effects of preexisting inequality. Thus, from a policy standpoint, the report naturally emphasizes the need to provide the resources and supports that will enable the least advantaged young adults to accomplish successful transitions to independent and productive lives as adults. The transcendent goal is preserving opportunity for *all* young adults.

Racial and Ethnic Disparities

Every domain of public policy in the United States is bedeviled by disparities in outcomes associated with race and ethnicity and by the challenges of eliminating these disparities. In the context of this report, the committee describes disparities in educational achievement, employment, health and health care outcomes, and participation in social service programs. However, further focused efforts are needed to provide in-depth analyses of the causes and consequences of disparities in each of these policy domains and to develop detailed policies to address them among young adults. A related topic of direct relevance to the committee's charge is the impact of experiencing prejudice and discrimination on the health and well-being of young adults. This topic is addressed briefly in Chapter 2 in the context of observations about the increasing diversity of American life and the prospects for eliminating prejudice and discrimination based on race and ethnicity. Appendix B explores this topic in somewhat greater detail, but the committee is convinced that it warrants a comprehensive review on its own.

Recommendations

The recommendations offered in this report focus primarily on federal and state agencies, as the study charge specifies; the committee was also authorized to direct recommendations to local governments and nongovernmental entities, including private employers. Our main aim in this report is to set the stage for informed policy making. At present, evidence in most areas is insufficient to permit firm recommendations. The most immediate tasks are to improve data and research and to make a concentrated effort to evaluate existing policies and programs at every level so as to achieve greater specificity and improve outcomes for young adults, while exploring new policies and programs. In the few contexts in which the evidence appears sufficient (e.g., education and employment), we recommend specific actions. In other areas, we recommend some preliminary strategies designed to promote coordination across currently fragmented program areas and to identify those areas that might be ripe for experimentation and innovation.

ORGANIZATION OF THE REPORT

The remainder of this report examines young adults' health, safety, and well-being within various domains. Chapter 2 provides a broad overview of the transitional challenges and opportunities of young adulthood. It summarizes developmental changes occurring during this period and examines the broader social and economic structures that impact young adults' health, safety, and well-being. The chapter concludes with key findings from this review of development and trends and their implications for policies and programs. Chapter 3 considers young adults' relationships with their parents, friends, and romantic partners. Chapter 4 focuses on young adults' education and employment; the discussion includes consideration of the bidirectional relationship between education/employment and health/well-being. Chapter 5 looks at young adults' civic engagement and participation in national service, including both national service programs and the military. Chapter 6 examines public health priorities, interventions, and programs for young adults, while Chapter 7 focuses on young adults within the health care system, including consideration of behavioral health. Chapter 8 addresses marginalized young adults and examines the government programs designed to support them. Finally, Chapter 9 provides a summary of the committee's suggested approach for enhancing young adults' health, safety, and well-being, including recommendations for policies and programs, as well as priorities for research.

REFERENCES

Arnett, J. J. 2004. *Emerging adulthood: The winding road from the late teens through the twenties.* New York: Oxford University Press.

Belfield, C. R., H. M. Levin, and R. Rosen. 2012. *The economic value of opportunity youth.* Washington, DC: Corporation for National and Community Service.

Carr, P., and M. Kefalas. 2009. *Hollowing out the middle: The rural brain drain and what it means for America.* Boston, MA: Beacon Press.

Daly, M., and H. Silver. 2008. Social exclusion and social capital: A comparison and critique. *Theory and Society* 37(6):537-566.

Danziger, S., and C. Rouse, eds. 2007. *The price of independence: The economics of early adulthood.* New York: Russell Sage Foundation.

Federal Interagency Forum on Child and Family Statistics. 2014. *America's young adults: Special Issue, 2014.* Washington, DC: U.S. Government Printing Office.

Furstenberg, F. F., Jr. 2010. On a new schedule: Transitions to adulthood and family change. *The Future of Children* 20(1):67-87.

HHS (U.S. Department of Health and Human Services). 2012. *Healthy people 2020: Core indicators for adolescent and young adults health.* http://www.healthypeople.gov/2020/learn/Draft_Core_Indicators_Web.pdf (accessed July 14, 2014).

HHS. 2014a. *HHS announces $99 million in new grants to improve mental health services for young people.* http://www.hhs.gov/news/press/2014pres/09/20140922a.html?utm_campaign=09%2F22%2F2014%20-%20news%20release%20-%20mental%20health%20grants&utm_medium=email&utm_source=hhs%20news%20releases&utm_content=text%20-%20title%20link (accessed October 1, 2014).

HHS. 2014b. *HHS FY2015 budget in brief.* http://www.hhs.gov/budget/fy2015-hhs-budget-in-brief/hhs-fy2015budget-in-brief-samhsa.html (accessed October 1, 2014).

IOM (Institute of Medicine) and NRC (National Research Council). 2013. *Improving the health and well-being of young adults: Workshop summary.* Washington, DC: The National Academies Press.

MacArthur. 2014. *About the network on transitions to adulthood.* http://transitions.s410.sureserver.com/about (accessed June 14, 2014).

Mathiesen, J., J. Popay, E. Enoch, S. Escorel, M. Hernandez, H. Johnston, and L. Rispel. 2008. *Social exclusion: Meaning, measurement and experiences and links to health inequalities. A review of literature.* WHO Social Exclusion Knowledge Network Background Paper 1. http://www.who.int/social_determinants/media/sekn_meaning_measurement_experience_2008.pdf (accessed September 5, 2014).

My Brother's Keeper Task Force. 2014. *My Brother's Keeper Task Force Report to the President.* Washington, DC: The White House. http://www.whitehouse.gov/sites/default/files/docs/053014_mbk_report.pdf (accessed June 14, 2014).

NRC and IOM. 2009. *Adolescent health services: Missing opportunities.* Washington, DC: The National Academies Press.

Obama, B. 2014. *Presidential memorandum—Creating and expanding ladders of opportunity for boys and young men of color*. February 27, 2014. Washington, DC: The White House. http://www.whitehouse.gov/the-press-office/2014/02/27/presidential-memorandum-creating-and-expanding-ladders-opportunity-boys- (accessed June 14, 2014).

Osgood, D. W., E. M. Foster, C. Flanagan, and G. R. Ruth, eds. 2005. *On your own without a net: The transition to adulthood for vulnerable populations*. Chicago, IL: University of Chicago Press.

Roisman, G. I., A. S. Masten, J. D. Coatsworth, and A. Tellegen. 2004. Salient and emerging developmental tasks in the transition to adulthood. *Child Development* 75(1):123-133.

SAMHSA (Substance Abuse and Mental Health Services Administration). 2011. *Leading change: A plan for SAMHSA's roles and actions 2011-2014*. http://store.samhsa.gov/shin/content/SMA11-4629/01-FullDocument.pdf (accessed June 15, 2014).

SAMHSA. 2014. *FY2014 funding for SAMHSA expands vital mental health services—especially for children and youth*. http://www.samhsa.gov/newsroom/advisories/1402112340.aspx (accessed August 21, 2014).

Sen, A. K. 2000. *Social exclusion: Concept, application, and scrutiny*. Manila, Philippines: Office of Environment and Social Development, Asian Development Bank.

Settersten, R. A., and B. Ray. 2010. *Not quite adults: Why 20-somethings are choosing a slower path to adulthood, and why it's good for everyone*. 1st ed. New York: Delacorte Press.

Settersten, R. A., Jr., F. F. Furstenberg, Jr., and R. G. Rumbaut, eds. 2005. *On the frontier of adulthood: Theory, research, and public policy*. Chicago, IL: University of Chicago Press.

Taylor, P., K. Parker, R. Kochhar, R. Fry, C. Funk, E. Patten, and S. Motel. 2012. *Young, underemployed and optimistic: Coming of age, slowly, in a tough economy*. Washington, DC: Pew Research Center.

U.S. Department of Education. 2014. *PROMISE: Promoting Readiness of Minors in Supplement Security Income*. http://www2.ed.gov/about/inits/ed/promise/index.html#about (accessed August 21, 2014).

Waters, M. C., P. J. Carr, M. J. Kefalas, and J. Holdaway. 2011. *Coming of age in America: The transition of adulthood in the twenty-first century*. Oakland: University of California Press.

The White House. 2013. *Now is the time*. http://www.whitehouse.gov/sites/default/files/docs/wh_now_is_the_time_full.pdf (accessed August 21, 2014).

WHO (World Health Organization). 2006. *Constitution of the World Health Organization*. http://apps.who.int/gb/bd/PDF/bd47/EN/constitution-en.pdf?ua=1 (accessed June 14, 2014).

2

Young Adults in the 21st Century

This chapter provides a foundation for the remainder of the report. It summarizes current knowledge regarding young adulthood as a critical developmental period in the life course; highlights historical patterns and recent trends in the social and economic transitions of young adults in the United States; reviews data on the health status of the current cohort of young adults; briefly summarizes the literature on diversity and the effects of bias and discrimination on young adults' health and well-being; presents the committee's key findings and their implications; and enunciates several key principles to guide future action in assembling data, designing research, and formulating programs and policies pertaining to the health, safety, and well-being of young adults. Many of the topics summarized in this chapter are discussed in greater depth in subsequent chapters.

BASIC PATTERNS OF DEVELOPMENT

Biologically and psychologically, young adulthood is fundamentally a period of maturation and change, although the degree of change may seem less striking than the changes that occurred during childhood and adolescence. As just one example, the physical changes of the transition from childhood into adolescence are transformative, with bodies growing in dramatic bursts and taking on secondary sex characteristics as puberty unfolds. As young people move from adolescence into adulthood, physical changes continue to occur, but they are more gradual. Individuals begin the steady weight gain that will characterize adulthood, but these changes are not as discontinuous as they are at the beginning of adolescence (Cole, 2003; Zagorsky and Smith, 2011).

In some ways, the tendency for the developmental change that happens during young adulthood to be gradual instead of dramatic may have led to the devaluation of young adulthood as a critical developmental period, but that developmental change should be not be underestimated. It is integral to transforming children and adolescents into adults. The psychological and brain development that occurs during young adulthood illustrates this point.

Psychological Development

Over the past two decades, research has elucidated some of the key features of adolescent development that have made this period of the life course unique and worthy of attention. These insights, in turn, have helped shape policy in major ways. These adolescent processes, and the increasing scientific and public attention they have received, provide a reference point for understanding the developmental importance of young adulthood.

In general, adolescence is a complex period characterized by substantial cognitive and emotional changes grounded in the unfolding development of the brain, as well as behavioral changes associated with basic psychosocial developmental tasks. In particular, adolescents are faced with the task of individuating from their parents while maintaining family connectedness to facilitate the development of the identities they will take into adulthood. At the same time, the overactive motivational/emotional system of their brain can contribute to suboptimal decision making (Crosnoe and Johnson, 2011). As a result, many adolescents tend to be strongly oriented toward and sensitive to peers, responsive to their immediate environments, limited in self-control, and disinclined to focus on long-term consequences, all of which lead to compromised decision-making skills in emotionally charged situations (Galván et al., 2006; Steinberg et al., 2008). This combination of characteristics is implicated in the heightened rates of risky behaviors and accidental death among adolescents (and young adults) relative to childhood and later stages of life, and awareness of these issues has reshaped policy responses to adolescent behavior in general and crime in particular (as described in the National Research Council [2013] report on juvenile justice).

Clearly, much social, emotional, and cognitive maturation needs to occur before adolescents are capable of taking on adult responsibilities and their many behavioral risks decline to adult-like levels. The ongoing development that occurs during young adulthood is what marks the transition from adolescence to adulthood. Again, this development is not necessarily discontinuous (such as the notable surge in risk taking that occurs during the transition from childhood into adolescence), but instead, it takes a more gradual and linear form, less obvious perhaps but no less important. Although findings from studies that directly compare adolescents and young adults on various cognitive tests and decision-making tasks are by no means uniform, the available research documents the slow and steady progress in self-regulation and related psychological capacities that takes place as adolescents transition into their 20s (see Cauffman et al., 2010). Compared with adolescents, young adults

- take longer to consider difficult problems before deciding on a course of action,
- are less influenced by the lure of rewards associated with behavior,
- are more sensitive to the potential costs associated with behavior, and
- have better developed impulse control.

In other words, the differences between adolescents and adults are stark, and the years between 18 and 26 are when young people develop psychologically in ways that bridge these differences. This development reflects many things, including the opportunities young people have to take on new roles and responsibilities and changes in their social contexts. It also reflects the similar gradual development of their brains.

Brain Development

The process of structural and functional maturation of the brain through adolescence to adulthood has garnered a great deal of attention, as neurobiological processes are believed to stabilize before declining with age. Maturation is of particular interest given the role of plasticity in affording opportunities for specialization, but also posing risks for abnormal development. Developmental neuroscientists, however, have traditionally assumed that adulthood is reached by age 18—hence the predominance of neurodevelopmental studies that compare children (under age 12) and adolescents (approximately 12-17) with adults (18-21 or extending and averaging through the mid-20s to the 30s). This approach has revealed many immaturities during the adolescent period, but much less is known about young adulthood. Discussions recently have emerged of the possibility of a prolonged brain maturational trajectory through young adulthood, as described below. Although the most significant qualitative changes in brain maturation have been found to occur from childhood to adolescence, emerging evidence does suggest that specialization of brain processes continues into the 30s, supporting both cognitive and motivational systems.

The primary mechanisms underlying brain maturation through adolescence into adulthood are synaptic pruning, myelination, and neurochemical changes. Synaptic pruning refers to the programmed elimination of synaptic connections between neurons believed to support specialization of brain processes based on experience. After a proliferation of synaptic connections through childhood, when the gray matter thickens, a decline in synaptic connections occurs through adolescence (Petanjek et al., 2011) and is believed to contribute to the thinning of gray matter that proceeds through adolescence (Gogtay et al., 2004). Magnetic resonance imaging (MRI) studies, which provide in vivo measurements of gray matter thickness, have focused predominantly on immaturities during adolescence and have considered adulthood to be established by the early 20s (Gogtay et al., 2004). MRI studies that sample a wider age range, however, indicate a prolonged period of gray matter thinning of prefrontal cortex that persists through the third decade of life (Sowell et al., 2003; see also Figure 2-1). Similar maturational trajectories have been observed in human postmortem studies that indicate a continued decrease in synaptic connections in the prefrontal cortex into the 30s (Petanjek et al., 2011). The prefrontal cortex is the region that supports abstract reasoning and planning. Through its extensive connectivity throughout the brain, it also supports executive function, providing control and modulation of behavior (Fuster, 2008). It plays a major role in decision making, and its maturation is believed to support cognitive development (Fuster, 2002; Luna, 2009).

Notably, despite continued specialization in the prefrontal cortex through the 20s, its engagement during executive tasks can appear adult-like as early as adolescence. Functional MRI (fMRI) studies of executive control through adolescence report both greater and lesser engagement of lateral prefrontal regions known to play a primary role in executive function (Luna et al., 2010). A recent longitudinal study was able to characterize developmental changes in core cognitive components of the ability to suppress impulsive responses by measuring the ability to stop a reflexive eye movement (Ordaz et al., 2013). Results suggest a *decrease* in prefrontal engagement through childhood stabilizing by adolescence. However, recruitment of the anterior cingulate cortex, a medial prefrontal region that is distinct from other prefrontal regions in supporting performance monitoring and error processing, increases during executive function processing through adolescence and young adulthood (Ordaz et al., 2013). These results suggest that processes distinct from prefrontal executive function that support monitoring behavior underlie cognitive development and continue to mature through young adulthood. The implication is that by young adulthood, prefrontal executive processes are at adult levels, but processes involved in monitoring behavior are still improving, which may affect decision making.

In addition to the maturation of prefrontal systems that support ex-

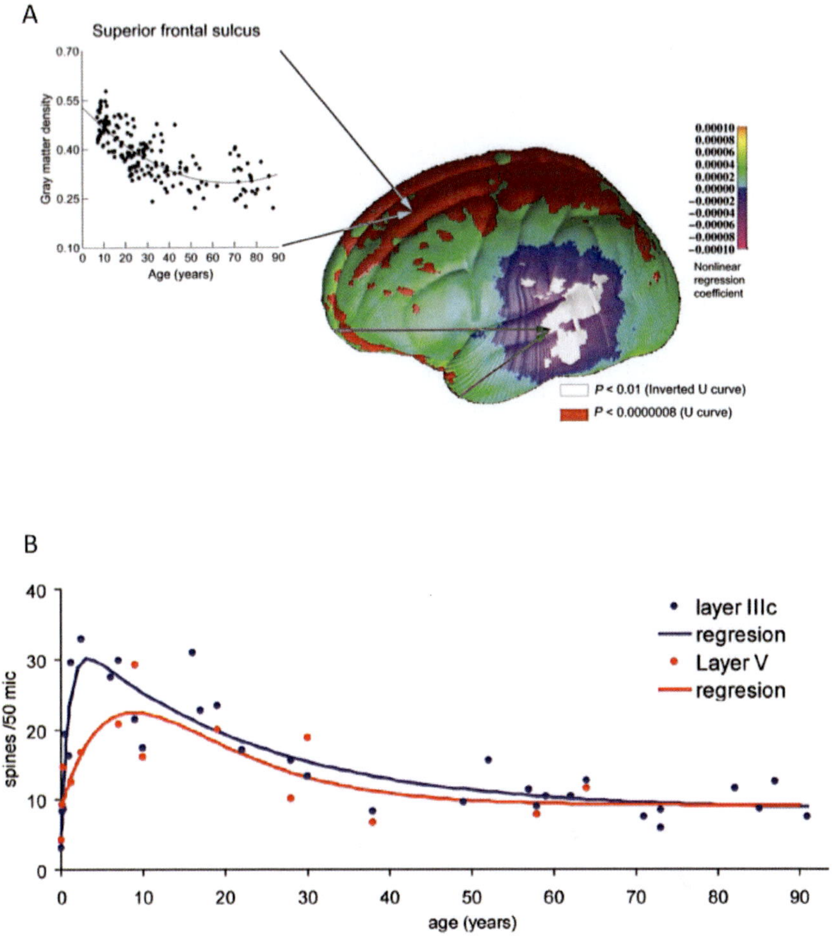

FIGURE 2-1 Continued maturation of prefrontal cortex through young adulthood evidenced from (A) in vivo MRI results showing thinning of cortical gray matter in prefrontal cortex and (B) postmortem evidence showing continued loss of synapses in prefrontal cortex into the 30s.
SOURCES: (A): Adapted from Sowell et al., 2003; (B): Petanjek et al., 2011; reprinted with permission.

ecutive function, motivational and emotional brain systems in limbic areas show a protracted development through adolescence and young adulthood. The striatum is a limbic region rich in dopaminergic innervation. Dopamine is the neurotransmitter that supports motivation and reward processing (Cools, 2008). Through its connectivity with prefrontal systems, it provides motivational modulation of behavior. MRI studies indicate that the striatum peaks in gray matter growth at an even later time than cortical regions through adolescence (Raznahan et al., 2014; Sowell et al., 1999; Wierenga et al., 2014). In addition, animal studies suggest a peak in the availability of dopamine, believed to play a role in increased sensation seeking beginning in adolescence (Padmanabhan and Luna, 2013; Spear, 2000; Wahlstrom et al., 2010). fMRI studies typically show a peak of increased recruitment of the striatum during monetary reward tasks in adolescence that decreases through young adulthood (Galván et al., 2006; Geier et al., 2010; van Leijenhorst et al., 2010). In particular, the presence of peers has significant salience in adolescence, engaging the reward circuitry to affect decision making (Chein et al., 2011). The trajectory of changes in reward processing through young adulthood, however, has not been directly investigated and in fact some studies have used young adults to represent all adults (van Leijenhorst et al., 2010). It is possible that developmental declines in striatal activity in response to rewards may be lower in young adulthood than in adolescence but still be greater than in later adulthood. Similarly, the amygdala, which supports emotional processing, has a peak in gray matter growth in the teen years, with a subsequent decrease in volume (Greimel et al., 2013; Scherf et al., 2013). The amygdala shows greater functional reactivity to emotional stimuli in adolescence (Blakemore, 2008; Hare et al., 2008), which may persist through young adulthood. Animal studies indicate that white matter fibers between the amygdala and cortex continue to increase into young adulthood (Cunningham et al., 2002). Despite this increase in structural connectivity, however, human neuroimaging indicates decreased functional connectivity into young adulthood, suggesting developmental increases in regulatory development with regard to the effects of emotion processing on behavior (Gee et al., 2013).

In parallel with decreases in gray matter in prefrontal and striatal regions are increases in white matter brain connectivity, which supports the ability for prefrontal executive systems to modulate reward and emotional processing. Postmortem studies indicate continued myelination—insulating of white matter connections—through adolescence and adulthood throughout cortical regions, including prefrontal systems (Lebel et al., 2008). Diffusion tensor imaging, which measures the integrity of white matter connections in vivo, indicates a hierarchical maturation of white matter, with tracts connecting cortical and limbic regions showing protracted development through adulthood (Lebel et al., 2008; Simmonds et al., 2013). During childhood to adolescence, a peak in white matter growth occurs throughout the brain, with continued growth of tracts as they reach cortical and limbic gray matter in young adulthood (Simmonds et al., 2013). Last to mature are the cingulum and uncinate fasciculus, which provide connectivity between cortical and limbic regions. The cingulum integrates *dorsal* frontal cognitive (e.g., anterior cingulate supporting performance monitoring) and limbic regions supporting emotion processing that continue to mature through the early 20s (Simmonds et al., 2013). The uncinate fasciculus, which integrates *ventral* frontal cortical (e.g., orbitofrontal cortex supporting motivation), amygdala (supporting emotion), hippocampus (supporting memory), and temporal cortical regions that form a circuit underlying socioemotional processing, continues to mature through the 20s (Simmonds et al., 2013). During young adulthood, therefore, connectivity that supports socioemotional processing is still immature but developing compared with later adulthood.

Within these maturation processes are unique gender differences that emerge in adolescence, are believed to be associated with earlier puberty in girls than in boys, and continue to dissociate through adulthood (Dorn et al., 2006; Ordaz and Luna, 2012). Young men have larger total brain volume, females show earlier cortical thinning and maturation of white matter integrity (Lenroot et al., 2007; Simmonds et al., 2013), and males show greater change in limbic regions (Giedd et al., 1997; Raznahan et al., 2014). These differences are believed to underlie gender differences in the emergence of different psychopathologies, including female predominance of depression and male predominance of antisocial personality disorders.

Taken together, the evidence demonstrates continuing maturation of limbic systems supporting motivation and reward processing and prefrontal executive systems. It has been proposed that the relative balance of maturation of motivational systems and prefrontal executive processing underlies the adolescent sensation seeking already discussed (Ernst et al., 2006; Smith et al., 2013; Somerville and Casey, 2010). In young adulthood, this imbalance diminishes but is still present. Brain systems supporting motivational and socioemotional processing are still maturing in young adulthood, influencing a more developed prefrontal executive system capable of more sophisticated and effective planning and resulting in unique influences on decision making, such as adaptive choices or risk-taking behavior. Overactive motivational systems may drive adult-like access to cognitive systems, resulting in planned responses that are driven by short-term rewards. Indeed, greater sensation seeking often persists into the mid-20s. This profile of decision making may also affect the attention given to choices regarding health, profession, and relationships, which are addressed in this and later chapters.

The Developmental Bottom Line

Overall, critical developmental processes clearly occur during young adulthood. Initial findings suggest that mature aspects of executive functioning are paired with continuing increased motivational/emotional influences affecting decision making. Still, more work is needed to fully understand young adulthood as a biologically and psychologically distinct and critical period of development and to relate these neurological changes to behavioral and social changes that typically occur during this period. Although these processes of maturation may sometimes appear as limitations on optimal decision making in young adulthood, the enhanced motivational processing that also occurs during this period plays an important adaptive role in supporting optimal learning and the ability and impetus to explore the environment and novel experiences.

HISTORICAL PATTERNS OF SOCIAL ROLES AND ACTIVITIES

The important psychological development experienced by young adults has not changed dramatically across generations, but their social functioning has (Steinberg, 2013). Social and behavioral scientists frequently discuss such social functioning in terms of five major role transitions of young adulthood—leaving home, completing school, entering the workforce, forming a romantic partnership, and transitioning into or moving toward parenthood (Schulenberg and Schoon, 2012; Shanahan, 2000). The focus on these social roles as the benchmark against which young adults from diverse segments of the population are compared can be critiqued as classist, ethnocentric, and heteronormative. These critiques certainly need to be acknowledged, but these role transitions do provide a useful structure for organizing the present discussion of young adulthood in the United States, especially if the significant diversity in these transitions among U.S. youth—both historically and in the contemporary era—is highlighted.

Two basic concepts—the timing and the sequencing of role acquisition—capture how the transition to these adult roles is taking more time and becoming more unpredictable (Settersten and Ray, 2010).

First, the *timing* of role acquisition in young adulthood is changing. In the long view, today's U.S. young adults are taking less time to undergo these role transitions relative to young adults in the distant past. Relative to more recent cohorts, however, they are taking more time. The timing of role acquisition is affected by, among other things, economic development and state investments that impose various signifiers of life transitions, such as legal rules on when youth are granted various privileges and allowed to enter certain statuses or, alternatively, when they age out of services or other protections (Modell et al., 1976; Shanahan, 2000).

Second, the *sequencing* of role acquisition (i.e., the order in which various roles are assumed) also is changing. Configurations of young adult statuses may change across cohorts. Recently, more diverse combinations of statuses have led to a "disordering" of the transition into adulthood, a term that seems pejorative but is not bad or good per se. The sequence of the roles assumed in the transition to adulthood increasingly is shaped by individual choices and actions rather than social structures. As discussed below, for example, young people partner and parent in different sequences because they have the freedom to do so now that the social stigma of nonmarital childbearing has diminished, and because economic or policy factors make various sequences more appealing and feasible than they used to be (Fussell and Furstenberg, 2005; Lichter et al., 2002; Rindfuss et al., 1987).

Family Roles

For many young adults, a major event is leaving the parental home to reside independently or with others of the same age. In some ways, leaving home is a rite of passage, which is why one main topic of interest concerning modern young adults in general and young adults during the Great Recession in particular is "boomerang" children—young adults who leave home to live independently but come back to reside with their parents (Stone et al., 2013). In truth, young adults living with their parents[1] in moderate to large numbers is not a new phenomenon in the United States or in other industrialized societies, and doing so is not inherently problematic or beneficial. In the United States, 32 percent of young adults aged 18-31 lived at home with their parent(s) in 1968, in 1981 31 percent did, and in 2012 36 percent did (Fry, 2013). How people assess young adults living with their parents instead of with peers or alone often reflects how they perceive (or misperceive) the past, including their own personal histories (Settersten and Ray, 2010; Stone et al., 2013).

Beyond leaving the parental home, many other noteworthy family events occur in the lives of today's young adults. In assessing the historical relevance of these contemporary patterns, one must keep in mind the importance of the comparison point. As with leaving home, contemporary young adult behaviors and statuses often seem so striking because they are viewed in the context of the post–World War II era, especially the 1950s. This era, however, was something of a historical outlier. What is going on today with young adults—especially in relation to family roles and responsibilities—appears to be less divergent, although still divergent, when compared against the full scope of the 20th century (Coontz, 2000).

Partnership and parenting are the core of family formation in the United States (see Chapter 3). How partnership is defined and how it connects to parenting have both evolved considerably in recent decades. Traditionally, partnership was defined in formal (i.e., legal) terms as marriage, especially among the white middle class. Today, partnership in young adulthood is most often viewed as a sequence from cohabitation—living with a

[1] Young adults may live with one or both parents.

romantic partner—to marriage (a transition from an informal to a formal partnership widely recognized by laws) or just as cohabitation itself. While most young Americans see cohabitation as a precursor to marriage, this has not always been the case. Many immigrant families from Latin America, for example, have a long tradition of cohabitation as a form of marriage, but the practice of cohabitation as a step toward marriage is new for most groups (Cherlin, 2009).

Figure 2-2 shows the percentages of young adults having engaged in at least one of three family formation behaviors—cohabitation, marriage, and parenting—by age 25 by gender, race/ethnicity, and level of education (high school or college graduate). In total, just under two-thirds of young adults have made at least one of these three family role transitions by age 25 (Payne, 2011). This proportion, however, fluctuates across the population. A larger proportion of women than men have made at least one of these role transitions (69 percent versus 53 percent), and family formation is less common among young adults who are white (59 percent) than among those who are not (66 percent for African Americans and 64 percent for Latino/as). There is also an educational gradient to family formation in young adulthood, with family role transitions becoming less common as

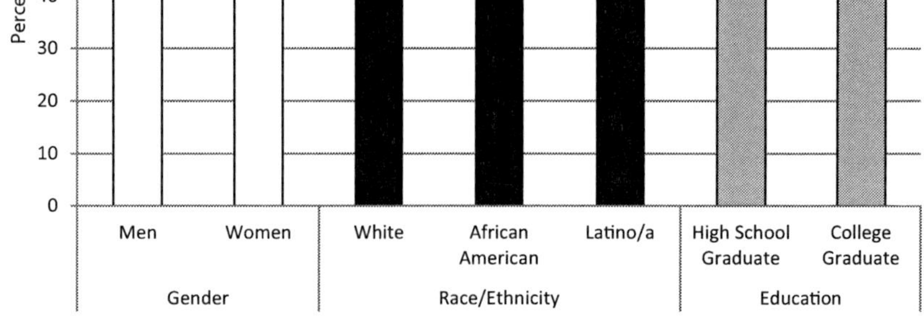

FIGURE 2-2 Percentage of young adults in the United States with at least one family formation behavior by age 25.
NOTE: The dotted line represents the overall sample average (61 percent).
SOURCE: National Longitudinal Study of Youth 1997 (see Payne, 2011).

educational attainment rises. Indeed, college graduates are the only segment of the population in which less than a majority of young adults have made at least one of the three family role transitions. Of these three transitions, the most common is cohabitation (47 percent), followed by becoming a parent (34 percent) and marrying (27 percent) (Payne, 2011).

One important caveat to keep in mind when considering these family formation patterns is that historically, tracking the family formation behaviors of lesbian, gay, bisexual, and transgender (LGBT) people has been exceedingly difficult. Because sexual relations between people of the same gender were outlawed in many states until recently, identifying the LGBT population was a challenge. Only within the past decade have same-sex couples been legally allowed to marry, and they may do so even now only within a minority of states (although the number is growing quickly). Thus, many LGBT young adults would have been classified as cohabiting in the past simply because they were legally barred from marrying. Moreover, innovations in reproduction technology and changes in adoption laws (domestically and internationally) have enabled these young adults to become parents without having to engage in an opposite-sex partnership before entering a same-sex partnership—long the most common path to parenthood for gays and lesbians. In states where same-sex marriage is legally recognized, same-sex parents are demonstrating patterns of union formation (and dissolution) similar to those of opposite-sex parents (Hunter, 2012; Parke, 2013; Seltzer, 2000).

In terms of timing, family formation is clearly showing signs of becoming a longer-term process. In short, young adults are taking more years to partner and become parents than they did in the past, especially compared with the last half of the 20th century. Today, the median age at first marriage—the age by which half of the population has married—is just under 27 for women, a nearly 5-year increase over the past 30 years and extending beyond the 18-26 age range used to define young adulthood in this report (Arroyo et al., 2013). A similar trend has occurred among men, although their median age at marriage has consistently been a year or so higher than that of women. This trend often is discussed in terms of "delay," but it is better thought of as part of the prolonged family formation process overall. As Americans live longer, they take more time to reach life-course milestones such as marriage. The transition to parenthood also tends to occur later in the life course, although the increase in median age at first birth over the last three decades has been less pronounced than the increase in median age at first marriage—about 3 years rather than 6 and just within our focal 18-26 age range (Arroyo et al., 2013).

These differences in the magnitude of the age increase in major family role transitions also speak to sequencing, or the growing tendency for transitions to cluster in heterogeneous ways. For most of American history (especially among the white middle class), marriage preceded parenthood. Yet the lesser increase in age at first birth compared with age at first marriage resulted in the two trends eventually converging (in 1991, to be precise). Since that point, median age at first marriage has been older than median age at first birth (Arroyo et al., 2013). The sequence (or order) of these transitions has become less predictable.

Breaking down partnerships into cohabitation and marriage when discussing major family role transitions of young adulthood also reveals evidence of changing sequencing. In line with the increasing prevalence of cohabitation in the population at large, the proportion of young adults who have cohabited by the age of 25 (47 percent) is higher than the proportion of young adults who have married (27 percent) (Payne, 2011). Three-fifths of all young adults who are married cohabited first, lending credence to the idea that cohabitation is now the modal pathway to marriage. Furthermore, one-third of young adults with children became parents before marrying or cohabiting. Just as with overall family formation patterns, these specific family patterns differ by gender, race/ethnicity, and educational attainment. For example, marriage without cohabitation is more common among whites and college graduates, but becoming a parent without partnering is far less common in these same two groups (Payne, 2011).

Overall, young adults (including LGBT young adults) in the United States are taking more time before entering into family roles that have long defined adulthood compared with their parents and grandparents, and they are sequencing these roles in multiple ways. This is particularly true for youth from white middle-class backgrounds.

Socioeconomic Roles

The transition from student to worker is a defining feature of young adulthood, given that Americans widely view financial independence from parents as a marker of becoming an adult. Yet young people are taking longer to become financially independent, and their school-work pathways are becoming more complex (Settersten and Ray, 2010). As with family formation, changes have been occurring in the timing and sequencing of the socioeconomic aspects of young adult role transitions. Chapter 4 gives a detailed accounting of how young people are faring in the educational system and in the labor market, but we highlight a few patterns in school-to-work transitions here in the context of the overall importance of studying young adults today.

Beginning with education, more young adults than in the past have been entering higher education in recent decades, but they are participating in higher education in many different ways and following diverse pathways (Fischer and Hout, 2006; Goldin and Katz, 2008; Patrick et al., 2013).

According to data from the National Longitudinal Study of Youth, in the United States, 59 percent of young adults have enrolled in some form of higher education by the time they reach age 25 (Payne, 2012). The overwhelming majority enrolled right after leaving high school, around age 18. Of those who enrolled, 33 percent enrolled in 2-year colleges and 44 percent in 4-year colleges and universities, with the remainder enrolling in both (Payne, 2012).

Of course, enrollment is not the same as graduation. The reality is that many young adults who enroll in higher education fail to earn a degree, at least while they are still young adults. Indeed, rates of completion of higher education in the United States have declined even as rates of enrollment have increased (Bailey and Dynarski, 2011; Bound et al., 2010), at least in part because enrollment rates have risen over time among those with less academic preparation in the K-12 years.

As with family role transitions, higher education patterns vary considerably across diverse segments of the population (Brock, 2010). Enrollment rates in both 2- and 4-year colleges are higher for women than for men and for whites than for nonwhites (Holzer and Dunlop, 2013; Payne, 2012). In fact, enrollment figures are at about 50 percent for African American and Latino/a young adults by the time they reach age 25 (compared with the population figure of 59 percent noted above), with even greater gender differences within these groups (Payne, 2012). The starkest disparities across these groups appear in graduation rates from 4-year colleges and universities, with women earning more bachelor's degrees than men and whites earning more bachelor's degrees than minorities (Payne, 2012). There are also growing disparities in educational attainment between young adults from poor and middle/upper-income families.

Thus, modal or average patterns of higher education enrollment and completion during young adulthood typically subsume a great deal of heterogeneity. This heterogeneity is clearly evident in the growing immigrant population, as many first- and second-generation immigrants have rates of college enrollment and graduation higher than those of the general population, while other immigrant groups (e.g., unauthorized immigrants, the children of Mexican immigrants) are significantly underrepresented in higher education (Baum and Flores, 2011).

Turning to employment, the increased enrollment of young adults in higher education has had a major impact on employment rates, as educational commitments often preclude substantial work commitments. Yet even taking into account the substitution of education for employment in the late teens and early 20s, a key feature of the employment status of young adults is unemployment, or being out of work when one wants to be working. Indeed, the unemployment rate for the under-25 population is twice that of the general population (Dennett and Modestino, 2013). This elevated unemployment among young adults is not altogether new; they have always struggled more than older adults to find and hold onto jobs. Still, this age-related disparity in unemployment has been growing in recent decades, and it has become especially marked since the start of the Great Recession in late 2007. Across all education levels and school enrollment statuses, young adult unemployment has increased significantly in the last several years relative to pre-recession years (Dennett and Modestino, 2013). Furthermore, among those who obtain jobs, many earn considerably less than similar demographic groups did in the past.

Another school-work scenario is "idleness"—when young adults are neither enrolled in higher education nor employed for pay. Many idle young adults are not just unemployed but have dropped out of the labor force altogether, sometimes for very long periods of time, in response to the lower wages and benefits now available to those with high school or less education, especially among young men (Dennett and Modestino, 2013). As discussed in Chapter 4, rates of idleness and labor force nonparticipation tend to be higher (and are becoming more so) for young African American men, who have been hit harder than other groups by broad changes in the economy and the labor market (Dennett and Modestino, 2013). Their lack of employment activity often becomes reinforced over time if they have a criminal record or if they are in arrears on child support they have been ordered to pay as noncustodial parents.

The sequencing of education and employment in young adulthood also is changing in important ways. A traditional school-work path was college enrollment and graduation in the late teens and early 20s, followed by full-time entry into the labor market in the mid-20s (with some pursuing more education and pushing back full-time employment). This primarily unidirectional path is related to higher economic returns throughout adulthood. Another traditional path was bypassing higher education altogether to enter the labor market directly after secondary schooling, a path related to higher earnings than those of other young adults in the short term but lower earnings in the long term.

In the contemporary economic climate of stagnant or lower real wages and generally higher costs of financing education (despite the rising availability of federal Pell grants to help low-income students pay for college), more young adults are trying to participate in higher education and employment at the same time or moving back and forth between the two. These mixed or bidirectional paths—which tend to be more common among young adults from more socioeconomically disadvantaged backgrounds—are one of several explanations for the lower odds of completing higher education among low-income or minority students (Bernhardt et al., 2001; Goldin and Katz, 2008).

Overall, young adults in the United States are attempting to gain more education, and more education improves employment prospects during young adulthood and beyond (not to mention affecting many nonemployment outcomes, such as civic engagement; see Chapters 4 and 5). Yet an unstable economic context and the high immediate costs of financing higher education mean that the process of gaining human capital to improve future job prospects and realize other benefits of education is not so simple, especially for some young adults from more disadvantaged socioeconomic and racial/ethnic groups.

Young adults' successes or failures in education and employment are integrally linked to their health. In general, the more educated a young adult becomes, the healthier she or he will be in adulthood, whereas lower educational attainment and occupational success is associated with poor health status, and involuntary loss of employment can have a negative impact on both physical and behavioral health. But the causal direction is also reversed in many cases: young adults with disabilities and chronic health conditions may find it significantly more difficult to obtain higher education and employment.

SOCIAL/ECONOMIC CHANGES AND THE REFASHIONING OF YOUNG ADULTHOOD

General physical and psychological development and the transition to major family and socioeconomic roles are personal experiences of individual young adults. Yet how these developmental and social processes unfold—and their timing and sequencing—is shaped by broader societal and historical forces (Shanahan, 2000). In other words, what is happening among young adults today reflects the larger context in which they find themselves, through no choice or fault of their own.

First, the U.S. economy has undergone substantial restructuring over the last several decades in ways that have radically altered the landscape of risk and opportunity in young adulthood. The traditional manufacturing and blue-collar sectors of the economy have shrunk, while the information and service sectors have grown. Even within these sectors, earnings inequality has increased dramatically, both across and within occupational categories. There are now broad strata of secure and stable professional and managerial jobs with benefits at the top of the labor market, and broad strata of insecure and unstable jobs with low wages and virtually no employer-provided benefits at the bottom (although these low wages can often be supplemented by a range of tax credits and publicly provided health care and child care benefits). The middle of the earnings distribution has diminished somewhat, however, especially in the production and clerical job categories that used to be accessible to high school graduates (and even dropouts in the manufacturing and blue-collar sectors).

As a result, the returns to higher education—how much more one earns over a lifetime by getting a college or graduate degree—have risen to historic levels, especially in specialized fields that support high-growth sectors of the economy. Increasingly, the way to achieve a middle-class level of earnings is to develop human capital by staying in school longer. A high school diploma, which used to be a ticket to the middle class, does not support mobility as it did in the past (Bernhardt et al., 2001; Goldin and Katz, 2008; Schneider, 2007); most jobs now require at least some postsecondary education or training, if not a bachelor's degree or higher. At the same time that the benefits of college enrollment have increased, however, the financial costs of enrolling (and staying enrolled) also have increased, as discussed in Chapter 4. Moreover, more students attend college without sufficient academic preparation and with very little knowledge or information about the world of colleges and universities. As a result, higher education is more economically necessary but also more difficult to attain for many young adults than in past decades.

Second, these socioeconomic changes have been accompanied by evolving norms and values regarding when young adults are expected to become independent of their parents and begin families of their own (Johnson et al., 2011; Roisman et al., 2004). Observers of modern social trends have noted that contemporary parents believe that their active parenting role extends further into their children's life courses than was the case for parents in the past (Fingerman et al., 2012). This new conceptualization of active and involved parenting as something that filters into children's 20s (and beyond) is often referred to as "helicopter" parenting (Fingerman et al., 2012). At the same time, Americans are less likely to view the early 20s as an appropriate time for family formation, especially having children, and young adults themselves tend to view marriage as unsuitable for this period of life (Teachman et al., 2000). Although this change in age norms has been most pronounced among the white middle class, it has pervaded diverse segments of the population in a process of cultural diffusion. Of course, changing age norms reflect changing behaviors (i.e., ideas about appropriate ages for a family transition change as people start making that transition at later ages), but age norms also shape how people view family transitions and, therefore, when they feel ready to make them (Cherlin, 2009; Teachman et al., 2000).

These macro-level trends are, of course, related. For example, the rising returns to and costs of higher education and the insecurity of the labor market for new workers mean that young people often concentrate on school and work in their late teens and early 20s rather than committing to a partner or starting a family. In this way, the economic changes that shape schooling and work alter age norms about family formation. This impact appears to be greater for marriage than for cohabitation or parenting, as many young adults have high economic standards for entering marriage that do not apply to these other family transitions (Edin and Kefalas, 2005; McLanahan, 2004). An economic consequence becomes a cultural influence. As discussed in Chapter 3, these trends are also raising questions about parental obligations to provide financial support for education and other costs during this transitional period.

Overall, young adults now focus more on socioeconomic attainment than on family formation, which is lengthening the time to financial independence and keeping them tied to their families of origin. For youth from socioeconomically advantaged backgrounds, this period can then become a time of freedom and exploration. For youth from more disadvantaged backgrounds, there is a higher potential for stagnation, with supposed freedoms masking scarcer opportunities and cultural norms and economic realities not always being well aligned (Arnett, 2004; Furstenberg, 2010). Both the timing and sequencing of young adult experiences, therefore, reflect the macro-level contexts in which young people are embedded and are closely connected to where they came from and where they are going.

A third important component of social change with implications for social roles and how they interact involves the advances in information technology in recent years. This technological revolution has reshaped American society as a whole and has been acutely felt among and driven by young adults. According to national data from the Pew Research Center, virtually all young adults use the Internet on a fairly regular basis, and nearly all have cell phones and use social media (Lenhart, 2013). Moreover, racial/ethnic and socioeconomic disparities in rates of usage are not large. In fact, information technology and social media pervade most aspects of daily life among most young adults (Lenhart, 2013). They are a central feature of school and work activities, keep young adults in closer contact with their parents compared with prior generations, allow young adults to greatly expand the reach of their social networks, serve as an increasingly popular venue for dating and union formation, provide new ways to increase health care access (and to improve health care delivery and facilitate the monitoring of personal health), and serve as a new context for political socialization and civic engagement (Chan-Olmsted et al., 2013; Clark, 2012; Kreager et al., 2014; Turkle, 2011; Wegrzyn, 2014). Indeed, young adults are driving much of the innovation and growth of social media (Lenhart, 2013). Consider a recent *Harvard Business Review* analysis (Frick, 2014), which reports that the modal age of founders of billion-dollar Silicon Valley startups is 20-24. Thus, young adults are both consumers and creators of the new media, and the ways in which they move toward, take on, and function within adult roles are changing as a result—a theme that is revisited repeatedly in subsequent chapters.

THE HEALTH OF YOUNG ADULTS

Thus far, the general developmental processes of young adulthood (unique in the life course if not historically specific) and the social activities and roles of young adulthood (unique in the life course and historically specific) have been discussed separately, but in reality, they are intertwined. One way to see this intertwining is to consider the health and health behaviors of young adults, which have physical, psychological, social, and structural underpinnings (Johnson et al., 2011).

Developmentally, young adults are continuing to accrue and refine cognitive skills and psychological competencies for mature decision making and self-regulation, and they face fewer natural threats to physical health compared with older adults. As a result, they should engage in less risky behavior than adolescents and be in better health than older adults, both of which are true to some extent. Socially, however, they tend to live more outside the purview of their parents relative to adolescents, and they are less governed by their family's lifestyle and health habits—with less parental monitoring of sleep, curfews, peer relations, physical activity, and diet (Harris et al., 2005). At the same time, compared with older adults, they are less likely to participate in work and family roles that serve as strong social controls on risk taking. And they often have less access to quality health care than younger adolescents or older adults. Consequently, some of the health advantages of young adulthood relative to adolescence or older adulthood may be undermined, and the period of vulnerability often associated with adolescence may be lengthened (Harris et al., 2006; Neinstein, 2013; Schulenberg and Maggs, 2002).

Health Behavior

Table 2-1 shows the top 10 causes of death among young adults in the United States. The top five are related in part to lifestyles, behaviors, and risk taking, especially the top three (injury, homicide, and suicide). The same is true of many other causes of death just below the top five, such as HIV. In this way, young adulthood has been described as a transitional period between behavioral causes of death in adolescence and health-related causes of death in later adulthood (Neinstein, 2013).

Looking more closely at the top two causes of death, rates of unintentional injury and homicide are higher among young adults—especially males—than among any other age group (CDC, 2012). Motor vehicle crashes account for the largest percentage of unintentional injuries, and young adults face the highest risk. Compared with those aged 26-34, young adults aged 18-25 are more likely to die or be injured in a motor vehicle crash and have more motor vehicle crash–related hospitalizations and emer-

TABLE 2-1 Leading Causes of Death in the United States (per 100,000 population), Ages 12-34

	Ages 12-17		Ages 18-25		Ages 26-34	
Rank	Cause of Death	No.	Cause of Death	No.	Cause of Death	No.
1	Unintentional Injury	11.9	Unintentional Injury	39.1	Unintentional Injury	27.1
2	Homicide	4.0	Homicide	14.5	Suicide	12.9
3	Suicide	3.8	Suicide	12.0	Homicide	11.0
4	Malignant Neoplasms	2.7	Malignant Neoplasms	4.4	Malignant Neoplasms	9.0
5	Heart Disease	1.1	Heart Disease	3.2	Heart Disease	8.3
6	Congenital Anomalies	0.9	Congenital Anomalies	1.1	HIV	2.5
7	Cerebrovascular	0.3	Diabetes Mellitus	0.6	Diabetes Mellitus	1.5
8	Chronic Lower Respiratory Disease	0.3	HIV	0.6	Cerebrovascular	1.4
9	Influenza & Pneumonia	0.3	Influenza & Pneumonia	0.6	Liver Disease	1.1
10	Benign Neoplasms	0.2	Cerebrovascular	0.5	Congenital Anomalies	0.9

SOURCE: Neinstein, 2013, reprinted with permission.

gency room visits (CDC, 2012). Young adults also are at greatest risk of injury due to firearms; young adult males have 10 times the risk of such an injury compared with young adult females (CDC, 2012).

With respect to basic health behaviors, Harris and colleagues (2006) tracked the health and health behavior of adolescents during their transition to young adulthood using National Longitudinal Study of Adolescent Health (Add Health) data. They examined 20 of the leading health indicators recognized in *Healthy People 2010*—the national public health agenda—as most critical to the development of healthy young people and tracked these indicators for the same cohort of individuals beginning when they were aged 12-18 until they were aged 19-26. Although there were some positives, the dominant pattern was declining health, seen most clearly in health behaviors and related health statuses. As these individuals entered their early and mid-20s, they were less likely to exercise, eat breakfast, and get regular physical checkups and dental checkups, and they were more likely to east fast food, contract sexually transmitted diseases, smoke cigarettes, binge drink, and use marijuana and hard drugs (Harris et al., 2006).

Substance use among young adults warrants special attention. The steady increase in substance use that begins in adolescence peaks during the young adult years (Johnston et al., 2014). Unlike many of the trends discussed in this report, this escalation of substance use tends to be as high or higher among middle-class whites relative to other groups (Johnston et al., 2014). Young adult rates and trajectories of substance use show considerable historical variation, reflecting cohort and period effects over the past 30 years (Johnston et al., 2014). Of particular concern, the rate of increase in use of alcohol and marijuana during this time period has become more rapid for more recent cohorts (Jager et al., 2013). At the same time, the general declines in substance use that characterize the rest of adulthood also tend to start in young adulthood; both sets of changes are associated with social role changes during this period (Bachman et al., 2001; Schulenberg and Maggs, 2002). Alcohol use and especially binge drinking generally peak in the early 20s before declining, a trajectory that is especially pronounced among college students (as discussed in Chapter 4); depending on the historical period, marijuana use tends to peak somewhat earlier (Johnston et al., 2014). Also depending on the historical period, annual and 30-day cigarette use tends to peak in the middle 20s and then decline; daily cigarette use, however, continues to increase with age across the 20s (Johnston et al., 2014). Thus, young adult health behavior is risky in many ways but also suggests a nascent positive trend. Another way of looking at these patterns is that young adulthood may be the last gasp of many of the behavioral risks of the early life course.

Along with these health risk behaviors, young adults also engage in health-promoting behaviors. For example, young adults (aged 18-24) are more likely than any other age group of adults to meet the recommended guidelines for physical activity (30 percent, compared with 24 percent of those aged 25-44 and 18 percent of those aged 45-54) (see HHS, 2011). In other words, young adulthood is a mix of positives and negatives when it comes to health behavior. Given that young adult health behavior is likely a foundation for lifelong health trajectories, these patterns are one important lens for understanding that young adulthood is a critical developmental period.

Health Conditions

Because young adults tend to be in better health than older adults, they are often thought to be in good health, but this is not necessarily true. Evidence suggests that the health status of young adults in the United States varies considerably. For example, overall obesity rates increase through adulthood, rising from 23 percent in those aged 20-24; to 35 percent among those in their late 20s, 30s, and early 40s; and to more than 40 percent at older ages (Harris, 2010). That being said, the rate among young adults is strikingly high (about one-quarter of the age group) and appears to be rising. In Add Health, a longitudinal study, obesity rates more than tripled from 11 percent in adolescence in 1995 to 37 percent by young adulthood in 2008 (Harris, 2010). Research documenting the emergence of the obesity epidemic has found that rising body mass indexes and obesity prevalence first occurred in the 1990s (particularly among adolescents and somewhat among children) (Lee et al., 2010, 2011), so current cohorts of young adults are entering adulthood with much higher obesity rates relative to previous cohorts of young adults and are the first generation to experience dramatically rising obesity rates in childhood and adolescence and they carry this health burden into adulthood. Importantly, the rate of increase in obesity across the age transition has been found to vary by educational experiences and expectations (Clarke et al., 2013).

In terms of obesity-related conditions, more than one in four young adults aged 24-32 in Add Health had hypertension, 69 percent were prehypertensive, 7 percent had diabetes, and 27 percent were prediabetic with impaired glucose tolerance or hyperglycemia (Gooding et al., 2014; Nguyen et al., 2011, 2014). Hypertension and diabetes are known risk factors for stroke, and the data reveal troubling increases in hospitalization for and prevalence of stroke among young adults over the past decade (George et al., 2011; National Center for Health Statistics, 2011). Alarmingly, because many of these conditions (e.g., high blood pressure, hyperglycemia) are asymptomatic and young adults typically are not exposed to routine screening systems or may not see a health care provider regularly, they often are unaware of ongoing and permanent damage caused by chronic conditions.

The levels of these health conditions suggest a higher than previously anticipated risk of cardiovascular disease in an age group often characterized as unburdened by chronic disease (Gordon-Larsen et al., 2004, 2010; Nguyen et al., 2011; Whitsel et al., 2011, 2012). Overall, the current generation of young adults appears to be at the forefront of the obesity epidemic and is vulnerable to experiencing its comorbid consequences.

Mental health among young adults also is cause for concern. Along with substance use, mental health disorders are the greatest source of disability among young adults in the United States. Indeed, nearly two-thirds of the burden of disability in young adults is associated with either mental health or substance use disorders (Davis, 2013), and by age 29, more than half of all individuals have experienced such a disorder (Kessler et al., 2005). The onset of the most serious mental health conditions—psychotic disorders—typically occurs in young adulthood (Seidman, 2013). Likewise, depression increasingly becomes a concern in young adulthood, as do suicidal thoughts, attempts, and deaths (recall the high placement of suicide in Table 2-1). Compared with those aged 25-34, young adults aged 18-25 have higher rates of serious psychological distress, and they are more likely to think about, plan for, and attempt suicide (SAMHSA, 2009). Compared with adolescents, young adults also are more likely to complete suicide (SAMHSA, 2009). Yet only a quarter of young adults with these experiences receive treatment or services, and they are more likely than older adults and adolescents to drop out of or discontinue treatment (SAMHSA, 2009). In many ways, they get lost within a health care system that treats them like adults even though they have special needs relative to other adults (Davis, 2013). That the specific mental health needs of young adults (relative to adolescents or all adults) rarely are studied on their own impedes the ability to serve this population.

In sum, the transition into adulthood is a critical period in health—despite the wide heterogeneity of experiences, health tends to worsen during this period and the higher levels of poor health in young adulthood tend to set the trajectories into adulthood with important consequences for future health (Harris, 2010). During the exploratory years of this transition, young adults as a group continue risk taking and poor (although improving) decision making that expose them to such health risks as unintended injury, unprotected sex, violence, binge drinking, motor vehicle accidents, suicide, and poor diet and nutrition, with potential adult consequences of liver and neurological disease, cardiac impairment, and stroke, as well as mortality (Clark et al., 2001; Johnston et al., 2014). As young adulthood comes to a close, there tend to be general improvements in health behavior.

The majority of young adults' health problems are preventable. The Affordable Care Act and other recent efforts to increase young adult health care coverage at the state level provide opportunities to enhance preventive care for young adults. However, efforts to provide them with preventive care are complicated by the lack of preventive guidelines for this age group and the fact that navigating the health care system during the transition from pediatric to adult providers is confusing and difficult, especially for those with behavioral health problems or a chronic disease (see Chapter 7).

Poor health in young adults has numerous negative impacts on individuals and on society at large. Beyond such obvious impacts as health care costs, it adversely affects national security, as reflected in the recruitment of military personnel. For example, estimates indicate that 12 percent of all age-eligible men and 35 percent of all age-eligible women were unable to meet U.S. Army standards for weight-to-height ratio and percent body fat in 2007-2008 (Cawley and Maclean, 2012). Furthermore, the Department of Defense reported that between 2006 and 2011, 62,000 individuals who arrived for military training failed their entrance physical because of their weight (Cutler and Miller, 2013).

Health Disparities

The health of young adults varies by race, ethnicity, sex, sexual identity, age, disability, education, socioeconomic position, and geographic location (Hudson et al., 2013; Mulye et al., 2009). Certain populations of young adults have higher rates of such risky behaviors as unhealthy eating, lack of physical activity, unprotected sexual activity, substance use, and unsafe driving. In addition, major gender differences exist, as well as considerable ethnic and racial disparities, with non-Hispanic black and American Indian/non-Hispanic Alaska Native young adults faring worse in many areas (Park et al., 2014). There are also gaps in knowledge about the health of certain groups, such as LGBT young adults and young adults living in poverty (for an overview of similar gaps in adolescent data, see Knopf et al., 2007). At the same time, it is important to note that the differences go both ways. Among young adults, for instance, black males have a higher homicide rate than white males (100.3 versus 11.4 homicides per 100,000) (Smith and Cooper, 2013), but black males have a lower rate of illicit substance use than white males from early adolescence to young adulthood (Chen and Jacobson, 2012).

DIVERSITY AND THE EFFECTS OF BIAS AND DISCRIMINATION ON YOUNG ADULTS' HEALTH AND WELL-BEING

The United States today is in the midst of "an explosion of diversity" (William Frey, quoted in Ohlemacher, 2006, p. 1). Based on the 2010 census count, one of every three Americans is a person of color (U.S. Census Bureau, 2010). If these demographic patterns continue, non-Hispanic European Americans will cease to be a majority population in the United States before 2050, and there will be no racial or ethnic majority (U.S. Census Bureau, 2012). These dramatic shifts in the "vanguard of America's new racial and ethnic diversity" are most evident in the booming population of minority youth (Johnson and Lichter, 2012, p. 32) and are likely, over time, to have a profound effect on the attitudes and experiences of adolescents and young adults as they are growing up, forming their group identities, and envisioning their place in the national community. Indeed, changes in the experiences of future cohorts of young adults will provide a useful measure of the extent to which coming of age in an increasingly diverse society affects the development of racial and ethnic identity, intergroup relations, and evolving conceptions of national identity.

In the meantime, however, many people of color continue to encounter systematic prejudice and discrimination that restrict opportunity and reduce well-being in pervasive ways and that contribute to the disparities in health and well-being of young adults documented throughout this report. Further, resistance to immigration in some parts of the country has heightened concerns about bias and discrimination based on ethnicity and religion (Cauce et al., 2011; Kim et al., 2013). Effects of bias and discrimination on health and well-being, as well as factors that protect or buffer young people against these effects, are briefly summarized here, considered throughout the report, and explored in greater depth in Appendix B.

The experience of being exposed to biased and discriminatory behavior has been characterized as a pervasive and normative stressor in the lives of people of color (García Coll et al., 1996). A 2013 national survey of adults by the Pew Research Center (2013a,b) indicates that 88 percent of non-Hispanic blacks and 57 percent of non-Hispanic whites believe that blacks are subject to "some"/"a lot" of discrimination in the United States. Among all adults, 73 percent say that Muslim Americans are subject to "some"/"a lot" of discrimination, while 65 percent hold this view of Hispanics.

Experiencing bias and discrimination has been linked to poorer outcomes in education and employment, worse physical and psychological outcomes, and acculturation stress. For example, African Americans and Hispanics are overrepresented among high school dropouts, and the associations between early school leaving and young adults' future outcomes, including joblessness, have been well established (see Chapter 4 of this report). Among the many interrelated family, social, and economic factors that contribute to educational disadvantage for minorities, it is widely acknowledged that the differential treatment of minority children in school classification and discipline policies plays a significant role (Alfaro et al., 2009; NRC, 2013; U.S. Department of Education and National Center for Education Statistics, 2014). Several systematic reviews (Lee et al., 2009; Priest et al., 2013; Williams and Williams-Morris, 2000; Williams et al.,

2003) have found strong associations between racial discrimination and mental health outcomes among all racial/ethnic groups. A recent meta-analytic review of experimental and correlational studies concludes that perceiving pervasive instances of discrimination negatively affects psychological well-being across a wide range of measures (Schmitt et al., 2014). Persistent exposure to race-related stress increases "allostatic load," and the accompanying heightened physiological responses are significant predictors of chronic diseases (Karlamangla et al., 2006).

Current patterns of discrimination are associated with structural factors (e.g., economic and/or residential segregation, institutional racism) that restrict opportunity and affect well-being in pervasive ways. However, it is also important to recognize that disadvantaged cultural groups have developed productive, adaptive means of coping with their deprivations and that individual resilience and family strengths play important roles in supporting the healthy development of ethnic minority young adults even in the face of societal stressors (García Coll et al., 1996). Several studies have identified factors that buffer, protect against, or reduce the impact of racism and discriminatory experiences on individuals (Luthar, 2006). These factors include social support, connections, feelings of belonging, and cultural socialization. For more detailed discussion, see Appendix B.

KEY FINDINGS AND IMPLICATIONS

The committee's key findings and their implications for the health, safety, and well-being of young adults are summarized below and discussed in greater detail in subsequent chapters of this report. Attention to these findings is intended to achieve progress toward ensuring the following key outcomes for young adults, with a particular focus on those young adults who are economically disadvantaged or otherwise marginalized:

- employment,
- education,
- housing stability,
- safety,
- health,
- healthy relationships and connections to responsible adults,
- civic engagement and community involvement, and
- effective parenting.

1. *Young adulthood is a critical developmental period.*

Like childhood and adolescence, young adulthood is a developmentally distinct period of the life course that can sensibly be viewed as a critical window of development with a strong effect on long-term trajectories. It is a time when individuals face significant challenges and are expected to assume new responsibilities and obligations. Success or failure in navigating these paths can set young adults on a course that will strongly affect the future trajectories of their adult lives. Early developmental and social trajectories may be reinforced or reversed, early risks may accumulate or be counteracted, new experiences can be turning points or sources of stagnation or thriving, and developmental tasks not completed may constitute a significant setback for the future.

Developmentally, young adulthood is a time of both opportunity and risk. The process of maturation is not suddenly completed when a young person turns 18. The brain is still maturing, and strengths and vulnerabilities continue to emerge. Thus, young adults continue to be strongly responsive to education and training and to incentives to create and contribute. Mistakes and failures can be reversed, and timely preventive interventions can reduce risks and ameliorate the consequences of injuries or disorders.

2. The world has changed in ways that place greater demands on young adults.

Although the normal course of physiological and biological development of young adults probably has not changed in generations, the world in which they live has changed greatly. Today's young adults live in a more global and networked world, marked by increased knowledge and information transfer, heightened risks, fairly low social mobility, and greater inequality. Economic restructuring, advances in information and communication technologies, and changes in the labor market have radically altered the landscape of risk and opportunity in young adulthood. Demands are higher, and there is less latitude for failure. Much of the burden of a restructured economy has been borne by the current cohort of America's young adults. Developmentally speaking, young people are resilient and adaptable, but many young adults are struggling to find a path to employment, economic security, and well-being.

3. Young adults today follow less predictable pathways compared with young adults in previous generations.

Beginning in the 1970s, several well-established patterns of social and economic transition that once defined young adulthood have been altered. In previous generations, the path for most young adults was predictable: graduate from high school, enter college or the workforce, leave home, find a spouse, and start a family (Fussell, 2002). While there were always exceptions, these established milestones provided structure and direction for young adults as they assumed adult responsibilities. Today, those pathways are considerably less predictable, often extended, and sometimes significantly more challenging, as the following examples illustrate:

- The cost of college has grown substantially, and many students have difficulty financing the investment or repaying the debt, yet prospects for well-paying jobs for high school graduates without some postsecondary credential are slim. Although many young adults enter college, dropout rates are high, and the number of years needed to finish degree programs has risen.
- Well-compensated entry-level jobs are becoming more difficult to find, even for young college graduates, and especially in the aftermath of the Great Recession. Many companies do not provide health insurance or other nonsalary economic benefits. Low earnings plague many young workers because they lack skills needed for higher-paying knowledge-based jobs, increasing numbers of the jobs available to them are part time, and institutions that have traditionally protected less-educated workers have been weakened.
- The estimate of a recent study is that 6.7 million youth and young adults aged 16-24—about 17 percent of the population in this age range—are neither in school nor working (Belfield and Levin, 2012). The rates are highest among African Americans and those aged 20-24, almost all of whom have left high school.
- Partnership and parenting patterns have shifted substantially. Many educated young adults live together for many years before marrying and having children, while many less-educated young adults have children outside of marriage before gaining the skills and income to support them. In addition, rapidly changing laws on same-sex marriage are providing new opportunities for family formation among LGBT young adults.
- The high cost of living independently has encouraged many young adults to move back into their parents' home, a pattern well documented among the "millennial" generation.[2]

4. Inequality can be magnified during the young adult years.

The disruption of established social and economic pathways has presented more choices and opportunities for some young adults while creating more barriers for others. The young adult population has diverse strengths, needs, social supports, and financial resources. Many young adults quickly

[2] A variety of age ranges are used to define the millennial generation. One example is those born between 1982 and 2003.

assume typical adult roles, although perhaps tenuously and continuing to need institutional support. Others reach the end of this period without assuming any adult roles and having few prospects, suggesting a lack of opportunities, experiences, skills, and/or maturity. These divergent trajectories reflect not only differences in psychological, social, and physical capacities but also differential opportunities rooted in economic and social inequality. Persistent prejudice and discrimination limit opportunities and mobility for racial, ethnic, and religious minorities, as well as individuals with disabilities and divergent sexual preferences, and can also have an adverse impact on health (see Appendix B).

In addition, marginalized young adults—such as those aging out of foster care, those in the justice system, those with disabilities, young parents, and children of low-income immigrants—are much less likely than other young adults to experience a successful transition to adulthood, although some of these young people ultimately fare very well as adults, and their hopes and aspirations are similar to those of their peers who have not been marginalized. Meeting the needs of marginalized groups not only improves their lives but also has the potential to help them become fully contributing members of society. In the absence of deliberate remedial action, however, this period of development is likely to magnify inequality, with lasting effects throughout adulthood.

5. *Young adults connect generations.*

As the children of prior generations and the parents of future generations, young adults are deeply embedded in family systems both at the level of individual families and at the population level. As a result, young adult experiences are shaped by the advantages and disadvantages their parents bring to their lives, and these experiences become the contexts for the parenting of their own children. The simultaneous proximity of young adults to being dependent children of parents and parents of dependent children creates both risks and opportunities.

6. *Young adults are at the forefront of social change.*

U.S. history is a story of sweeping economic, demographic, social, and technological changes, and young adults have long been at the leading edge of these changes. People in this age group tend to be highly interested in the broader world, their place in it, and how they can and do make a difference. They are greatly affected by global economic change, tend to be less conflicted than older adults about divisive cultural debates concerning behavioral norms and values, and are early adopters of new technologies—digital and social media being the most salient current example. They also are the leading edge of "an explosion of diversity" (William Frey, quoted in Ohlemacher, 2006, p. 1) that will change the face of the nation, which, if current demographic trends continue, will have no racial or ethnic majority by 2050. As a result, adults who conduct research and design policies in any one era cannot simply extrapolate their own young adult experiences to those of the current cohort of young adults.

7. *Young adults are surprisingly unhealthy.*

Young adulthood is a critical period for protecting health, not just during the transitional years but over the life course. Despite some positives, however, the dominant pattern among young adults today is declining health, seen most clearly in health behaviors and related health statuses such as the following:

- As adolescents age into their early and mid-20s, they are less likely to eat breakfast, exercise, and get regular physical and dental checkups, and more likely to eat fast food, contract sexually transmitted diseases, smoke cigarettes, use marijuana and hard drugs, and binge drink.
- In many areas of risky behavior, young adults show a worse health profile than both adolescents and older adults. Thus, young adulthood is when many risky behaviors peak, but it is also the time when involvement in risky behaviors begins to decline. Across this time period are many opportunities for prevention and early intervention.
- Early adulthood is a time of heightened psychological vulnerability and onset of serious mental health disorders, a problem compounded by failure to recognize illness or to seek treatment.
- The current generation of young adults appears to be at the forefront of the obesity epidemic and is more vulnerable than previous generations to obesity-related health consequences in later years.

The higher levels of poor health in young adulthood have important consequences for future health, educational attainment, and economic well-being. Rapid technological changes, economic challenges, and a prolonged transition to adulthood appear to be contributing to the health problems of young adults by increasing their stress and sedentary habits while making them less likely to participate in work and family roles that serve as strong social controls on risk taking. Therefore, these worrisome trends in young adult health can be expected to continue or worsen.

PRINCIPLES TO GUIDE ACTION

Young adults are different from both adolescents and older adults, yet they often are combined with one or the other in statistical reporting and research design, as well as in policy and program classification. As a result, not enough is known about the special strengths and vulnerabilities of this population, as well as the ways in which socioeconomic and demographic disparities during this period of the life course contribute to disparities in the population at large. Likewise, little is known about the relative importance of young adulthood and other periods of the life course for long-term health and well-being. Furthermore, because of historical changes in how young adults live and what is expected of them, one cannot easily extrapolate from past research or policy traditions to today. An active, productive, and resilient population of young adults will benefit not only these young people but all members of U.S. society and the nation as a whole. Using the above findings and implications as a foundation, we offer corresponding principles to guide action that will help achieve this goal and that structure the discussion in the chapters to follow. Subsequent chapters provide an in-depth discussion of policies and programs in key domains for young adults' health and well-being, along with specific recommendations for key actors.

Principle 1: Pay specific attention to young adults in research and policy.

Given the critical nature of young adulthood within the life course, it needs to be studied on its own rather than as an extension of adolescence or as a fungible period of adulthood. At the same time, long-term studies that embed this period within the life course are needed to elucidate both the independent and interconnected roles of young adult experiences in long-term life-course outcomes. Young adults often are cut off from child/adolescent services they may still need and are treated the same as older adults in adult services. Policy makers should ensure that outcomes are measured specifically for young adults and that programs take account of relevant differences between young and older adults.

Principle 2: Create economic opportunities for young adults.

A shrinking number of well-paying jobs for young adults without a college education, the cost of higher education, and the prolonged period of transition to adult roles, exacerbated by economic volatility, pose an underlying threat to young adults' healthy adjustment and functioning. Taking action to improve prospects for social mobility can address the fundamental risks these young people face in modern society, risks that themselves have implications for the overall stability and progress of the nation.

Principle 3: Allow flexibility in policies and programs for young adults.

Given the absence of clear normative pathways during this period of the life course, the transitions and subsequent trajectories of young adults depend on both the individual characteristics of young adults and the environments in which they are embedded. Thus, efforts to serve this population through policies and programs need to be tailored to the various subpopulations of young adults, defined not just developmentally but also demographically and socioeconomically. Age alone during this period of life should not necessarily define needs and dictate programming. Flexibility is needed in defining eligibility criteria and program requirements.

Principle 4: Invest in the least advantaged young adults.

The prolonged period of educational attainment, together with its increasing costs, poses substantial burdens for the vast majority of families. But these challenges are especially daunting for the least advantaged families and the most marginalized young adults. Both research and policy should focus not just on increasing absolute levels of health, educational attainment, or other desired outcomes for young adults as a group, but also on making the investments needed to increase the productivity, health, and well-being of the many who are being left behind, as well as rectifying persistent racial and ethnic disparities.

Principle 5: Use multigenerational strategies to support young adults and their children.

Multigenerational investments and interventions are a promising trend in policy and practice that needs to receive greater attention. Supporting the human capital and workforce development of young parents is likely an investment in the long-term developmental trajectories of their children, and programs focused on the early health and education of young children provide an opportunity to reach their parents, many of whom are young adults. Targeting the connections between generations, therefore, offers two ways to serve young adults, with ripple effects over time.

Principle 6: Empower and engage young adults in policies and programs.

Young adults need to be at the table when decisions that affect them are being made, both because they deserve to be involved and because their input will contribute to better decision making. Their interest in such involvement is likely to be strong given their expanding perspective on the world. The influence of social media on young adult development and functioning is not yet fully understood, and the potential for social media to facilitate the implementation of policies and programs, especially in public health and health care, has not been fully tapped. Both research and policy agendas need to integrate social media and related information technologies. Because young adults typically are more expert in social media than many researchers and policy makers, the incorporation of social media into these agendas would be an example of the broader value of giving young adults a voice in the process.

Principle 7: Invest in preventive approaches to improve the health of young adults.

Traditionally, the nation's health system has underemphasized preventive health services for young adults. Young adults' lack of health care insurance coverage often precludes them from seeking health care services, including the provision of preventive screening and services, although this gap has been somewhat alleviated by the Affordable Care Act and Medicaid expansion in some states. The role of families in ensuring continuity with a health care provider that offers preventive services also is diluted as young adults age out of their pediatrician's practice. Yet many of the risk behaviors in which young adults engage can be addressed by population-based interventions, as well as earlier screening and referrals, for example, for clinical and behavioral interventions. The Affordable Care Act, as one example, incorporates preventive health services as part of health insurance coverage. Given the act's emphasis on preventive services in such areas as reproductive health, substance abuse, and mental health, which reflect many of the health care needs of young adults, those young adults who enroll can clearly benefit from this newly available care.

CONCLUSION

The stability and progress of society at large depend on how any cohort of young adults fares as a whole. The same can be said of each cohort of children and adolescents, of course, but it is the transition to adulthood that reflects the end of trial periods and the beginning of more consequential actions. Young adults' successful transition to independent and healthy adulthood, entry into the workforce, continued productivity, and successful parenting can help ensure the security and well-being of the nation. A healthy and productive generation of young adults nurtures the next generation and provides the worker replacement needed to support the retiring generation.

Focusing on the health and well-being of the current cohort of young adults (those becoming adults in the first third of the 21st century) is especially important because of the powerful (and perhaps transformative) economic and social forces now at work. One is the rapidly increasing "elder dependency ratio" (i.e., the ratio of individuals in the population aged 65 and older to the working-age population). This ratio has been increasing rapidly in all advanced industrial countries while the fertility rate has been declining, leaving the current cohort of working-age adults to support increasing numbers of retiring elders. In the United States, the elder dependency ratio increased from about 1 elder to 10 workers (0.1) in 1950 to 0.2 in 2000 and is expected to increase to 0.35 by 2050 (Fussell, 2002). This demographic shift led Elizabeth Fussell to call for renegotiating the "intergenerational contract" to couple building human capital through collective investments in young adults with increasing the age of eligibility for retirement support (Fussell, 2002). A similar collective renegotiation may already be occurring, explicitly or implicitly, when parents invest in education and support for young adults well into their 20s.

Another transformative social and economic change now under way is the substantial increase in immigration to the United States. This trend has helped replenish the workforce and attenuate the rise in the elder dependency ratio (which is expected to increase, on average, to about 0.45 in other developed countries by 2050) while also changing the very face of U.S. society (Fussell, 2002). This dramatic change is likely, over time, to have a profound effect on attitudes and experiences of adolescents and young adults as they are growing up, forming group identities, and envisioning their place in the national community. Indeed, changes in the experiences of future cohorts of young adults will provide a useful measure of the extent to which coming of age in an increasingly diverse society affects intergroup relations and evolving conceptions of national identity.

In sum, healthy, productive, and skilled young adults are critical for the nation's workforce, global competitiveness, public safety, and national security. Providing more of the educational, economic, social, and health supports needed by *all* young adults—particularly those whose background and characteristics put them at risk of experiencing the greatest struggles—will ensure equal opportunity, erase disparities, and enable more young adults to successfully embrace adult roles as healthy workers, parents, and citizens.

REFERENCES

Alfaro, E. C., A. J. Umaña-Taylor, M. A. Gonzales-Backen, M. Y. Bámaca, and K. H. Zeiders. 2009. Latino adolescents' academic success: The role of discrimination, academic motivation, and gender. *Journal of Adolescence* 32(4):941-962.

Arnett, J. J. 2004. *Emerging adulthood: The winding road from the late teens through the twenties*. New York: Oxford University Press.

Arroyo, J., K. K. Payne, S. L. Brown, and W. D. Manning. 2013. *Crossover in median age at first marriage and first birth: Thirty years of change*. Bowling Green, OH: National Center for Family and Marriage Research.

Bachman, J. G., P. M. O'Malley, J. E. Schulenberg, L. D. Johnston, A. L. Bryant, and A. C. Merline. 2001. *The decline of substance use in young adulthood: Changes in social activities, roles, and beliefs*. New York: Psychology Press.

Bailey, M. J., and S. M. Dynarski. 2011. *Gains and gaps: Changing inequality in U.S. college entry and completion*. Cambridge, MA: National Bureau of Economic Research.

Baum, S., and S. Flores. 2011. Higher education and children in immigrant families. *The Future of Children* 21:171-193.

Belfield, C., and H. Levin. 2012. *The economics of investing in opportunity youth*. New York: Civic Enterprises.

Bernhardt, A., M. Morris, M. S. Handcock, and M. A. Scott. 2001. *Divergent paths: Economic mobility in the new American labor market*. New York: Russell Sage Foundation.

Blakemore, S.-J. 2008. The social brain in adolescence. *Nature Reviews Neuroscience* 9(4): 267-277.

Bound, J., M. F. Lovenheim, and S. Turner. 2010. Why have college completion rates declined? An analysis of changing student preparation and collegiate resources. *American Economic Journal-Applied Economics* 2(3):129-157.

Brock, T. 2010. Young adults and higher education: Barriers and breakthroughs to success. *The Future of Children* 20(1):109-132.

Cauce, A. M., R. Cruz, M. Corona, and R. Conger. 2011. The face of the future: Risk and resilience in minority youth. In *Health disparities in youth and families*. New York: Springer. Pp. 13-32.

Cauffman, E., E. P. Shulman, L. Steinberg, E. Claus, M. T. Banich, S. Graham, and J. Woolard. 2010. Age differences in affective decision making as indexed by performance on the Iowa gambling task. *Developmental Psychology* 46(1):193-207.

Cawley, J., and J. C. Maclean. 2012. Unfit for service: The implications of rising obesity for U.S. military recruitment. *Health Economics* 21(11):1348-1366.

CDC (Centers for Disease Control and Prevention). 2012. *Nonfatal injury report, 2001-2012*. http://webappa.cdc.gov/sasweb/ncipc/nfirates2001.html (accessed July 22, 2014).

Chan-Olmsted, S., H. Rim, and A. Zerba. 2013. Mobile news adoption among young adults: Examining the roles of perceptions, news consumption, and media usage. *Journalism & Mass Communication Quarterly* 90:126-147.

Chein, J., D. Albert, L. O'Brien, K. Uckert, and L. Steinberg. 2011. Peers increase adolescent risk taking by enhancing activity in the brain's reward circuitry. *Developmental Science* 14(2):F1-F10.

Chen, P., and K. C. Jacobson. 2012. Developmental trajectories of substance use from early adolescence to young adulthood: Gender and racial/ethnic differences. *Journal of Adolescent Health* 50(2):154-163.

Cherlin, A. J. 2009. *The marriage-go-round*. New York: Random House LLC.

Clark, D. B., K. G. Lynch, J. E. Donovan, and G. D. Block. 2001. Health problems in adolescents with alcohol use disorders: Self-report, liver injury, and physical examination findings and correlates. *Alcoholism-Clinical and Experimental Research* 25(9):1350-1359.

Clark, L. S. 2012. *The parent app: Understanding families in the digital age*. New York: Oxford University Press.

Clarke, P. J., P. M. O'Malley, J. E. Schulenberg, H. Lee, N. Colabianchi, and L. D. Johnston. 2013. College expectations in high school mitigate weight gain over early adulthood: Findings from a national study of American youth. *Obesity* 21(7):1321-1327.

Cole, T. J. 2003. The secular trend in human physical growth: A biological view. *Economics & Human Biology* 1(2):161-168.

Cools, R. 2008. Role of dopamine in the motivational and cognitive control of behavior. *The Neuroscientist* 14(4):381-395.

Coontz, S. 2000. Historical perspectives on family studies. *Journal of Marriage and Family* 62(2):283-297.

Crosnoe, R., and M. K. Johnson. 2011. Research on adolescence in the twenty-first century. *Annual Review of Sociology* 37:439-460.

Cunningham, M. G., S. Bhattacharyya, and F. M. Benes. 2002. Amygdalo-cortical sprouting continues into early adulthood: Implications for the development of normal and abnormal function during adolescence. *Journal of Comparative Neurology* 453(2):116-130.

Cutler, T., and G. A. Miller. 2013. *Retired military generals: Recruits dismissed for obesity cost $1.1 billion a year*. http://www.mlive.com/news/index.ssf/2013/09/retired_military_generals_recr.html (accessed August 21, 2014).

Davis, M. 2013. *Young adult mental health*. Presentation at IOM/NRC Workshop on Improving the Health, Safety, and Well-Being of Young Adults, Washington, DC. http://www.iom.edu/~/media/Files/Activity%20Files/Children/ImprovingYoungAdultsHealth/Davis%20Presentation.pdf (accessed October 10, 2014).

Dennett, J., and A. S. Modestino. 2013. *Uncertain futures? Youth attachment to the labor market in the United States and New England*. Boston, MA: New England Public Policy Center.

Dorn, L. D., R. E. Dahl, H. R. Woodward, and F. Biro. 2006. Defining the boundaries of early adolescence: A user's guide to assessing pubertal status and pubertal timing in research with adolescents. *Applied Developmental Science* 10(1):30-56.

Edin, K., and M. Kefalas. 2005. *Promises I can keep: Why poor women put motherhood before marriage*. Oakland: University of California Press.

Ernst, M., D. S. Pine, and M. Hardin. 2006. Triadic model of the neurobiology of motivated behavior in adolescence. *Psychological Medicine* 36(3):299-312.

Fingerman, K. L., Y. P. Cheng, E. D. Wesselmann, S. Zarit, F. Furstenberg, and K. S. Birditt. 2012. Helicopter parents and landing pad kids: Intense parental support of grown children. *Journal of Marriage and Family* 74(4):880-896.

Fischer, C. S., and M. Hout. 2006. *Century of difference: How America changed in the last one hundred years*. New York: Russell Sage Foundation.

Frick, W. 2014. How old are Silicon Valley's top founders? Here's the data. *Harvard Business Review,* April 3.

Fry, R. 2013. *A rising share of young adults live in their parents' home*. Philadelphia, PA: Pew Research Center.

Furstenberg, Jr., F. F. 2010. On a new schedule: Transitions to adulthood and family change. *The Future of Children* 20(1):67-87.

Fussell, E. 2002. Youth in aging societies. In *The future of adolescent experience: Societal trends and the transition to adulthood*, edited by J. Mortimer and R. Larson. New York: Cambridge University Press. Pp. 18-51.

Fussell, E., and F. Furstenberg. 2005. The transition to adulthood during the 20th century: Race, nativity and gender. In *On the frontier of adulthood: Theory, research, and public policy*, edited by R. Settersten, F. Frustenberg, and R. Rumbaut. Chicago, IL: University of Chicago Press. Pp. 29-75.

Fuster, J. M. 2002. Frontal lobe and cognitive development. *Journal of Neurocytology* 31(3-5):373-385.

Fuster, J. M. 2008. *The prefrontal cortex*. 4th ed. Oxford, UK: Elsevier Ltd.

Galván, A., T. A. Hare, C. E. Parra, J. Penn, H. Voss, G. Glover, and B. Casey. 2006. Earlier development of the accumbens relative to orbitofrontal cortex might underlie risk-taking behavior in adolescents. *The Journal of Neuroscience* 26(25):6885-6892.

García Coll, C., G. Lamberty, R. Jenkins, H. P. McAdoo, K. Crnic, B. H. Wasik, and H. Vázquez García. 1996. An integrative model for the study of developmental competencies in minority children. *Child Development* 67(5):1891-1914.

Gee, D. G., K. L. Humphreys, J. Flannery, B. Goff, E. H. Telzer, M. Shapiro, T. A. Hare, S. Y. Bookheimer, and N. Tottenham. 2013. A developmental shift from positive to negative connectivity in human amygdala-prefrontal circuitry. *Journal of Neuroscience* 33(10):4584-4593.

Geier, C., R. Terwilliger, T. Teslovich, K. Velanova, and B. Luna. 2010. Immaturities in reward processing and its influence on inhibitory control in adolescence. *Cerebral Cortex* 20(7):1613-1629.

George, M. G., X. Tong, E. V. Kuklina, and D. R. Labarthe. 2011. Trends in stroke hospitalizations and associated risk factors among children and young adults, 1995-2008. *Annals of Neurology* 70(5):713-721.

Giedd, J. N., F. X. Castellanos, J. C. Rajapakse, A. C. Vaituzis, and J. L. Rapoport. 1997. Sexual dimorphism of the developing human brain. *Progress in Neuro-Psychopharmacology and Biological Psychiatry* 21(8):1185-1201.

Gogtay, N., J. N. Giedd, L. Lusk, K. M. Hayashi, D. Greenstein, A. C. Vaituzis, T. F. Nugent, D. H. Herman, L. S. Clasen, and A. W. Toga. 2004. Dynamic mapping of human cortical development during childhood through early adulthood. *Proceedings of the National Academy of Sciences of the United States of America* 101(21):8174-8179.

Goldin, C. D., and L. F. Katz. 2008. *The race between education and technology*. Cambridge, MA: Belknap Press of Harvard University Press.

Gooding, H.C., S. McGinty, T. K. Richmond, M. W. Gillman, and A. E. Field. 2014. Hypertension awareness and control among young adults in the National Longitudinal Study of Adolescent Health. *Journal of General Internal Medicine* 29(8):1098-1104.

Gordon-Larsen, P., L. S. Adair, M. C. Nelson, and B. M. Popkin. 2004. Five-year obesity incidence in the transition period between adolescence and adulthood: The National Longitudinal Study of Adolescent Health. *American Journal of Clinical Nutrition* 80(3):569-575.

Gordon-Larsen, P., N. S. The, and L. S. Adair. 2010. Longitudinal trends in obesity in the United States from adolescence to the third decade of life. *Obesity (Silver Spring)* 18(9):1801-1804.

Greimel, E., B. Nehrkorn, M. Schulte-Rüther, G. R. Fink, T. Nickl-Jockschat, B. Herpertz-Dahlmann, K. Konrad, and S. B. Eickhoff. 2013. Changes in grey matter development in autism spectrum disorder. *Brain Structure and Function* 218(4):929-942.

Hare, T. A., N. Tottenham, A. Galván, H. U. Voss, G. H. Glover, and B. J. Casey. 2008. Biological substrates of emotional reactivity and regulation in adolescence during an emotional go-nogo task. *Biological Psychiatry* 63(10):927-34.

Harris, K. M. 2010. An integrative approach to health. *Demography* 47(1):1-22.

Harris, K. M., R. B. King, and P. Gordon-Larsen. 2005. Healthy habits among adolescents: Sleep, exercise, diet, and body image. In *What do children need to flourish?* New York: Springer. Pp. 111-132.

Harris, K. M., P. Gordon-Larsen, K. Chantala, and J. R. Udry. 2006. Longitudinal trends in race/ethnic disparities in leading health indicators from adolescence to young adulthood. *Archives of Pediatrics & Adolescent Medicine* 160(1):74-81.

HHS (U.S. Department of Health and Human Services). 2011. *Healthy people 2020*. http://www.healthypeople.gov/2020/default.aspx (accessed July 22, 2014).

Holzer, H. J., and E. Dunlop. 2013. *Just the facts, ma'am: Postsecondary education and labor market outcomes in the US*. Bonn, Germany: IZA (Institute for the Study of Labor).

Hudson, D. L., E. Puterman, K. Bibbins-Domingo, K. A. Matthews, and N. E. Adler. 2013. Race, life course socioeconomic position, racial discrimination, depressive symptoms and self-rated health. *Social Science & Medicine* 97:7-14.

Hunter, N. D. 2012. Introduction: The future impact of same-sex marriage: More questions than answers. *Georgetown Law Journal* 100(6):1855-1879.

Jager, J., J. E. Schulenberg, P. M. O'Malley, and J. G. Bachman. 2013. Historical variation in drug use trajectories across the transition to adulthood: The trend toward lower intercepts and steeper, ascending slopes. *Development and Psychopathology* 25(2):527-543.

Johnson, K. M., and D. T. Lichter. 2012. Rural natural increase in the new century: America's third demographic transition. In *International handbook of rural demography*, edited by L. J. Kulcsár and K. J. Curtis. The Netherlands: Springer. Pp. 17-34.

Johnson, M. K., R. Crosnoe, and G. H. Elder. 2011. Insights on adolescence from a life course perspective. *Journal of Research on Adolescence* 21(1):273-280.

Johnston, L. D., P. M. O'Malley, J. G. Bachman, J. E. Schulenberg, and R. A. Miech. 2014. *Monitoring the future national survey results on drug use, 1975-2013. Volume II: College students and adults ages 19-50.* Ann Arbor: Institute for Social Research, University of Michigan.

Karlamangla, A. S., B. H. Singer, and T. E. Seeman. 2006. Reduction in allostatic load in older adults is associated with lower all-cause mortality risk: MacArthur studies of successful aging. *Psychosomatic Medicine* 68(3):500-507.

Kessler, R. C., W. T. Chiu, O. Demler, and E. E. Walters. 2005. Prevalence, severity, and comorbidity of 12-month DSM-IV disorders in the national comorbidity survey replication. *Archives of General Psychiatry* 62(6):617-627.

Kim, S. Y., Q. Chen, Y. Wang, Y. Shen, and D. Orozco-Lapray. 2013. Longitudinal linkages among parent-child acculturation discrepancy, parenting, parent-child sense of alienation, and adolescent adjustment in Chinese immigrant families. *Developmental Psychology* 49(5):900-912.

Knopf, D. K., M. J. Park, C. D. Brindis, T. P. Mulye, and C. E. Irwin, Jr. 2007. What gets measured gets done: Assessing data availability for adolescent populations. *Maternal and Child Health Journal* 11(4):335-345.

Kreager, D. A., S. E. Cavanagh, J. Yen, and M. Yu. 2014. Where have all the good men gone? Gendered interactions in online dating. *Journal of Marriage and Family* 76(2):387-410.

Lebel, C., L. Walker, A. Leemans, L. Phillips, and C. Beaulieu. 2008. Microstructural maturation of the human brain from childhood to adulthood. *NeuroImage* 40(3):1044-1055.

Lee, H., D. Lee, G. Guo, and K. M. Harris. 2011. Trends in body mass index in adolescence and young adulthood in the United States: 1959-2002. *Journal of Adolescent Health* 49(6):601-608.

Lee, J. M., S. Pilli, A. Gebremariam, C. C. Keirns, M. M. Davis, S. Vijan, G. L. Freed, W. H. Herman, and J. G. Gurney. 2010. Getting heavier, younger: Trajectories of obesity over the life course. *International Journal of Obesity* 34(4):614-623.

Lee, S., H. S. Juon, G. Martinez, C. E. Hsu, E. S. Robinson, J. Bawa, and G. X. Ma. 2009. Model minority at risk: Expressed needs of mental health by Asian American young adults. *Journal of Community Health* 34(2):144-152.

Lenhart, A. 2013. *Young adults, mobile phones and social media: Technology and the transition to adulthood.* Presentation at IOM/NRC Workshop on Improving the Health, Safety, and Well-Being of Young Adults, Washington, DC. http://www.iom.edu/~/media/Files/Activity%20Files/Children/ImprovingYoungAdultsHealth/Lenhart%20Presentation.pdf (accessed October 10, 2014).

Lenroot, R. K., N. Gogtay, D. K. Greenstein, E. M. Wells, G. L. Wallace, L. S. Clasen, J. D. Blumenthal, J. Lerch, A. P. Zijdenbos, and A. C. Evans. 2007. Sexual dimorphism of brain developmental trajectories during childhood and adolescence. *NeuroImage* 36(4):1065-1073.

Lichter, D. T., D. K. McLaughlin, and D. C. Ribar. 2002. Economic restructuring and the retreat from marriage. *Social Science Research* 31(2):230-256.

Luna, B. 2009. Developmental changes in cognitive control through adolescence. *Advances in Child Development and Behavior* 37:233-278.

Luna, B., A. Padmanabhan, and K. O'Hearn. 2010. What has fMRI told us about the development of cognitive control through adolescence? *Brain and Cognition* 72(1):101-113.

Luthar, S. S. 2006. Resilience in development: A synthesis of research across five decades. In *Developmental psychopathology*, Vol. 3, 2nd ed., edited by D. Cicchetti and D. J. Cohen. Hoboken, NJ: Wiley. Pp. 739-795.

McLanahan, S. 2004. Diverging destinies: How children are faring under the second demographic transition. *Demography* 41(4):607-627.

Modell, J., F. F. Furstenberg, and T. Hershberg. 1976. Social-change and transitions to adulthood in historical-perspective. *Journal of Family History* 1(1):7-32.

Mulye, T. P., M. J. Park, C. D. Nelson, S. H. Adams, C. E. Irwin, Jr., and C. D. Brindis. 2009. Trends in adolescent and young adult health in the United States. *Journal of Adolescent Health* 45(1):8-24.

National Center for Health Statistics. 2011. *Health, United States, 2011*. Washington, DC: U.S. Government Printing Office.

Neinstein, L. 2013. *The new adolescents: An analysis of health conditions, behaviors, risks and access to services among young adults*. Los Angeles: University of Southern California.

Nguyen, Q. C., J. W. Tabor, P. P. Entzel, Y. Lau, C. Suchindran, J. M. Hussey, C. T. Halpern, K. M. Harris, and E. A. Whitsel. 2011. Discordance in national estimates of hypertension among young adults. *Epidemiology* 22(4):532-541.

Nguyen, Q. C., E. A. Whitsel, J. W. Tabor, C. C. Cuthbertson, M. H. Wener, A. J. Potter, C. T. Halpern, L. A. Killeya-Jones, J. M. Hussey, C. Suchindran, and K. M. Harris. 2014. Blood spot-based measures of glucose homeostasis and diabetes prevalence in a nationally representative population of young U.S. adults. *Annals of Epidemiology* (published online ahead of print). http://dx.doi.org/10.1016/j.annepidem.2014.09.010 (accessed October 22, 2014).

NRC (National Research Council). 2013. *Reforming juvenile justice: A developmental approach*. Washington, DC: The National Academies Press.

Ohlemacher, S. 2006. *Diversity grows in 49 of 50 states*. Associated Press. http://seattletimes.com/html/nationworld/2003199276_diversity15.html (accessed October 16, 2014).

Ordaz, S., and B. Luna. 2012. Sex differences in physiological reactivity to acute psychosocial stress in adolescence. *Psychoneuroendocrinology* 37(8):1135-1157.

Ordaz, S. J., W. Foran, K. Velanova, and B. Luna. 2013. Longitudinal growth curves of brain function underlying inhibitory control through adolescence. *Journal of Neuroscience* 33(46):18109-18124.

Padmanabhan, A., and B. Luna. 2013. Developmental imaging genetics: Linking dopamine function to adolescent behavior. *Brain and Cognition* 89(0):27-38.

Park, M. J., J. T. Scott, S. H. Adams, C. D. Brindis, and C. E. Irwin, Jr. 2014. Adolescent and young adult health in the United States in the past decade: Little improvement and young adults remain worse off than adolescents. *Journal of Adolescent Health* 55(1):3-16.

Parke, R. D. 2013. *Future families: Diverse forms, rich possibilities*. Hoboken, NJ: John Wiley & Sons.

Patrick, M. E., J. E. Schulenberg, and P. M. O'Malley. 2013. High school substance use as a predictor of college attendance, completion, and dropout: A national multicohort longitudinal study. *Youth & Society* 1-23.

Payne, K. 2011. *FP-11-11. On the road to adulthood: Sequencing of family experiences*. http://scholarworks.bgsu.edu/ncfmr_family_profiles/10 (accessed July 22, 2014).

Payne, K. 2012. *FP-12-04. School enrollment and completion*. http://scholarworks.bgsu.edu/ncfmr_family_profiles/17 (accessed July 22, 2014).

Petanjek, Z., M. Judaš, G. Šimić, M. R. Rašin, H. B. Uylings, P. Rakic, and I. Kostović. 2011. Extraordinary neoteny of synaptic spines in the human prefrontal cortex. *Proceedings of the National Academy of Sciences of the United States of America* 108(32):13281-13286.

Pew Research Center. 2013a. *After Boston, little change in views of Islam and violence*. Washington, DC: Pew Research Center. http://www.people-press.org/2013/05/07/after-boston-little-change-in-views-of-islam-and-violence/ (accessed October 15, 2014).

Pew Research Center. 2013b. *For African Americans, discrimination is not dead*. Washington, DC: Pew Research Center. http://www.pewresearch.org/fact-tank/2013/06/28/for-african-americans-discrimination-is-not-dead/ (accessed September 26, 2014).

Priest, N., Y. Paradies, B. Trenerry, M. Truong, S. Karlsen, and Y. Kelly. 2013. A systematic review of studies examining the relationship between reported racism and health and wellbeing for children and young people. *Social Science & Medicine* 95:115-127.

Raznahan, A., P. W. Shaw, J. P. Lerch, L. S. Clasen, D. Greenstein, R. Berman, J. Pipitone, M. M. Chakravarty, and J. N. Giedd. 2014. Longitudinal four-dimensional mapping of subcortical anatomy in human development. *Proceedings of the National Academy of Sciences of the United States of America* 111(4):1592-1597.

Rindfuss, R. R., C. G. Swicegood, and R. A. Rosenfeld. 1987. Disorder in the life course—how common and does it matter. *American Sociological Review* 52(6):785-801.

Roisman, G. I., A. S. Masten, J. D. Coatsworth, and A. Tellegen. 2004. Salient and emerging developmental tasks in the transition to adulthood. *Child Development* 75(1):123-133.

SAMHSA (Substance Abuse and Mental Health Services Administration). 2009. *Results from the 2008 National Survey on Drug Use and Health: National findings*. Rockville, MD: SAMHSA.

Scherf, K. S., J. M. Smyth, and M. R. Delgado. 2013. The amygdala: An agent of change in adolescent neural networks. *Hormones and Behavior* 64(2):298-313.

Schmitt, M. S., N. R. Branscombe, T. Postmes, and A. Barcia. 2014. The consequences of perceived discrimination for psychological well-being: A meta-analytic review. *Psychological Bulletin* 140:921-948.

Schneider, B. 2007. *Forming a college-going community in U.S. public high schools*. Lansing: Michigan State University.

Schulenberg, J. E., and J. L. Maggs. 2002. A developmental perspective on alcohol use and heavy drinking during adolescence and the transition to young adulthood. *Journal of Studies on Alcohol* 14:54-70.

Schulenberg, J. E., and I. Schoon. 2012. The transition to adulthood across time and space: Overview of special section. *Longitudinal and Life Course Studies* 3(2):164-172.

Seidman, L. J. 2013. *Mental health—psychotic disorders*. Presentation at IOM/NRC Workshop on Improving the Health, Safety, and Well-Being of Young Adults, Washington, DC. http://www.iom.edu/~/media/Files/Activity%20Files/Children/ImprovingYoungAdults Health/Seidman%20Presentation.pdf (accessed October 10, 2014).

Seltzer, J. A. 2000. Families formed outside of marriage. *Journal of Marriage and Family* 62(4):1247-1268.

Settersten, R. A., and B. Ray. 2010. *Not quite adults: Why 20-somethings are choosing a slower path to adulthood, and why it's good for everyone*. 1st ed. New York: Delacorte Press.

Shanahan, M. J. 2000. Pathways to adulthood in changing societies: Variability and mechanisms in life course perspective. *Annual Review of Sociology* 26:667-692.

Simmonds, D., M. N. Hallquist, M. Asato, and B. Luna. 2013. Developmental stages and sex differences of white matter and behavioral development through adolescence: A longitudinal diffusion tensor imaging (DTI) study. *NeuroImage* 92:356-368.

Smith, A. R., J. Chein, and L. Steinberg. 2013. Impact of socio-emotional context, brain development, and pubertal maturation on adolescent risk-taking. *Hormones and Behavior* 64(2):323-332.

Smith, E. L., and A. Cooper. 2013. *Homicide in the U.S. known to law enforcement, 2011.* Washington, DC: Bureau of Justice Statistics.

Somerville, L. H., and B. Casey. 2010. Developmental neurobiology of cognitive control and motivational systems. *Current Opinion in Neurobiology* 20(2):236-241.

Sowell, E. R., P. M. Thompson, C. J. Holmes, T. L. Jernigan, and A. W. Toga. 1999. In vivo evidence for post-adolescent brain maturation in frontal and striatal regions. *Nature Neuroscience* 2(10):859-861.

Sowell, E. R., B. S. Peterson, P. M. Thompson, S. E. Welcome, A. L. Henkenius, and A. W. Toga. 2003. Mapping cortical change across the human life span. *Nature Neuroscience* 6(3):309-315.

Spear, L. P. 2000. Neurobehavioral changes in adolescence. *Current Directions in Psychological Science* 9(4):111-114.

Steinberg, L. 2013. *Psychological development in young adulthood.* Presentation at IOM/NRC Workshop on Improving the Health, Safety, and Well-Being of Young Adults, Washington, DC.

Steinberg, L., D. Albert, E. Cauffman, M. Banich, S. Graham, and J. Woolard. 2008. Age differences in sensation seeking and impulsivity as indexed by behavior and self-report: Evidence for a dual systems model. *Developmental Psychology* 44:1764-1778.

Stone, J., A. Berrington, and J. Falkingham. 2013. Gender, turning points, and boomerangs: Returning home in young adulthood in Great Britain. *Demography* 51:257-276.

Teachman, J. D., L. M. Tedrow, and K. D. Crowder. 2000. The changing demography of America's families. *Journal of Marriage and Family* 62(4):1234-1246.

Turkle, S. 2011. *Together alone: Why we expect more from technology and less from each other.* New York: Basic Books.

U.S. Census Bureau. 2010. *Foreign-born population in the United States, 2010.* Washington, DC: U.S. Department of Commerce. http://www.census.gov/prod/2012pubs/acs-19.pdf (accessed October 10, 2014).

U.S. Census Bureau. 2012. *2012 national population projections.* http://www.census.gov/population/projections/data/national/2012.html (accessed October 16, 2014).

U.S. Department of Education and National Center for Education Statistics. 2014. *The condition of education 2014* (NCES 2014-083). http://nces.ed.gov/pubs2014/2014083.pdf (accessed October 10, 2014).

van Leijenhorst, L., B. G. Moor, Z. A. Op de Macks, S. A. Rombouts, P. M. Westenberg, and E. A. Crone. 2010. Adolescent risky decision-making: Neurocognitive development of reward and control regions. *NeuroImage* 51(1):345-355.

Wahlstrom, D., P. Collins, T. White, and M. Luciana. 2010. Developmental changes in dopamine neurotransmission in adolescence: Behavioral implications and issues in assessment. *Brain and Cognition* 72(1):146-159.

Wegrzyn, C. 2014. *Social media and information technology.* Presentation at IOM/NRC Workshop on Improving the Health, Safety, and Well-Being of Young Adults: State Policies and Programs and Social Media and Information Technology, Washington, DC.

Whitsel, E. A., Q. C. Nguyen, C. Suchindran, J. M. Hussey, L. A. Killeya-Jones, J. W. Tabor, C. S. Fitzgerald, S. P. Hallquist, C. T. Halpern, and K. M. Harris. 2011. Value added quality, quantity, and diversity of national blood pressure data on young adults. *Epidemiology* 22(4):544-545.

Whitsel, E. A., Q. C. Nguyen, C. Suchindran, J. W. Tabor, C. C. Cuthbertson, M. H. Wener, A. J. Potter, L. Killeya-Jones, J. M. Hussey, C. T. Halpern, and K. M. Harris. 2012. Dried capillary whole blood spot-based hemoglobin A1c, fasting glucose, and diabetes prevalence in a nationally representative population of young U.S. adults: Add Health, wave IV. *Circulation* 125:AP010.

Wierenga, L., M. Langen, S. Ambrosino, S. van Dijk, B. Oranje, and S. Durston. 2014. Typical development of basal ganglia, hippocampus, amygdala and cerebellum from age 7 to 24. *NeuroImage* 96:67-72.

Williams, D., and R. Williams-Morris. 2000. Racism and mental health: The African American experience. *Ethnicity and Health* 5(3-4):243-268.

Williams, D. R., H. W. Neighbors, and J. S. Jackson. 2003. Racial/ethnic discrimination and health: Findings from community studies. *American Journal of Public Health* 93(2): 200-208.

Zagorsky, J. L., and P. K. Smith. 2011. The freshman 15: A critical time for obesity intervention or media myth? *Social Science Quarterly* 92(5):1389-1407.

3

Relationships

Key Findings

- Young adulthood is a critical period for the formation of formal and informal romantic relationships that can have implications for the life course and many consequences for future mental and physical health and well-being.
- Relationship patterns and trends vary by gender, race, ethnicity, and socioeconomic position. These variations can lead to health disparities and differing patterns of social and achievement role transitions across the life course.
- Increasingly diverse levels of social networks that develop from family relations, romantic/sexual partners, peers, work, community, and educational institutions and other organizations have direct and indirect impacts on the health, safety, and well-being of young adults.
- Delays in childbearing have been taking place at the population level, together with an increasing proportion of nonmarital births occurring within cohabitation and increases in multiple-partner births. These trends vary by race and socioeconomic position, with health consequences for children and young adult parents.
- Changing demographic patterns of adult children are complex, and findings are mixed on the long-term implications of parental support for the development of young adults.

- Incarceration can impact relationship patterns and quality, family life, parenting, and children's development.

This chapter considers the relationships that make up the social lives of young adults, which comprise many of the most salient contexts and developmental tasks of young adulthood and have profound consequences for future adult emotional, physical, and mental health (House et al., 1988; Schulenberg and Maggs, 2002; Umberson et al., 2010b). In childhood and early adolescence, family and peer relationships are the primary contexts in which emotional ties, social support, and social interactions take place (Furman et al., 1999). Throughout adolescence, developmental tasks include gaining autonomy from parents, bonding with peers, and exploring romantic interests. During the transition from adolescence into young adulthood, young people explore new lifestyles and experience diverse environments that expand their social relationships. Developmental tasks shift to renegotiating parent-child relationships, expanding networks of peers, and pursuing romantic connections (Furstenberg et al., 2005; Shanahan, 2000). The family of origin remains a central relationship context, but young adults experience growing and more diverse social networks of friends, peers, classmates, workmates, neighbors, community members, and sexual and romantic partners (Bucx and van Wel, 2008). Indeed, central to the life course of young adults is developing more permanent romantic relationships, forming their own families, and potentially becoming parents and forging relationships with their own children.

"Relationships can't be built overnight. Young adults need to have someone they are generally able to engage with who can serve as a mentor within school or the neighborhood they live in."*

The discussion in this chapter is guided by a socioecological framework that integrates three prominent theoretical perspectives on human development in general and the transition from adolescence into adulthood in particular (Lerner, 2006): life-course theory (Elder, 1998), human ecology (Bronfenbrenner and Morris, 1998), and systems-based developmental psychopathology (Sameroff, 2010). This framework encompasses several basic tenets that are woven into the discussion throughout this chapter:

* Quotations are from members of the young adult advisory group during their discussions with the committee.

- Healthy development is a product of dynamic transactions between the individual and his or her close relationships within safe, prosocial, and supportive contexts.
- Individuals, their close relationships, and the transactions between them unfold over time within diverse social contexts.
- Social contexts can range from the concrete proximate settings of daily life (e.g., peers, schools, communities) to more abstract and distal social systems and structures (e.g., media, legal, political, cultural).
- The socially embedded role of relationships in healthy development can change dramatically across time and place.
- Public policy and programmatic efforts aimed at serving individuals can use relationships and the contexts in which they are embedded as intervention points.

Although this socioecological framework applies to the full life course, it is particularly relevant to young adulthood, a time of dynamic change and diversity in social relationships and the contexts in which they occur.

This chapter examines in turn four broad areas of relationship development in the lives of young adults: social relationships, romantic relationships and union formation, the transition to parenthood, and intergenerational relationships. Within these areas, we examine trends and patterns of relationship development as they relate to the themes of young adulthood described in Chapter 2. Given the centrality of family relationships during young adulthood—both the creation of one's own family through union formation and childbearing and intergenerational relationships—they are the primary focus of this chapter. We emphasize the protective nature of relationships; factors that inhibit or facilitate their development; and their link to health, safety, and well-being. We also examine the heterogeneity of these trends and patterns by gender, race, ethnicity, and socioeconomic position and the implications for disparities in health and achievement across the life course. In addition, we highlight topics in young adult relationships that have as yet received little research attention, as well as topics especially relevant to policies and programs that would improve the health, safety, and well-being of young adults. Chapter 9 includes a discussion of policies and programs for young adults who are parents.

> "In transitioning from college to work, you have to fit yourself into a new community. It can be really challenging. It can be very isolating."

SOCIAL RELATIONSHIPS

Social relationships are integral to physical and mental health and well-being. In contemporary societies, social relationships are articulated in the form of social networks (e.g., Simmel, 1950; Wasserman and Faust, 1994; Wellman and Berkowitz, 1997)—social structures that evolve out of dyadic relationships emerging from family relations, peership, friendship, work, groups, and organizations. It is within this web of affiliations that individuals self-actualize, and opportunities for and constraints on health and well-being present themselves.

Research suggests that a wide range of behaviors related to health and well-being develop and spread within networks. For example, research has shown that people are likely to be happier if they have close ties with happy people (Christakis and Fowler, 2009); by contrast, if people are depressed, their networks are more likely to be populated by depressed people (Rosenquist et al., 2010a). In addition, people closely connected within the same network tend to have similar health-related habits, such as smoking, alcohol drinking, and behaviors related to obesity (Rosenquist et al., 2010b). This similarity reflects a complex process by which individuals select networks and network members that share characteristics, attitudes, behaviors, and even genetic makeup within structural constraints often defined by socioeconomic position, race, ethnicity, and geography, and in which network influence is bidirectional (Boardman et al., 2012; Cohen-Cole and Fletcher, 2008).

Communication technologies expand the ability of people to preserve a variety of social ties and connect with a variety of networks. Media multiplexity theory builds on Granovetter's (1973) work to posit that those in stronger relationships tend to use more media with greater frequency than those in weaker relationships, although media are also helpful in activating and maintaining connections with weaker but potentially helpful social ties (Haythornthwaite, 2005; Haythornthwaite and Wellman, 1998). This theory has enabled researchers to connect social media use to relational strength (Baym and Ledbetter, 2009; Ledbetter, 2009) and also to growth in network size and diversity (Hampton et al., 2011). In other words, if one thinks of networks as the everyday neighborhoods people occupy (Rainie and Wellman, 2012), social and mobile media make these neighborhoods more accessible and interconnect people beyond the confines of geographic proximity. Reflecting a general theme of this report, young adults are at

> "Social media can be a tool to extend someone's social network for good or bad."

the forefront of this technological reshaping of social and interpersonal contexts.

Social and mobile media not only extend but also converge social networks, providing a rich sociocultural context for maintaining existing and cultivating new interpersonal relationships. Through this relational context, two main avenues for enhancing health and well-being present themselves: connection and expression.

Connection

The interconnected structure of social and mobile networks provides avenues for the sharing of information in ways that blend the potential of mass broadcasting with the immediacy of interpersonal conversation. This sociotechnical environment is enhanced by being constructed out of overlapping and interwoven social relations, weak or strong. People access a number of valuable resources through social relations, including information, advice, emotional support, and general forms of feedback (Baym, 2010), and social and mobile networks amplify potential points of social contact.

Not all points of contact have equal value for networked individuals. Social capital refers to the benefits that can be attained from the connections people maintain through their networks (Putnam, 2001). Depending on their nature, social ties are variably equipped to offer opportunities for different forms of social capital (Burt, 1992). Weak ties often work as "bridges," connecting "otherwise disparate groups of individuals" and thus exposing them to heterogeneous groups and a wider and more diverse range of information (Ellison et al., 2011, p. 128; Granovetter, 1973). Strong ties, on the other hand, consist of close friends and family, lending themselves to *bonding* forms of social capital and therefore potentially being capable of offering more substantive forms of support. Social and mobile media make it easier for individuals to maintain a larger network of weak ties. They make ephemeral connections persistent, lower barriers to initial interaction, and help people seek both information and support from both weak and strong social ties (Baym, 2010; Boyd, 2014; Ellison et al., 2011; Humphreys, 2005, 2010; Quinn and Papacharissi, 2014).

> "I have talked to people who say, 'Oh, I know that person from Facebook,' but they don't talk to them."

Expression

The sociotechnical environments resulting from the convergence of social and mobile networks invite people to connect further with others by disclosing information about themselves and their everyday lives. This form of self-disclosure has most recently been described as *lifestreaming*: "the ongoing sharing of personal information to a networked audience, the creation of a digital portrait of one's actions and thoughts" (Marwick, 2013, p. 208). These daily exercises in self-disclosure, self-documentation, and self-representation are a way for people to frame and maintain a coherent story of who they are, where they have been, and where they are headed in the face of modern challenges that constantly require them to adjust their personal boundaries (Gergen, 1991; Giddens, 1991; Papacharissi, 2012; Rettberg, 2013).

The process of lifestreaming is relevant in the present context because it allows people to share stories about health and well-being and to present their own point of view—to tell their own story in their own terms. This potentially empowering act also allows people to affiliate with a particular culture, not just telling their own story but engaging with others and their stories in the process. The networking enabled by social and mobile media thus provides new places where relationships can evolve, while the stories shared through these networks afford connection that permits these relationships to flourish in supportive ways.

ROMANTIC RELATIONSHIPS AND UNION FORMATION

Young adulthood is a critical period in the formation of romantic unions. Young adults engage in a wide variety of romantic activities during their early 20s, but the nature of these activities has changed considerably over time. A century ago, most Americans in the young adult age range were already married; today, that is no longer the case (Sassler, 2010). Today, changes such as gender role fluctuations, birth control access, social capital for marriage and unions, and the importance attached to single-generation households in mainstream U.S. culture may be creating a new set of expectations and values relative to traditional romantic union pathways. Reflecting the theme of different pathways that runs throughout this report, the idea of a normative path to romantic union has increasingly come to seem unrealistic.

> "There is a lot of pressure on young adults to be in relationships, and this is impacting their daily lives and mental health."

Generally, romantic unions—which represent more significant and durable ties than dating—fall into two categories: formal and informal. Marriage is a formal union, defined by a government-sanctioned and legally binding contract. Cohabitation is the most common form of informal union, denoting couples in an intimate relationship who live together but are not legally married. Although cohabitation was long stigmatized as "living in sin," it is now both common and widely accepted, such that most young Americans view it as a logical and expected step in the evolution of a relationship (Smock, 2000). As will be discussed shortly, same-sex unions could occur only in the context of cohabitation for most of U.S. history, as these unions were not legally recognized by the state. Today, moving from an informal to a formal union is now possible for same-sex couples, at least in some states (Hunter, 2012).

Despite the increased heterogeneity of the young adult population, efforts to disentangle racial and ethnic differences in this area are quite sparse. The majority of today's young adults form formal or informal unions before turning 25, with higher rates for African American and Hispanic young adults (across levels of education) and lower rates for college students and graduates (across races/ethnicities). Early cohabitation patterns are strongly influenced by early sexual debut, school dropout, and early parenthood (Hofferth and Goldscheider, 2010). Family stability (e.g., married parents, parents with more than high school education) appears to decrease the chances of early cohabitation (Hofferth and Goldscheider, 2010). Nearly 50 percent of young adults in the United States have cohabited by the time they turn 25, while only about a quarter have married. Among those who marry by age 25, the overwhelming majority (three-fifths) cohabit first (Payne, 2011). Racial/ethnic minority young adults are somewhat less likely to fit this pattern (although most do) (63 percent of whites cohabited before marriage compared with 57 percent of African Americans and 53 percent of Hispanics); those with a General Educational Development (GED) credential most often cohabited before marriage (77 percent), while those with a bachelor's degree or higher were least likely to cohabit before getting married (12 percent) (Payne, 2011). In other words, the modern style of union formation (cohabitation that may or may not be followed by marriage) tends to be less common in historically disadvantaged segments of the population (Payne, 2011).

These contemporary patterns are manifestations of much longer-term trends. Specifically, lower rates of marriage among young adults do not necessarily imply that marriage is becoming less common overall. Instead, they reflect a delay in marriage: young adults will get married eventually, but not during their early 20s. The median age at first marriage (the age by which half of the population has married) generally has increased over the last century. Today the median age is 29.4 for men and 27.4 for women

(U.S. Census Bureau, 2013). Thus the median age of marriage now falls outside of the 18-26 age range that is the focus of this report. Moreover, it is now older than the median age at first birth, meaning that on average, young adults become parents before marrying. They still form unions, just not formal unions, or at least not yet (Arroyo et al., 2013; Payne, 2012). The most common explanations for these trends are economic: American youth have high expectations for where they need to be economically before getting married but have more trouble getting there; in addition, getting to that point now requires greater investments in education and career development, especially among women, than was previously the case. Cultural explanations include an attitudinal shift away from the traditional exchange system of marriage toward women's economic independence and two-career households (Settersten and Ray, 2010; Teachman et al., 2000).

Even as cohabitation becomes a normative part of young adult pathways, its meaning and role in the social lives of young adults differ widely, reflecting this report's theme of population heterogeneity and diverse pathways. Family demographers Casper and Bianchi (2002) propose a basic typology of cohabitation that is not specific to young adulthood but is highly relevant to this period of the life course. Some young adults may cohabit as an *alternative to marriage*; they expect the relationship to endure but do not expect to make it legal—a marriage in all aspects but name. Another type of cohabitation is a *precursor to marriage*, a preliminary step on the road to getting married, almost like part of the engagement. A *trial marriage* is when a couple cohabits as practice, to explore whether they are compatible and whether marriage may make sense in the future. Finally, some young adults may use cohabitation as a form of *coresidential dating*—not wanting to get married but not wanting to be alone, so that they live together while dating without expecting that the arrangement will lead anywhere.

Although cohabitation as an alternative to marriage has a long tradition in Latin America (and, therefore, among Latin American immigrants in the United States) (see Frank and Wildsmith, 2005), it is relatively uncommon overall in this country. The other three types of cohabitation are much more common in the United States. The prevalence of these three types helps explain why cohabitation among Americans, including young adults, is a temporary state with a typical duration of about 1 year. Couples either move to marriage, decide that they are not marriage material, or just drift apart (Smock, 2000). In a comparison with dozens of other Western developed countries, Heuveline and Timberlake (2004) found that the most prototypically American form of cohabitation was akin to the alternative to singlehood as described above, a reflection of ample housing and widespread birth control in the United States, and indicative of short relationships without children.

As noted, same-sex couples often have been difficult to classify in terms of marriage and cohabitation. Many same-sex couples (including young adults) lived together, but because of heterosexual definitions of legal marriage, one could not know whether they were more like a cohabiting couple (and if so, what type) or a married couple. Unlike opposite-sex couples, they had no choice in the matter (Gates, 2013). Over the past decade, some states began to recognize same-sex marriage legally, through either court decisions or legislative deliberations, and some states grant some marriage-like status to same-sex couples (e.g., civil unions). In June 2013, the U.S. Supreme Court rendered a decision in *United States v. Windsor* holding that the federal government is obligated to recognize any marriage granted by a state, regardless of whether it is between a same-sex or opposite-sex couple (Hunter, 2012).[1]

When same-sex marriage is legal, same-sex and opposite-sex couples tend to follow similar union formation (and dissolution) patterns (Hunter, 2012). How these dramatic legal changes will affect young adults is currently unknown. Given that young adulthood is an important period in union formation and that young adults are by far among Americans the most supportive of same-sex marriage (Dimock et al., 2013), this is an important topic for future research as more data on same-sex relationships become available.

The distinctions among formal and informal unions, same-sex or opposite-sex, are significant in light of the considerable evidence showing that romantic unions, especially formal unions, bring many benefits, including greater economic security, more social support, and better health. These patterns often are conditional on the duration of formal and informal unions throughout adulthood. Yet simply transitioning into a romantic partnership can have implications for the life course, as union formation itself can facilitate healthier and more prosocial behavior (Umberson et al., 2010b). Consistent with this report's theme of social change and social network activities being concentrated in young adulthood, it is not surprising that union formation is increasingly taking place online. Popular dating sites need to be better understood as contexts for romantic partnerships, cohabitation, and even marriage (Kreager et al., 2014).

Union Formation and Health

One of the recurring themes of this report concerns the high stakes of pathways forged during young adulthood—a theme clearly evident when one considers how patterns of union formation shape lifelong health trajectories. Decades of research have documented the health benefits of marriage for men and women, including reduced health risk behaviors, improved

[1] *United States v. Windsor*, 570 U.S. 12 (2013).

access to health insurance, and improved physical health and psychosocial well-being (Umberson and Montez, 2010; Waite, 1995; see the review and synthesis of research by Wood et al., 2007). Notable in this research is the attempt to disentangle health selection from the protective effects of marriage on health. Health selection occurs when underlying processes operate to increase the chances that healthier people enter marriage, leaving less healthy individuals unmarried or in cohabiting relationships. For example, observed differences in socioeconomic position and, in turn, better health are important selection factors that give individuals a higher probability of being married and of having better health over their life course (Goldman, 1993; Haas, 2006). On the other hand, marriage may have a causal protective effect, over and above health selection, that improves the health of married individuals (Hughes and Waite, 2002; Zhang and Hayward, 2006). In general, evidence indicates that both selection and protection operate in the health advantages of marriage, with protection effects being greater for men than for women (Goldman, 1993; Wood et al., 2007).

In comparison with effects of other role transitions, including parenthood and employment, marriage tends to be more predictive of greater health and decreased involvement with the justice system during early adulthood (Duncan et al., 2006; Sampson et al., 2006; Staff et al., 2010). Marriage is consistently associated with declines in alcohol and other drug use (Bachman et al., 2002; Duncan et al., 2006; Leonard and Eiden, 2007; Staff et al., 2010), although this effect is limited when both partners are heavy substance users (Merline et al., 2008). Criminal involvement also tends to decrease with marriage (Sampson et al., 2006).

Beneficial health effects also are found for cohabitation, although to a limited degree. Research in Europe and Canada, where cohabitation has a longer history than in the United States, has found that single individuals report the lowest levels of health, while cohabiters' self-reported health typically falls in the middle of that of married and single persons (Joung et al., 1995; Mastekaasa, 1994; Ren, 1997). Other Canadian research shows that a variety of physical health measures are improved equally for those who cohabit or marry compared with those who remain single (Wu et al., 2003), or are unaffected by entry into cohabitation (Wu and Hart, 2002). With respect to mental health in the United States, some research shows that it is not associated with cohabitation (Booth et al., 2008; Horwitz and White, 1998; Kim and McKenry, 2002; Lamb et al., 2003), some shows that it is similar for those who cohabit and marry (Ross, 1995), and some shows that cohabitation compared with marriage is associated with greater depression (Brown, 2000; Brown et al., 2005). Much of this prior research, however, suffers from limited health indicators and controls or small or unrepresentative samples, or is based on cross-sectional data or otherwise fails to account for selection effects, making it difficult to separate the effects of selection into unions from the protective effects of union status. Furthermore, the broader societal context and prevalence of cohabitation have changed in the past few decades, suggesting that the meaning and health effects of cohabitation have changed as well, and may continue to do so.

Recent longitudinal research by Pollard and Harris (2013) examines a wide array of health indicators, including general health status, mental health, health behavior (regular physical exam, binge drinking, tobacco use, physical exercise), and body mass index among cohabiting versus married and single young adult men and women, controlling for health selection prior to union formation. Consistent with some of the previous research, the authors report mixed findings. They find that cohabitation does not benefit the health of young adult women who report poorer physical and mental health than married or single young adult women. Although cohabiting young adult women engage in less problem drinking behavior, they have lower levels of physical activity and more frequent use of tobacco than single adult women. Cohabiting young adult men experience more health benefits, with improved mental health and less problem drinking. Selection plays an important role in health differentials by union status. In general, young adults with worse mental health and poorer health behaviors appear to be selected into cohabitation compared with remaining single. Despite this selection, however, the protective effects of a union are the likely cause of any benefits found, especially for men. The presence of a cohabiting partner likely increases social support, benefiting the mental health of men in particular (Kessler and Cleary, 1980; Thoits, 1983).

THE TRANSITION TO PARENTHOOD

Parenthood has been a common role transition during young adulthood throughout U.S. history, but the age pattern and union context of childbearing have changed dramatically with the changes in union formation described above. Consonant with the delay in marriage has been a delay in childbearing at the population level. The average age at first childbearing has been increasing since the 1970s and currently stands at 26 for women and 28 for men (Martin et al., 2013; Mathews and Hamilton, 2009). While the 20s remain the peak years for childbearing, the rates of childbearing have been declining slightly for women aged 20-29 and increasing slightly for women over age 30, and teen childbearing rates have been declining since 1991 (Martin et al., 2013). What is most notable about childbearing among young adults is that it occurs predominantly outside of marriage.

With the increasing prevalence of cohabitation and delayed marriage—demographic trends concentrated among young adults—a growing proportion of births to young adults have been occurring outside of marriage. The trend in nonmarital childbearing among young adults is due in part to couples delaying marriage but not delaying childbearing by an equal or greater number of years, and shows persistent racial, ethnic, and socioeconomic position gradients. The percentage of births that occur outside of marriage has increased for all young adults in America, although the rates by race and ethnicity still differ markedly. Among young adult women aged 20-24, blacks have the highest rate of nonmarital fertility (103.5 births per 1,000 unmarried black women), followed by Hispanics (96.5), whites (46.6), and Asians/Pacific Islanders (22.0) (Martin et al., 2013). Thus 88.2 percent of all births to black women aged 20-24 are outside of marriage, compared with 66.6 percent among Hispanic women, 54.8 percent among white women, 76.6 percent among American Indian/Alaska Native women, and 45.5 percent among Asian/Pacific Islander women in that age group (Martin et al., 2013).

In addition, young adults who bear children outside of marriage often are more disadvantaged, both before and after birth, in comparison with married young adults that have children. Compared with married young adult mothers, unmarried young adult mothers usually have lower incomes and education levels, and they are more likely to receive public assistance (Driscoll et al., 1999; Lichter et al., 2003; Mincieli et al., 2007; Smock and Greenland, 2010), and these patterns hold across race and ethnicity. Similarly, the majority of nonmarital births to young adults are reported to be unintended (Smock and Greenland 2010; Wildsmith et al., 2011). "Unintended births are those that, at the time of conception, were either mistimed (the mother wanted the pregnancy to occur earlier or later than it did) or unwanted (at that time or any time in the future)" (Wildsmith et al., 2011, p. 4). Estimates vary, but a recent study reviewing data from the Early Childhood Longitudinal Study-Birth Cohort found that while 20 percent of births to married women are reported to be unintended, this is the case for 65 percent of births to women who are not married or cohabiting with the child's father and 50 percent of births to women who are cohabiting with the child's father (Wildsmith et al., 2011). Note, however, that the "unintendedness" status of births is a subjective and typically retrospective assessment. Qualitative studies indicate that some women may report a birth as "unintended" when in fact they knowingly made no effort to avoid unintended pregnancy through the use of birth control (Edin and Kefalas, 2005). Thus survey estimates of unintended births may be overstated.

Another important trend in the transition to parenthood among young adults is the increasing proportion of nonmarital births that occur within cohabitation, which varies by race and ethnicity. Sixty-one percent of white and 65 percent of Hispanic nonmarital births occur among women who are cohabiting, while fewer than 30 percent of nonmarital births occur among cohabiting black women (Mincieli et al., 2007). Perhaps the most important distinction in childbearing patterns by race and ethnicity is that births to young adult black women occur predominantly outside of unions.

In sum, patterns of the transition to parenthood vary by socioeconomic position (Ellwood and Jencks, 2001; Smock and Greenland, 2010). Many young adult couples are waiting to have children in order to follow career goals, and consequently, many have smaller families (Hines, 2008), but these women are primarily of higher socioeconomic position, with higher levels of education and eventual income. Young adults of higher socioeconomic position from all racial and ethnic groups delay childbearing until their late 20s or 30s (Sassler and Cunningham, 2008; Smock and Greenland, 2010). Young adults who are making the transition to parenthood tend to come from a lower socioeconomic background, with fewer years of completed education and lower potential household income. Young adults of lower socioeconomic position tend to have children early in young adulthood (i.e., before the average age of first childbearing in America), and most of their births occur outside of marriage. Both quantitative and qualitative research has documented this pattern of delaying marriage but not delaying childbearing (Edin and Kefalas, 2005; Gibson-Davis et al., 2005; Smock and Greenland, 2010; Sweeney, 2002). Because racial and ethnic minority women tend to come from lower socioeconomic backgrounds and face higher risks of poverty, rates of early, nonmarital, and unintended childbearing are higher for black and Hispanic women, but the primary driver of early childbearing patterns in young adulthood remains socioeconomic position.

Explanations for this pattern of childbearing among young adult women of low socioeconomic position include the low opportunity costs associated with childbearing (i.e., because employment and career opportunities are lower for these women, they do not suffer a loss of opportunities due to childbearing) and a lack of marriageable men, together with the increasing economic independence of women and deteriorating economic fortunes of men in their occupational and economic stratum (Edin and Kefalas, 2005; Oppenheimer, 2003; Wilson, 1987). Another important factor behind the rise in nonmarital childbearing at all socioeconomic levels is the dramatic shift in attitudes toward women's roles in the workplace and family, including increasing acceptance of working mothers and single-mother families (Casper and Bianchi, 2002; Edin and Kefalas, 2005).

Multiple-Partner Fertility

Another trend that varies by race and socioeconomic position is the dramatic increase in the number of women having multiple-partner births, a phenomenon termed multiple-partner fertility (MPF). This phenomenon underscores two major themes of this report: population diversity (i.e., group differences in the prevalence of MPF) and intergenerational connections (i.e., family influences on MPF and its implications for children). Having children by more than one partner is an overlooked yet important component of family formation and family structure. According to Guzzo and Furstenberg (2007), the phenomenon is fairly common among low-income individuals and differs remarkably by race. Based on national survey data, the rate of MPF is nearly 7 percent for black women aged 19-25, more than twice the rate for white or Hispanic women. MPF is seen most commonly among those who are young and unmarried at first birth and have conflicted and weak relationships with current or previous partners. Switching to another partner and having additional children in that relationship often is prompted by the hope of improving prospects for having a stable relationship. Women following such relationship trajectories frequently experience depression and substance use, which increases the likelihood that their partners will raise their own biological children solo because of the destabilizing factors in their relationships with the mothers of their children.

Manlove and colleagues (2008) contend that the combination of increased marital dissolution and nonmarital fertility may contribute to the rising rates of MPF and that the phenomenon may become even more prevalent in the future, "fostering intergenerational trends in disadvantage and in disconnected families" (p. 547). Anderson (1999) has suggested that high rates of uncommitted sexual relationships in disadvantaged communities may be caused by a shortage of financial opportunities.

Another important issue in understanding the complexities of MPF families is the extent to which women bearing children with romantic partners who have additional children by other women influences childrearing and parenting patterns. Burton and Hardaway (2012) pose the question of whether such women serve as "other-mothers" to the children of their current or past romantic partners. Other-mothering has a long-standing tradition in African American and Latino families. Findings from Burton and Hardaway's study of low-income women reveal that the majority of MPF women were overwhelmed with the day-to-day management of their own households; very few were serving as other-mothers. Alarmingly, half of the women had been medically diagnosed with depression and/or anxiety, often associated with their contentious relationships with romantic partners and the lack of resources from the biological father(s) of their children. Many of the women sought new partners or continued relationships with former partners knowing that the men had children with multiple women. Additional research is needed to inform practice and policies aimed at meeting the mental health and parenting needs of women involved in MPF, including enhancing their ability to manage relational stress and conflict with their romantic partners.

Because of the increasing rate of MPF and the potential negative consequences for children, research also is needed to identify ways of encouraging fathers to support their children from concurrent or previous relationships. Doing so will require programs and policies that facilitate school completion so as to increase employment, and perhaps diversion programs that reduce incarceration to increase men's marriage potential. Finally, in light of the declining birth rate among teenagers and rising nonmarital birth rates among young adults in their 20s, efforts designed to reduce nonmarital and unintended pregnancies previously targeting teenagers need to be expanded to include young adult men and women.

Childbearing and Health

The consequences of nonmarital fertility for the health of children have received considerable research attention. Most of the research on the health of unmarried mothers comes from European settings where single mothers report worse health than married or cohabiting mothers (e.g., Elstad, 1996; Shouls et al., 1999; Westin and Westerling, 2006). Other research on representative U.S. samples has examined the health consequences of nonmarital childbearing among women in mid-life (age 40) (Williams et al., 2011) and the long-term consequences among elderly women in their 60s and 70s (Henretta, 2007). Likewise, research examining the birth and health outcomes of children born to never-married mothers finds greater risks to their health and well-being compared with children born to married mothers (e.g., Albrecht et al., 1994; Bennett, 1992; Bennett et al., 1994; Chomitz et al., 1995; Williams et al., 2013). However, there is less research on the consequences for the young adult mothers and absent fathers.

The large literature on marriage and health described above is relevant, however, to the health consequences of nonmarital fertility among young adult mothers. Health operates as an important selection factor associated with nonmarital fertility, if only through the process of nonmarriage, but more importantly because relationship and childbearing decisions often are made jointly (Edin and Kefalas, 2005; Musick, 2007; Upchurch et al., 2002). As noted above, despite the increasing prevalence of nonmarital childbearing in the mainstream young adult population, there remain significant differences by socioeconomic position, with nonmarital childbearing being more common among women with lower levels of education and income and disadvantaged parental backgrounds (Lichter and Qian, 2008; Lichter et al., 1992). These selection differences are correlated with health prior to nonmarital childbearing and matter for the health consequences of nonmarital fertility. Thus, preconception and preunion health is an important factor in understanding how a nonmarital birth is related to the subsequent health of a young adult mother. Recent research by Wagner and Harris (2014) taking preconception and preunion health into account finds an additional negative health impact among women who have births outside of marriage, especially those who are not in cohabiting or highly committed relationships. Although research has yet to uncover the mechanisms through which this additional health disadvantage operates, the stress experienced by single mothers and the disadvantaged environments in which nonmarital births occur are likely explanations (Williams et al., 2011). As with the health effects of cohabitation, however, the broader societal context and prevalence of nonmarital fertility have changed in recent decades, suggesting that the significance and health effects of such births for both parents and children have changed. Multicohort research therefore is needed to examine historical variation in the effects of nonmarital fertility.

Young Adult Parents

Given the contexts in which young adults experience childbearing, as described above, it is not surprising that research has focused on the number of challenges they face as they become parents. Reflecting one of the themes of this report—that the stakes of young adulthood are high—pathways that include childbearing have profound consequences for the health and well-being of young adults and their families (Amato, 2005; Demo and Cox, 2000; Gibson-Davis, 2008; Haveman et al., 2001). While those consequences include both costs and benefits, the balance of research finds that having children is more costly than rewarding for young adults in terms of economic security, daily stress, social relationships, and psychological well-being (Nomaguchi and Milkie, 2003; Thomas and Sawhill, 2005; Umberson et al., 2010a). However, this general finding is dependent on the gender and marital status of the young adult (Umberson and Williams, 1999). In particular, women and the unmarried tend to experience greater risks of low family income and poverty, and as a result, greater distress and lower psychological well-being relative to men or married young adults. Unmarried young adult mothers living alone and raising young children lack economic, social, and emotional resources and face the challenges of providing for their family and parenting young children alone.

Grandparents can play important roles in helping their young adult children with childrearing. Over the past several decades, a growing number of grandparents have been taking care of grandchildren. In 2010, approximately 10 percent of children (7.5 million) were living with a grandparent, and 4.9 million of them lived in the grandparent's home (U.S. Census Bureau, 2010). Fully 82 percent of such households are three-generation households; in the remainder, neither of the grandchild's parents is in the household (Wilson, 2012). Caregiving by coresident grandparents occurs disproportionately among families who are poor and among racial/

ethnic minorities (Wilson, 2012). When the parents are absent, grandparents act as "surrogate parents" and role models, supporting and guiding their grandchildren's development and imparting cultural and family values (Burton, 1992). Empirical findings show that caregiving can be beneficial for the grandparents, the young adult parents, and the grandchildren. It also can improve the developmental outcomes of children raised by poor single parents, most of whom are young (Burton, 1992; Dunifon and Kowaleski-Jones, 2007; Hayslip and Kaminski, 2005). On the other hand, in many cases, caregiving grandparents—African American grandmothers in particular—report physical, mental, and financial burdens associated with caregiving (Fuller Thomson, 2000). Further, a significant proportion of grandparents experience stress-related health problems that they believe contributed to the onset of various chronic illnesses (e.g., diabetes, hypertension) (Burt, 1992).

A wealth of data has documented the increased risks of economic insecurity and poverty associated with single motherhood, and nonmarital childbearing in particular, in young adulthood (e.g., Ellwood and Jencks, 2001; Garfinkel and McLanahan, 1986; McLanahan and Sandefur, 1994). Children create substantial demands on parents' time and physical and emotional energy, but these demands generally take a greater toll on parents' well-being when economic security, social resources, and emotional support are lacking. Marriage tends to increase family economic stability, emotional well-being, and psychological health, which in turn lead to higher-quality relationships and positive parenting behaviors (Brown and Booth, 1996; Lerman, 2002; Nock, 1995). Cohabitation provides some of these resources, but the lack of institutionalization of expectations, norms, and legal supports for parenting, as well as the shorter duration and instability of such unions, makes this union context less beneficial to the well-being of young adult parents (Cherlin, 2004; Manning et al., 2004).

The overload all parents experience from combining family responsibilities with employment and job responsibilities and having to find child care is particularly stressful in the context of family poverty and/or single motherhood (Gibson-Davis, 2008; Umberson et al., 2010a). The lack of a partner's potential resources and of social networks within the world of work further isolates poor and low-educated single mothers in particular. The stressors experienced by these young adults as a consequence of being uneducated and having limited skills with which to obtain gainful employment not only inhibit their ability to support themselves but also affect their children. Raising children in poverty diminishes parents' ability to meet the basic needs of their children while producing multiple strains for both parents and children that can have long-lasting consequences.

These strains often manifest through harsh and inconsistent parenting, elevated family conflict and violence, and depleted emotional energy.

The chronic stress associated with facing the daily difficulties of economic insecurity and providing and caring for children erodes mothers' physical and mental health, undermining effective parenting and connections with the extended family that might provide some support (Avison et al., 2007; Evenson and Simon, 2005). The stress experienced by disconnected parents also is heightened by living in crowded, substandard housing, often located in high-crime and socially disorganized neighborhoods. Krieger and Higgins (2002) characterize housing as one of the determinants of health, with poor living conditions being linked with anxiety; depression; psychological distress, including irritability; and social intolerance. Children who reside in poor housing are at increased risk for numerous health problems, such as respiratory infections, asthma, lead poisoning, and injuries (Krieger and Higgins, 2002).

The risks faced by young adults who become parents and their children require policy attention and program intervention. However, interventions can be effective only if the causes of early and nonmarital childbearing and its consequences are identified. Research aimed at understanding the elevated risks to young adult and child functioning among unmarried parents and poor families has identified two major explanations: selection and structural constraints (Biblarz and Raftery, 1999; Gibson-Davis, 2008).

The preponderance of this research examines selection efforts. This evidence indicates that the poorer outcomes of young adult parents and their children are due to preexisting differences in family background (primarily lower socioeconomic position) compared with those who do not become parents in young adulthood and delay both marriage and childbearing (Oesterle, 2013). For example, Amato and Kane (2011) found that college-bound women who delayed family formation rated their health higher, were less depressed, and had higher self-esteem in their mid-20s compared with single mothers, who ranked the lowest on all of these measures; however, these same differences were evident in adolescence before the women followed divergent pathways into young adulthood. This evidence suggests that the disadvantaged outcomes experienced by young adult parents are due more to their disadvantaged backgrounds in childhood and adolescence than to the process of becoming a parent in young adulthood.

There is some evidence that having limited social, economic, and emotional resources undermines parenting behaviors, as well as parents' health and well-being. For example, the lack of a spouse or partner reduces such resources for single mothers, as well as the social capital associated with the father's extended family (McLanahan and Sandefur, 1994). However, research examining parenting styles and parent-child relationships by family structure has not found significant differences in positive engagement, harsh parenting behaviors, or parental aggravation among married, cohabiting, and single mothers once preexisting differences in family background and adolescent well-being are taken into account (Gibson-Davis, 2008), thus further supporting the importance of selection factors.

In sum, social stratification in the United States tends to reinforce disadvantaged pathways by which young adults enter parenthood, cope with the stressors of work and family, and parent the next generation of children. Early exposure to adversities among the children of these disadvantaged young parents disrupts brain development; impedes learning; and increases the likelihood of low academic performance, repeated grades, school disengagement, and early dropout from school—a cycle that is repeated as those who experience these adversities have children. The problems associated with growing up in a hazardous environment are compounded as individuals attempt to manage their life circumstances. Specifically, feeling helpless, hopeless, distressed, anxious, depressed, and unable to change one's life course may lead to maladaptive coping strategies (e.g., alcohol/substance use, risky sexual practices) (Murry et al., 2013).

Two-Generation Programs: Saving a Generation of At-Risk Children by Investing in Their Young Parents

Various programs targeting either young mothers or their children have failed to yield the desired results (Chase-Lansdale and Brooks-Gunn, 2014). A promising policy trend therefore involves investing in both generations at the same time—an approach that reflects the theme of this report of connecting generations. The ultimate goal of this investment is to move the young adult onto a pathway that leads to self-sufficiency and economic independence. Programs currently being designed with this goal explicitly target low-income parents and their children. "For children, two-generation programs can include health and education services such as home visiting, early childhood education, and interventions for those exposed to trauma. Services for parents can involve parenting, literacy, learning the English language, earning a General Educational Development (GED) credential, obtaining a postsecondary education, receiving treatment for mental health problems, and receiving counseling aimed at preventing child abuse and domestic violence, as well as case management and workforce development" (Chase-Lansdale and Brooks-Gunn, 2014, p. 14).

Two-generation programs are not new. The two-generation concept was fundamental to the launch of Head Start in 1965. In the early 1990s, the Foundation for Child Development described two-generation programs that involved two strategies: embedding some self-sufficiency programs for parents in early childhood education programs and adding child care to education and employment services for parents (Smith, 1995). Other two-generation programs in the 1980s and 1990s were focused on adolescent mothers on welfare. Their main goal was to promote life skills, high school graduation or GED attainment, employment, and reductions in long-term welfare use (Zaslow et al., 2002). A few services for children also were provided—mainly child care, with little attention to its quality. Although these early two-generation programs took a fresh approach to the problems of both young parents and children in low-income families, the impetus to expand such programs was lost because several large demonstration programs for adolescent mothers yielded disappointing results (e.g., Duncan and Magnuson, 2004; Granger and Cytron, 1999; Moore and Brooks-Gunn, 2002), and because work-first policies instituted through welfare reform began to dominate the human capital focus for poor young parents (Shaw et al., 2005).

The mid-2000s saw a resurgence of interest in two-generation programs, led primarily by foundation support and initiatives. For example, The Bill & Melinda Gates Foundation launched an ambitious postsecondary education program for low-income students in 2008; the Foundation for Child Development added a two-generation component to its PreK-3rd initiative; the Annie E. Casey Foundation launched an initiative to expand and study implementation strategies for two-generation human capital interventions (see Box 3-1); the W.K. Kellogg Foundation is foster-

BOX 3-1
Examples of Two-Generation Programs

The Annie E. Casey Foundation has an initiative to strengthen programs that link family economic success with high-quality early childhood education for children (Murrell, 2012). The strategy for this initiative is to identify barriers to the implementation of two-generation programs while working with programs that combine parent and child services in order to develop creative ways of improving implementation. The foundation has funded the implementation of programs at four sites (the Community Action Project [CAP] of Tulsa, the Atlanta Partnership, the Educational Alliance, and the Garrett County Community Action Committee). Two of these sites are discussed below. An evaluation will focus on the challenges and best practices in the implementation of two-generation programs, as well as short-term parent and child indicators (Chase-Lansdale and Brooks-Gunn, 2014).

Career*Advance*®, a program of CAP Tulsa, is the first fully operating two-generation sectoral training program in the United States. It is an education and training program in the health care sector (nursing and medical technology) for parents of young children enrolled in CAP Tulsa's early childhood education centers. The health care profession was identified as a source of family-supporting wages in Tulsa. In partnership with community colleges, Career*Advance* offers a sequence of programs that enable participants to obtain a certificate so they can enter the workplace with a credential; participants also can return for further advancement. Partnerships are maintained with a range of organizations—including community colleges, employers, public schools, GED and English as a second

BOX 3-1 Continued

language programs, and the Tulsa Workforce Board—that implement the workforce intermediary approach. Innovations include GED preparation that is specific to health care terms and concepts, and a number of support components including career coaches, financial incentives, and peer group meetings. The program is tuition free and covers all expenses. A quasi-experimental evaluation of Career*Advance*, begun in 2010, will continue until 2015. The evaluation is using a mixed-methods longitudinal design that compares participants in Career*Advance* with a matched group of families in which the children are enrolled in CAP Tulsa's early childhood education centers, but the parents are not enrolled in Career*Advance*.

The Annie E. Casey Foundation's Atlanta Partnership merges adult and child programs and comprises the foundation's Atlanta Civic Site, the Sheltering Arms Early Learning and Resource Center, an elementary school, and the Center for Working Families. These programs have achieved national recognition and are located on the same campus in Atlanta. The Center for Working Families, for example, "provides a combination of comprehensive education and workforce development services, as well as coaching and leadership training, in one location so residents can compete in the workforce. The two-generation program specifically targets parents of children in Sheltering Arms" (Chase-Lansdale and Brooks-Gunn, 2014, p. 32). An implementation study and a short-term outcomes study are in progress.

In addition to these programs, the Annie E. Casey Foundation, together with the Open Society, Kresge, Paul Allen, and Kellogg Foundations, as well as the National Institutes of Health and the Department of Health and Human Services, funded the Urban Institute's launch of a Housing Opportunity and Services Together (HOST) program in Chicago and Portland, Oregon. HOST is a whole-family or dual-generations program that establishes partnerships with various community organizations and coordinates services and programs for parents and children in public and mixed-income housing. The program uses a case management approach to prepare families in low-income neighborhoods to overcome barriers to self-sufficiency. At the parent level, the focus is on pathways to completing education and training that will lead to certification and employment. Career services and life skills development, as well as programs and services addressing both physical and mental health concerns, also are available. At the child level, programs and services are designed to promote academic success and school completion and to reduce risky behaviors. Programs also target family-level improvements, with emphasis on connecting young adults to support networks and relationships through neighborhood organizations. Preliminary findings show great promise, as case managers are reporting fewer lease violations, higher employment rates, increased civic engagement among residents, and improvement in youth school and extracurricular activities, and some families have begun saving to purchase a home or start a business. The overall goal is to utilize housing as a platform for addressing numerous challenges that confront the most vulnerable residents by bridging public housing authorities, private developers, and federal policy makers (Scott et al., 2013).

The promise shown by these initiatives suggests the need for more funding to expand the offerings of evidence-based two-generation interventions.

ing innovative family engagement programs; and the Aspen Institute has established a broad two-generation investment in policy, practice, research philanthropy, and the media (Two Generations, One Future). These initiatives have a renewed and explicit focus on promoting the human capital of low-income parents and children in the same program. For parents, education and training go beyond adult basic education and obtaining a GED to include postsecondary education and certification, thus responding to the rising need for credentials and skills in a service-oriented and technological workplace and preparing parents for jobs that will lead to family-supporting wages. These programs also capitalize on new directions in job training by including "workforce intermediaries" (discussed below). For children, the programs reflect the evidence that high-quality childhood education centers can have significant short- and long-term benefits. The current two-generation approach also has expanded to encompass the full range of low-income families, not just those on welfare or teen parents.

Most two-generation programs are still in the pilot stages, exploring various innovations, but the theory behind these initiatives suggests and their leaders strongly believe that two-generation programs will be more effective than single-generation programs (Chase-Lansdale and Brooks-Gunn, 2014). There are two primary reasons for this optimism. First, designers of intensive education and training programs for parents are situating their programs in organizations where the children are—in high-quality early-childhood education centers and prekindergarten programs. This collocation strategy promotes social capital and networking among parents, children, teachers, program leaders, and family support staff (Small, 2009). As parents see their children thriving and learning, they are more motivated to improve their own education and economic standing and tend to be more committed to and persistent in their education and training programs. Second, the early-childhood education centers have become key partners that serve as workforce intermediaries for low-income parents (an approach called "sectoral training"). This approach entails bringing together employers and workers and private and public funding streams. In essence, low-income parents are linked directly to partners such as employers and community colleges that offer peer support, coaching, and other services (King et al., 2009).

INTERGENERATIONAL RELATIONSHIPS

The changes discussed thus far in social relationships, union formation, and the transition to parenthood among young adults have been occurring in the context of another notable change: the delays in leaving home and the return to the parental home of adult children.

Living Arrangements Among Young Adults

Even as the social maturation of children is occurring more rapidly than in previous generations as a result of the increased influence of television and the Internet, "many young adults are seeking to capture their lost childhoods" by delaying the uptake of responsibilities and milestones commonly associated with the transition into adulthood (Hines, 2008, p. 20). Hines (2008) coined the terms "rejuveniles" or "kidults" for these young adults. The former are those who have left home and returned to live with their parents, while the latter have never left.

Studies have shown that patterns of leaving and returning home among young adults are complex. For example, early home leaving is more common among children growing up in low-income families and those with personal or family problems. Delayed home leaving is seldom related to relationship quality but usually is economically linked, in particular the consequence of continued financial dependency of adult children (Ward and Spitze, 2007). Delayed leaving has been associated with positive outcomes, such as prolonged access to financial and network support from parents that provides social capital young adults would not be able to attain on their own (Swartz, 2009). Further, delayed home leavers have substantially higher educational attainment at every level through college graduation. Those whose home leaving is facilitated by military service also fare well compared with those leaving home early to enter marriage or cohabit (White and Lacy, 1997).

A notable difference between delayed and early home leaving is that parents report feeling less emotionally close to children who have left home and view independent-living children as less supportive than those remaining at home. What appears to be key to continued parent-adult child connections is the quality of the relationship during adolescence and into adulthood, the social role milestones of adult children, and time engaged in interactional activities (Aquilino, 1997).

Adult children who return home to live with their parents are often called "boomerangers" (Hines, 2008, p. 20). These children frequently have more negative relations with parents before leaving compared with those who never leave. Returning home is a common response to the economic needs of adult children, regardless of the prior relationship quality.

Intergenerational Relationship Quality, Social Support, and Parenting

Young adults can be both children and parents at the same time, so they represent a major connector of family generations—a theme of this report. Their relationships with parents and children, however, evolve over time, and what happens during young adulthood is a critical window into their social trajectories across the life course—another important theme of the report. Studies designed to understand the nature and context of multigenerational families focus in several areas. One area of focus is the pathways through which affective ties and instrumental support between adult children and parents are sustained across generations (Rossi, 1990). Another focus links intergenerational inequalities in the United States to differential transference of skills and socioeconomic resources from parents to children (Behrman et al., 1995; Lee, 1998). Still another area of focus is whether romantic relationship formation, stability, and satisfaction, as well as parenting patterns, are transmitted across generations. Before summarizing relevant research studies, we emphasize that longitudinal studies following respondents from childhood to older ages are rare. Consequently, while this field of research has greatly expanded in recent years, it has yielded insufficient data with which to draw conclusions about the transmission of family patterns across generations (Elder et al., 1986).

Close, positive, and supportive family relationships during childhood and adolescence make key contributions to development and psychological adjustment. For example, families that are highly stressed and conflicted tend to rely on coercive control as a management strategy in the home (Fosco et al., 2012). This environment often creates anger and resentment among youth that not only disrupt and undermine their development but may cause them to seek support from nonconforming peers, do poorly in school, and engage in risky behaviors (Fosco et al., 2012). Conversely, growing up in a warm and socially connected family creates a sense of security, comfort, and safety. Such youth are more likely to seek advice, guidance, and support from their parents when confronted with stressful or demanding life circumstances, which in turn may offer opportunities to develop proactive coping behaviors.

Fosco and colleagues (2012) contend that a supportive, warm family environment serves a critical role in children's development and mastery of skills needed to respond to demands they encounter, which in turn promotes overall well-being and decreases their vulnerability to emotional distress and aggressive behavior. These proactive adaptive coping behaviors and emotional management skills have been characterized as "effortful control" (Derryberry and Reed, 2002; Eisenberg et al., 2009). The protective nature of effortful control per se has not been studied beyond adolescence, with the exception of Fosco and colleagues (2012). Their longitudinal, developmental study of a diverse sample of 17-year-old adolescents and their parents over a 6-year period yielded several important findings. First, the parent-adolescent relationship plays a pivotal role in the maintenance of effortful control, with implications for adolescents' development and adjustment as they transition into young adulthood. Second, adaptive coping, or exercising control to manage emotions and behaviors, increases one's capacity to navigate pressure associated with deviant peer affiliations (Goodnight et al., 2006) as youth transition from adolescence to young adulthood (Rueda et al., 2011; Silk et al., 2003). Third, effortful control appears to be protective in multiple domains of young adult development necessary to prepare for and adapt to adult social roles (O'Connor et al., 2011), and reduces the likelihood of psychological maladjustment (Côté et al., 2010) and the risk of psychopathology (Clements and Bailey, 2010).

One of the major limitations of research on parent-child relationships is that studies often are based on data obtained from particular parent-child dyads instead of examining patterns across multiple parent-child relationships. Further, studies of parents' interactions with children over the life course are quite rare. To fill this gap, Ward and colleagues (2009) examined the relationships of middle-aged parents with multiple adult children, including adult stepchildren. They found that having more children was associated with more positive relationships but also lower-quality relationships and less contact with at least one child. Relational patterns differed by gender and the presence of stepchildren in the household. In terms of gender, mothers compared with fathers reported more positive and better-quality relationships and more contact with their biological adult children. Mothers compared with fathers reported more problematic relationships with adult stepchildren. Better health outcomes were associated with positive relationships between parents and adult children, but frequency of contact was not a contributing factor to overall health. This finding, in particular, warrants further exploration.

Balancing Parental Support and Autonomy

Recent years have seen increased interest in the long-term implications of parental support for young adults' development. Fingerman and colleagues (2012) examine the extent to which parents' intense support promotes or hampers positive adjustment and development in their children. Their findings are mixed. Both the intensely supportive parents and their young adult children perceived the support as "too much." Yet the children also reported better psychological adjustment and life satisfaction compared with their counterparts who received less frequent and intense support from their parents.

Providing instrumental support that extends into adulthood may create ambivalent feelings in families and may strain parent-child relationships (Connidis and McMullin, 2002). Specifically, having a dependent adult child runs counter to U.S. society's notion of individualism and to the life-course norms and expectations that parents may have for their adult children. In addition, a lack of reciprocity between parents and adult children may strain their relationship (Fingerman et al., 2012). Parents may perceive their grown children as needing too much support. Intensely supportive parents in particular tend to report greater financial and emotional strain, poorer life satisfaction, and less satisfaction with overall well-being compared with parents providing less support to their grown children (Fingerman et al., 2012). This issue may be especially important as parents of young adults age and their health deteriorates.

> "Some parents are very sheltering and aren't okay with their kids making mistakes, and I see many kids in college who are not able to cope with things very well. There are some things young adults just have to learn themselves."

While intergenerational families are an important source of support for young adults, the prolonged direct transmission of support by aging family members to the younger generation is shifting two major developmental, life-course patterns—extending the parenting years and delaying the transition of adult children to the assumption of adult social roles and responsibilities. Future research is needed to understand more clearly the developmental and life-course consequences of these changes across generations, using longitudinal data to document how these relationships fare over time.

Evidence on the effects of parental support on relationships between young adults and their parents comes primarily from research on white, middle-class parents (Furstenberg, 2010; Goldscheider et al., 2001). However, there is some evidence that middle-class and more affluent minorities are following the same patterns (Lareau, 2004; Settersten and Ray, 2010). What is clear now is that differential access to family capital and the older generation's aggregated resources and investments is increasing disparities and inequalities among young adults. While many young adults get some financial support from their family, young adults receive approximately 70 percent more material assistance when their parents are in the top 25 percent of the income distribution compared with their young adult counterparts whose families are in the bottom 25 percent (Schoeni and Ross, 2005). Young adults from families of higher socioeconomic position are more likely to receive assistance from their parents to purchase a home or advance their education, which in turn influences their subsequent standard of living and ability to become self-sufficient (Semyonov and Lewin-Epstein, 2001).

Under current law in most states, parents have no formal legal obligation to provide financial support to their children once the children reach the age of majority unless they have disabilities that preclude gainful employment (NCSL, 2014a,c). Even without a legal obligation to do so, however, many parents in intact families do provide continuing support within their means, especially for the costs of higher education (Settersten and Ray, 2010). By contrast, it is well established that divorced or separated parents provide less support, even for higher education, than married parents with similar incomes (López Turley and Desmond, 2011). Moreover, postmajority assistance for children of divorced or separated parents is provided more often by mothers than by fathers (Emery, 2013). Even fathers who are legally obligated to provide support while their child is a minor often do not continue to do so after the child reaches the age of majority unless they have entered into a binding agreement or are under a judicial order to assist with college expenses in those jurisdictions that authorize such orders (Wallerstein and Lewis, 2004). No state currently authorizes a judicial order for financial support other than college expenses once a child reaches the age of majority (NCSL, 2014b). The net result is that the burden of supporting young adults in families with divorced or separated parents falls disproportionately on mothers, and young adult children of divorced or separated parents typically have lower rates of attending and graduating from college than young adult children of married parents of similar means (Emery, 2013; Ginther and Pollak, 2004). Goldfarb (2014) proposes that child support orders covering educational expenses as well as other types of financial support be made more broadly available for young adults who are over the age of majority. State legislatures could consider whether current laws governing support obligations for divorced or separated parents need to be modified to take adequate account of the rising costs of higher education and the other financial challenges faced by many young adults over the age of majority.

Young adults' access to family resources until they can support themselves financially may be especially important in light of the social and economic challenges currently confronting young adults. It is important to acknowledge, however, that access to family financial support is not available to all young adults. For this reason, it is not surprising that stark differences are seen in the developmental trajectories of young adults based on whether their families can afford them this luxury. A large proportion of young adults grow up in families that cannot (Wickrama et al., 2012), and they are particularly vulnerable to becoming disconnected. Such young adults also are more likely to experience diminished life opportunities that have long-term consequences for their ability to become self-sufficient. This pattern occurs among many racial/ethnic minorities, but most notably among African Americans.

Compared with other racial/ethnic groups, African American young adults have consistently lower earnings and assets at every level of education, a situation that has changed little since the civil rights movement (Murry and Li, 2014). In contrast, young adult Asian Americans and

Cuban Americans attain higher incomes, assets, and job quality relative to Caucasians irrespective of community and family characteristics (Wickrama et al., 2012). Wickrama and colleagues (2012) attribute these differential patterns to the high aspirations, fields of employment and education, family support, and immigrant status that collectively constitute high human capital for these ethnic minorities. Nonetheless, that economic and employment disparities persist for African Americans, regardless of family income, parental education, or community context, suggests that these differences may be attributable in part to systematic discrimination experienced by this population (Brody et al., 2006).

Transmission of Parenting Practices Across Generations

Studies examining the transmission of parenting practices across generations have just begun to illuminate the mechanisms through which those practices are internalized, carried forward, and reactivated in later generations by adult children who become parents (Kohn et al., 1986). Findings from intergenerational studies of the transmission of both parenting practices and externalizing behavior across generations are mixed (Bailey et al., 2009). Thus, the extent to which parenting patterns are transmitted across multiple generations is an issue requiring additional longitudinal research.

> "There is a need to take into consideration how various cultures impact families. For example, my parents didn't go through school or college, so they thought I would just get a job at the end of high school."

A developing line of research demonstrates that constructive parenting can influence parenting over three generations to promote socioemotional development (Kerr et al., 2009). Two hypotheses have been proposed to explain this phenomenon. The modeling hypothesis contends that adult children imitate their own parents' behavior and practices, and views the transmission as a psychological process of internalizing and subsequently engaging in familiar behavior when similar circumstances arise. The second hypothesis posits reworking or compensatory transmission processes whereby adult children attempt to modify and improve the parenting of their own children so as not to repeat dysfunctional patterns they experienced with their own parents (Gaunt and Bassi, 2012; Guzzo, 2011). Findings from a national survey of two-generation families revealed that men who described their fathers as warm were more likely to model their own parenting after their father and perceived themselves as good parents (Hofferth et al., 2012).

Men who reported being raised by harsh fathers were more likely to rework their fathers' parenting strategies so as to utilize positive parenting practices, and likewise perceived themselves as good parents. Those whose fathers were perceived to be uninvolved, neither warm nor harsh, struggled most as parents and were less able to develop parenting approaches that worked effectively with their own children (Hofferth et al., 2012). Future research is needed to understand the role of fathering in the transmission of parenting dynamics. In addition, while fathering programs often target those perceived to be "at risk," consideration needs to be given to recruiting all fathers.

Other studies examining the transmission of constructive parenting across generations have found only modest intergenerational continuity (Chen and Kaplan, 2001). When continuity is observed, it appears to occur through interpersonal relationships and social interactions that facilitate opportunities to model the behavior. Whereas Simons and colleagues (1993) found that modeling was the strongest predictor of intergenerational transmission of constructive parenting, young adults' perception of their upbringing did not affect their subsequent reports of their own parenting practices in middle adulthood. Further, studies have shown that parental education, poverty, and family structure are not strong predictors of the transmission of constructive parenting across generations (Chen and Kaplan, 2001; Kohn et al., 1986).

Another line of research attempts to extend the notion of modeling of parenting behaviors to the development of social skills that promote good parenting. Children who are exposed to positive parenting are socialized to have successful interpersonal relationships that range from relationships with peers to relationships with their own children (Furman et al., 2002; Shaffer et al., 2009). Social skills are sustained by cognitive representations of positive, stable, trusting relationships. Peers may contribute to the development of social skills and the capabilities to form and maintain relationships. Developing social competence in relationships with peers may in turn contribute to improved parenting skills and parent-child relationships. Further, Ehrensaft and colleagues (2011) found that observing one's own parents' socioemotional and relationship functioning may be important in predicting parenting patterns across generations.

Parenting and Incarceration

Incarceration in the United States has continued to increase. As of 2012, 1 in every 108 adults was incarcerated, and an estimated 1 in 50 adults were on probation or parole (Glaze and Herberman, 2013). Among males in 2012, African Americans were 6 times and Hispanics 2.5 times more likely than whites to be incarcerated, and 18- to 19-year-old African

Americans were approximately 9.5 times more likely to be incarcerated than their white counterparts (Carson and Golinelli, 2013). It is worth noting that most of those incarcerated are parents (more than 1.7 million children under 18 had a parent in prison in 2007). The majority of incarcerated parents are males (744,200 male versus 65,500 female inmates in 2007) of low socioeconomic position, and many of those men (46 percent) are African American (Glaze and Maruschak, 2008). Among inmates aged 25-34, 64 percent in state prisons and 74.1 percent in federal prisons have minor children, compared with 44.1 percent in state prisons and 45.8 percent in federal prisons under age 24 (Glaze and Maruschak, 2008).

While incarcerated fathers are embedded in social networks that include their family of origin, relatives, romantic partners, children, and friends, studies examining this population focus primarily on the incarcerated individuals. Yet incarceration makes families fragile, and diminishes the financial resources and well-being of intimate partners/wives and children who are left behind.

Arditti and colleagues (2003) contend that having an incarcerated family member has detrimental social, economic, and health consequences for children and other family members. Many families feel personal shame and experience marginalization and stigma associated with the incarceration. To manage and cope with the shame, a code of silence or conspiracy of silence may be created in families whereby mothers hide a father's incarceration from their children. Arditti and colleagues (2003) note that while most families of incarcerated fathers were suffering economically prior to the incarceration, they became even more vulnerable afterwards. The imprisonment not only created physical and emotional distance between mothers and their incarcerated partners but also increased parental strain, emotional stress, and concerns about children's loss of contact and involvement with their incarcerated parent. Being incarcerated is consistently associated with disrupted and damaged romantic relationships, often resulting from stigma associated with having a partner who is incarcerated and problems that emerge from time spent apart (Apel et al., 2010; Lopoo and Western, 2005; Massoglia et al., 2011). Reentering family life under these conditions can exacerbate instability in an already unstable romantic relationship and may negatively impact fathers' involvement with their children. This inability to engage with their children may lead in turn not only to long-term desertion but also to reduced contact with other relatives (Massoglia et al., 2011), creating a disconnect between the individual and important social support systems. Thus, imprisonment has a corrosive effect on families, contributes to relational breakups, exacerbates preexisting behavioral and psychological problems in children, and adds to the economic and relational deficits of children and families that were already struggling prior to the father's incarceration (Comfort, 2007; Lewis et al., 2007).

Because of the increased number of incarcerated parents, many fatherhood initiatives have been implemented in recent years to reconnect incarcerated fathers with their children and families; many parenting programs have been implemented in prisons. However, few such programs have been evaluated, and those that have yielded mixed results (Cabrera and Peters, 2000; Martinson and Nightingale, 2008). Although fatherhood intervention programs for incarcerated men may be effective, only four such programs were considered effective according to a recent review (Bronte-Tinkew et al., 2008). There is as yet no evidence suggesting what characteristics contribute to a program's overall success, and few programs found to be effective have been replicated (Bronte-Tinkew et al., 2008; Loper and Tuerk, 2006).

Longitudinal research is needed to document the intergenerational patterns and consequences of incarceration in families, such as the extent to which parents' criminality and incarceration influence their children's behavior and adjustment over time. Further, more work is needed to document ways in which criminal justice policies and practices impact family functioning, including parents' abilities to fulfill their roles as mothers and fathers and a father's sense of familial obligations (Hairston, 2009).

CONCLUSIONS AND RECOMMENDATION

The developmental and social contexts of young adult relationships in contemporary American society have changed dramatically relative to earlier generations of young adults. Advances in communication and social media have had a profound impact on the context, access, and interactions of social relationships and social networks among young adults. More advanced educational credentials and job skills are needed for successful employment trajectories in the predominantly service-oriented and high-tech occupations of the 21st century. Those who come from advantaged family backgrounds can meet these demands by investing in their education and career development and delaying marriage and childbearing to their late 20s and early 30s, enabling them to achieve greater employment, family, and financial stability into adulthood. Those from economically disadvantaged backgrounds may need to curtail their education and tend to work at low-skilled jobs, choosing instead, or by default, to initiate their family pathways in young adulthood by having children outside of marriage or in cohabiting relationships.

The stakes for these pathway choices in young adulthood are high, with consequences for health, safety, and well-being. Those who initiate the family pathway with early, nonmarital, unintended childbearing or multiple-partner fertility experience greater stress, less social and economic support from a committed spouse or partner and extended family, precarious economic circumstances, and poor physical and mental health. Those who invest in the education and career development pathway and delay family formation beyond young adulthood tend to experience more family and work supports, greater financial security—or at least the promise of financial security—greater family and employment stability, and better physical and mental health. Some health advantages and disadvantages precede these diverging pathways, as those from backgrounds of higher socioeconomic position have better health in childhood and adolescence, which leads to more options for young adult pathways involving relationships, education, employment, and stable and supportive contexts for family formation and, in turn, health.

> "The media needs to emphasize the positive aspects of young adults instead of the negatives. This impacts how young adults think about themselves and see themselves in society."

In young adulthood, increasingly diverse social networks develop from family relations, romantic/sexual partners, peers, work, community, and educational institutions and other organizations. Although most young people are immersed in these social networks, many feel isolated, without the human contact or individual support needed to cope with psychological and emotional problems common to this life stage. One of the committee's young adult consultants poignantly told us of how alone and desperate she felt in dealing with mental illness, not knowing where to turn for help despite multiple connections to peer, family, and community networks. Intergenerational relations can serve as vital sources of resources and support, especially for young parents, but the changing demographic patterns of adult children are complex, and the long-term implications of parental support for the development of young adults can be mixed. As detailed throughout this chapter, moreover, relationship patterns and trends vary by gender, race/ethnicity, and socioeconomic position, which can lead to health disparities and differing patterns of social and achievement role transitions across the life course. Social relationships, union formation, the transition to parenthood, and intergenerational relationships have direct and indirect impacts on the health, safety, and well-being of young adults.

There have been many debates about the role of government programs and policies aimed at strengthening relationships and parenting, and a variety of initiatives with this aim have been implemented. Some evidence suggests that marriage programs can reduce conflict and increase parenting and communication skills, marital happiness, and stability (Fagan et al., 2002). Likewise, some interventions designed to improve the transition into parenthood have had positive effects on parents and their relationships, such as increasing self-esteem, marital satisfaction, and stability (Cowan and Cowan, 1995, 2000). A few programs have shown enhanced development in children as well (Cowan and Cowan, 1995, 2000). Such initiatives, however, have traditionally focused on married couples in favorable socioeconomic and relationship circumstances (Cowan and Cowan, 1995), and have not always addressed issues relevant to low-income individuals. Some programs have been created for the latter individuals, but they have not yet been assessed (Dion, 2005; Roulet, 2009). The fatherhood initiatives discussed above are an exception to this general pattern; they target diverse audiences and provide a wide variety of services.

While some programs designed to strengthen relationships and marriage and help families have shown positive effects, moreover, many have had small or no effects. The Healthy Marriage Initiative, for example, launched in 2002, established several national efforts aimed at encouraging or supporting marriage. One of these was the Building Strong Families program, which was designed to promote relationships between couples with a new baby or about to have a child and to help those desiring marriage to achieve it (Brown, 2010; Roulet, 2009). An evaluation of this program, which followed more than 4,000 couples, found that it did not succeed in improving the couples' relationship or the quality of coparenting or in enhancing father involvement (Wood et al., 2014). No difference in major outcomes was found between the control and program couples in eight sites (Donahue et al., 2010). In fact, in one of the sites, the program had modest negative effects on some of the outcomes, including lower coparenting quality, less father involvement, and more severe domestic violence (Donahue et al., 2010). On the other hand, in another site, the program did have positive effects on African American couples with respect to reduced infidelity, family violence, and destructive behaviors and enhanced coparenting and ability to manage conflict.

In sum, social, romantic, and family relationships are central to the lives of young adults. And young adulthood clearly is a period entailing some of the highest rates of disadvantage defining risks, including nonmarital, unintended childbearing and multiple-partner fertility; poverty and material hardship; incarceration; alienation and loss of extended family support; social isolation; and social and economic disconnection. However, existing social policy research does not provide a sufficient evidence base for extensive policy recommendations in this area. Mechanisms linking marriage, socioeconomic position, and child outcomes still are not fully understood, and several programs are being evaluated to determine whether they can facilitate healthy relationships and marriage (Brown, 2010). Overall, most programs and initiatives that have been evaluated have shown small, inconsistent, or no effects. This may be because of the substantial diversity in relationship development, contexts, and statuses during young adulthood, as documented in this chapter. Young adulthood is a fluid period, and thus far there is insufficient evidence to show what works in fortifying and supporting young adult relationships and for whom these programs work. Our review of existing research on the social lives of young adults revealed a number of areas in which the development of such policies and programs would benefit from more research, as highlighted throughout this chapter.

The results of evaluations of the two-generation programs discussed in this chapter are promising and could be monitored closely, with successful programs being expanded to new sites. Findings from recent two-generation programs implemented as part of early-childhood interventions show potential for enhancing the outcomes experienced by young adults. It is important for two-generation programs to value the parents as individuals in addition to the vital role the programs play in relation to the children. Accordingly, the committee makes the following recommendation:

> **Recommendation 3-1: In funding the implementation and evaluation of two-generation programs, philanthropic funders and federal government agencies should actively monitor the outcomes of the young parent participants in addition to early childhood outcomes. Doing so would be valuable for programs that target primarily health and well-being (such as home visiting programs), as well as those that target primarily human capital development.**

Our findings also suggest a number of additional intervention points and possible directions for policy makers for such policies and programs:

- Socially isolated young adults are more likely than their peers to be disconnected from systems that can serve as key sources of support for health care, parenting, or early-childhood development. Research is needed to understand how social media could be used to identify potential vulnerabilities of these young adults, including mental illness and depression, and respond with interventions that can reduce their vulnerabilities, increase their social integration, and link them to needed resources and contexts for support.
- Rising rates of incarceration among young adults have destabilized intergenerational family patterns, which may suggest the need for more concerted efforts to devise rehabilitation programs. The U.S. Department of Health and Human Services and the U.S. Department of Justice could follow up on the report of the Federal Interagency Working Group for Children of Incarcerated Parents (2013) to improve efforts in the following areas: (1) ensure that prison visiting conditions are sensitive to the needs of children;

(2) give incarcerated parents opportunities to improve their parenting capacities; (3) facilitate parents' involvement in their children's schooling during incarceration; and (4) provide appropriate services for improving parenting skills during reentry.

- As many young people delay or are thwarted in making a successful and stable transition to adulthood, the parents of young adults continue carrying out their parenting roles and serving as sources of support. This changing nature of parenting young adults has implications for privacy laws under the Health Insurance Portability and Accountability Act of 1996; eligibility for programs; and the straining of economic, social, and emotional resources across generations.
- Shoring up the economic circumstances of at-risk families can help promote entry into the education and career development pathway over the early family formation pathway in young adulthood. As discussed in Chapter 4, for disadvantaged youth who cannot meet demands for increased educational credentials and high-tech job skills, vocational training can help open up alternative pathways into adulthood that provide the economic security needed to form families within stable, committed relationships.

REFERENCES

Albrecht, S. L., M. K. Miller, and L. L. Clarke. 1994. Assessing the importance of family structure in understanding birth outcomes. *Journal of Marriage and Family* 56(4):987-1003.

Amato, P. R. 2005. The impact of family formation change on the cognitive, social, and emotional well-being of the next generation. *The Future of Children* 15(2):75-96.

Amato, P. R., and J. Kane. 2011. Life-course pathways and the psychosocial adjustment of young adult women. *Journal of Marriage and Family* 73(1):279-295.

Anderson, E. 1999. *Code of the street: Decency, violence, and the moral life of the inner city*. New York: W.W. Norton & Company.

Apel, R., A. A. Blokland, P. Nieuwbeerta, and M. van Schellen. 2010. The impact of imprisonment on marriage and divorce: A risk set matching approach. *Journal of Quantitative Criminology* 26(2):269-300.

Aquilino, W. S. 1997. From adolescent to young adult: A prospective study of parent-child relations during the transition to adulthood. *Journal of Marriage and Family* 59(3):670-686.

Arditti, J. A., J. Lambert-Shute, and K. Joest. 2003. Saturday morning at the jail: Implications of incarceration for families and children. *Family Relations* 52(3):195-204.

Arroyo, J., K. K. Payne, S. L. Brown, and W. D. Manning. 2013. *Crossover in median age at first marriage and first birth: Thirty years of change*. Bowling Green, OH: National Center for Family and Marriage Research.

Avison, W. R., J. Ali, and D. Walters. 2007. Family structure, stress, and psychological distress: A demonstration of the impact of differential exposure. *Journal of Health and Social Behavior* 48(3):301-317.

Bachman, J. G., P. M. O'Malley, J. E. Schulenberg, L. D. Johnston, A. L. Bryant, and A. C. Merline. 2002. *Why substance use declines in young adulthood: Changes in social activities, roles, and beliefs*. Mahwah, NJ: Lawrence Erlbaum Associates.

Bailey, J. A., K. G. Hill, S. Oesterle, and J. D. Hawkins. 2009. Parenting practices and problem behavior across three generations: Monitoring, harsh discipline, and drug use in the intergenerational transmission of externalizing behavior. *Developmental Psychology* 45(5):1214-1226.

Baym, N. 2010. *Personal connections in the digital age*. Cambridge, UK: Polity Press.

Baym, N. K., and A. Ledbetter. 2009. Tunes that bind? Predicting friendship strength in a music-based social network. *Information, Communication & Society* 12(3):408-427.

Behrman, J. R., R. A. Pollak, and P. Taubman. 1995. The wealth model: Efficiency in education and distribution in the family. In *From parent to child: Intrahousehold allocations and intergenerational relations in the United States,* edited by J. R. Behrman, R. A. Pollak, and P. Taubman. Chicago, IL: University of Chicago Press. Pp. 113-138.

Bennett, T. 1992. Marital status and infant health outcomes. *Social Science & Medicine* 35(9):1179-1187.

Bennett, T., P. Braveman, S. Egerter, and J. L. Kiely. 1994. Maternal marital status as a risk factor for infant mortality. *Family Planning Perspectives* 26(6):252-256, 271.

Biblarz, T. J., and A. E. Raftery. 1999. Family structure, educational attainment, and socioeconomic success: Rethinking the "pathology of matriarchy." *American Journal of Sociology* 105(2):321-365.

Boardman, J. D., B. W. Domingue, and J. M. Fletcher. 2012. How social and genetic factors predict friendship networks. *Proceedings of the National Academy of Sciences of the United States of America* 109(43):17377-17381.

Booth, A., E. Rustenbach, and S. McHale. 2008. Early family transitions and depressive symptom changes from adolescence to early adulthood. *Journal of Marriage and Family* 70(1):3-14.

Boyd, D. 2014. *It's complicated: The social lives of networked teens.* New Haven, CT: Yale University Press.

Brody, G., Y.-F. Chen, V. Murry, X. Ge, R. Simons, F. Gibbons, M. Gerrard, and C. E. Cutrona. 2006. Perceived discrimination and the adjustment of African American youths: A five year longitudinal analysis with contextual moderation effects. *Child Development* 77(5):1170-1189.

Bronfenbrenner, U., and P. A. Morris. 1998. The ecology of developmental processes. In *Handbook of child psychology,* 5th ed., Vol. 1, edited by W. Damon and R. M. Lerner. New York: Wiley. Pp. 993-1028.

Bronte-Tinkew, J., M. Burkhauser, K. Mbwana, A. Metz, and A. Collins. 2008. *Elements of promising practice in programs serving fathers involved in the criminal justice system.* Gaithersburg, MD: National Responsible Fatherhood Clearinghouse.

Brown, S. L. 2000. The effect of union type on psychological well-being: Depression among cohabitors versus marrieds. *Journal of Health and Social Behavior* 41(3):241-255.

Brown, S. L. 2010. Marriage and child well-being: Research and policy perspectives. *Journal of Marriage and Family* 72(5):1059-1077.

Brown, S. L., and A. Booth. 1996. Cohabitation versus marriage: A comparison of relationship quality. *Journal of Marriage and Family* 58(3):668-678.

Brown, S. L., J. R. Bulanda, and G. R. Lee. 2005. The significance of nonmarital cohabitation: Marital status and mental health benefits among middle-aged and older adults. *The Journals of Gerontology Series B: Psychological Sciences and Social Sciences* 60(Suppl. 1): S21-S29.

Bucx, F., and F. van Wel. 2008. Parental bond and life course transitions from adolescence to young adulthood. *Adolescence* 43(169):71-88.

Burt, R. S. 1992. *Structural holes: The social structure of competition.* Cambridge, MA: Harvard University Press.

Burton, L., and C. R. Hardaway. 2012. Low-income mothers as "othermothers" to their romantic partners' children: Women's coparenting in multiple partner fertility relationships. *Family Process* 51(3):343-359.

Cabrera, N., and H. E. Peters. 2000. Public policies and father involvement. *Marriage & Family Review* 29(4):295-314.

Carson, E. A., and D. Golinelli. 2013. *Prisoners in 2012*. Washington, DC: Bureau of Justice Statistics.

Casper, L. M., and S. M. Bianchi. 2002. *Continuity and change in the American family*. Thousand Oaks, CA: Sage Publications.

Chase-Lansdale, P. L., and J. Brooks-Gunn. 2014. Two-generation programs in the twenty-first century. *The Future of Children* 24:13-40.

Chen, Z., and H. B. Kaplan. 2001. Intergenerational transmission of constructive parenting. *Journal of Marriage and Family* 63(1):17-31.

Cherlin, A. J. 2004. The deinstitutionalization of American marriage. *Journal of Marriage and Family* 66(4):848-861.

Chomitz, V. R., L. W. Cheung, and E. Lieberman. 1995. The role of lifestyle in preventing low birth weight. *The Future of Children* 5(1):121-138.

Christakis, N. A., and J. H. Fowler. 2009. *Connected: The surprising power of our social networks and how they shape our lives*. New York: Hachette Book Group.

Clements, A. D., and B. A. Bailey. 2010. The relationship between temperament and anxiety: Phase I in the development of a risk screening model to predict stress-related health problems. *Journal of Health Psychology* 15(4):515-525.

Cohen-Cole, E., and J. M. Fletcher. 2008. Is obesity contagious? Social networks vs. environmental factors in the obesity epidemic. *Journal of Health Economics* 27(5):1382-1387.

Comfort, M. 2007. *Doing time together: Love and family in the shadow of the prison*. Chicago, IL: University of Chicago Press.

Connidis, I. A., and J. A. McMullin. 2002. Sociological ambivalence and family ties: A critical perspective. *Journal of Marriage and Family* 64(3):558-567.

Côté, S., A. Gyurak, and R. W. Levenson. 2010. The ability to regulate emotion is associated with greater well-being, income, and socioeconomic status. *Emotion* 10(6):923.

Cowan, C. P., and Cowan, P. A. 1995. Interventions to ease the transition to parenthood: Why they are needed and what they can do. *Family Relations* 44(4):412-423.

Cowan, C. P., and Cowan, P. A. 2000. *When partners become parents: The big life change for couples*. Hillsdale, NJ: Lawrence Erlbaum Associates.

Demo, D. H., and M. J. Cox. 2000. Families with young children: A review of research in the 1990s. *Journal of Marriage and Family* 62(4):876-895.

Derryberry, D., and M. A. Reed. 2002. Anxiety-related attentional biases and their regulation by attentional control. *Journal of Abnormal Child Psychology* 111(2):225-236.

Dimock, M., C. Doherty, and J. Kiley. 2013. *Growing support for gay marriage: Changed minds and changing demographics*. Washington, DC: Pew Research Center.

Dion, M. R. 2005. Healthy marriage programs: Learning what works. *The Future of Children* 15(2):139-156.

Donahue, E., I. Garfinkel, R. Haskins, S. McLanahan, and R. B. Mincy. 2010. *Strengthening fragile families*. Social Genome Project Research Brief 11. Washington, DC: The Brookings Institution.

Driscoll, A. K., G. K. Hearn, V. J. Evans, K. A. Moore, B. W. Sugland, and V. Call. 1999. Nonmarital childbearing among adult women. *Journal of Marriage and Family* 61(1):178-187.

Duncan, G., and K. Magnuson. 2004. Individual and parent-based intervention strategies for promoting human capital and positive behavior. In *Human development across lives and generations: The potential for change*, edited by P. L. Chase, K. Kiernan, and R. Friedman. Cambridge, UK: Cambridge University Press. Pp. 93-135.

Duncan, G. J., B. Wilkerson, and P. England. 2006. Cleaning up their act: The effects of marriage and cohabitation on licit and illicit drug use. *Demography* 43(4):691-710.

Dunifon, R., and L. Kowaleski-Jones. 2007. The influence of grandparents in single-mother families. *Journal of Marriage and Family* 69(2):465-481.

Edin, K., and M. Kefalas. 2005. *Promises I can keep: Why poor women put motherhood before marriage.* Oakland: University of California Press.

Ehrensaft, M. K., H. M. Knous-Westfall, and P. Cohen. 2011. Direct and indirect transmission of relationship functioning across generations. *Journal of Family Psychology* 25(6):942-952.

Eisenberg, N., C. Valiente, T. L. Spinrad, J. Liew, Q. Zhou, S. H. Losoya, M. Reiser, and A. Cumberland. 2009. Longitudinal relations of children's effortful control, impulsivity, and negative emotionality to their externalizing, internalizing, and co-occurring behavior problems. *Development and Psychopathology* 45(4):988-1008.

Elder, G. H. 1998. The life course as developmental theory. *Child Development* 69(1):1-12.

Elder, G., A. Caspi, and G. Downey. 1986. Problem behavior and family relationships: Life course and intergenerational themes. In *Human development and the life course: Multidisciplinary perspectives*, edited by A. B. Sorenson, F. E. Weinert, and L. R. Sherrod. Hillsdale, NJ: Lawrence Erlbaum Associates. Pp. 293-340.

Ellison, N., C. Lampe, C. Steinfield, and J. Vitak. 2011. With a little help from my friends: Social network sites and social capital. In *A networked self: Identity, community and culture on social network sites*, edited by Z. Papacharissi. New York: Routledge. Pp. 124-145.

Ellwood, D. T., and C. Jencks. 2001. *The growing differences in family structure: What do we know? Where do we look for answers.* http://www.russellsage.org/sites/all/files/u4/Ellwood%26Jencks.pdf (accessed August 6, 2014).

Elstad, J. I. 1996. Inequalities in health related to women's marital, parental, and employment status—a comparison between the early 70s and the late 80s, Norway. *Social Science & Medicine* 42(1):75-89.

Emery, R. E. 2013. *Cultural sociology of divorce: An encyclopedia.* Thousand Oaks, CA: Sage Publications, Inc.

Evenson, R. J., and R. W. Simon. 2005. Clarifying the relationship between parenthood and depression. *Journal of Health and Social Behavior* 46(4):341-358.

Fagan, P. F., R. W. Patterson, and R. E. Rector. 2002. *Marriage and welfare reform: The overwhelming evidence that marriage education works.* Backgrounder Executive Summary 1606. Washington, DC: The Heritage Foundation.

Federal Interagency Working Group for Children of Incarcerated Parents. 2013. *Promoting social and emotional well-being for children of incarcerated parents.* http://csgjusticecenter.org/wp-content/uploads/2013/06/Promoting-Social-and-Emotional-Well-Being-for-Children-of-Incarcerated-Parents.pdf (accessed September 10, 2014).

Fingerman, K. L., Y.-P. Cheng, E. D. Wesselmann, S. Zarit, F. Furstenberg, and K. S. Birditt. 2012. Helicopter parents and landing pad kids: Intense parental support of grown children. *Journal of Marriage and Family* 74(4):880-896.

Fosco, G. M., A. S. Caruthers, and T. J. Dishion. 2012. A six-year predictive test of adolescent family relationship quality and effortful control pathways to emerging adulthood and emotional health. *Journal of Family Psychology* 26(4):565-575.

Frank, R., and E. Wildsmith. 2005. The grass widows of Mexico: Migration and union dissolution in a binational context. *Social Forces* 83(3):919-947.

Furman, W., B. B. Brown, and C. Feiring. 1999. *The development of romantic relationships in adolescence.* New York: Cambridge University Press.

Furman, W., V. A. Simon, L. Shaffer, and H. A. Bouchey. 2002. Adolescents' working models and styles for relationships with parents, friends, and romantic partners. *Child Development* 73(1):241-255.

Furstenberg, F. F., Jr. 2010. On a new schedule: Transitions to adulthood and family change. *The Future of Children* 20(1):67-87.

Furstenberg, F. F., Jr., R. A. Settersten, Jr., and R. G. Rumbaut. 2005. *On the frontiers of adulthood: Theory, research, and public policy*. Chicago, IL: University of Chicago Press.

Garfinkel, I., and S. S. McLanahan. 1986. Single mothers and their children: A new American dilemma. *Journal of Policy Analysis and Management* 7(2):388-394.

Gates, G. J. 2013. Demographics and LGBT health. *Journal of Health and Social Behavior* 54(1):72-74.

Gaunt, R., and L. Bassi. 2012. Modeling and compensatory processes underlying involvement in child care among kibbutz-reared fathers. *Journal of Family Issues* 33(6):823-848.

Gergen, K. 1991. *The saturated self: Dilemmas of identity in contemporary life*. New York: Basic Books.

Gibson-Davis, C. M. 2008. Family structure effects on maternal and paternal parenting in low-income families. *Journal of Marriage and Family* 70(2):452-465.

Gibson-Davis, C. M., K. Edin, and S. McLanahan. 2005. High hopes but even higher expectations: The retreat from marriage among low-income couples. *Journal of Marriage and Family* 67(5):1301-1312.

Giddens, A. 1991. *Modernity and self-identity: Self and identity in the late modern age*. Cambridge, UK: Polity Press.

Ginther, D., and R. Pollak. 2004. Family structure and children's educational outcomes: Blended families, stylized facts, and descriptive regressions. *Demography* 41(4):671-696.

Glaze, L. E., and E. J. Herberman. 2013. *Correctional populations in the United States, 2012*. Washington, DC: Bureau of Justice Statistics.

Glaze, L. E., and L. M. Maruschak. 2008. *Parents in prison and their minor children*. Washington, DC: Bureau of Justice Statistics.

Goldfarb, S. F. 2014. Who pays for the "boomerang generation"?: A legal perspective on financial support for young adults. *Harvard Journal of Law and Gender* 37:45.

Goldman, N. 1993. Marriage selection and mortality patterns: Inferences and fallacies. *Demography* 30(2):189-208.

Goldscheider, F. K., A. Thornton, and L.-S. Yang. 2001. Helping out the kids: Expectations about parental support in young adulthood. *Journal of Marriage and Family* 63(3):727-740.

Goodnight, J. A., J. E. Bates, J. P. Newman, K. A. Dodge, and G. S. Pettit. 2006. The interactive influences of friend deviance and reward dominance on the development of externalizing behavior during middle adolescence. *Journal of Abnormal Child Psychology* 34(5):573-583.

Granger, R. C., and R. Cytron. 1999. Teenage parent programs a synthesis of the long-term effects of the new chance demonstration, Ohio's learning, earning, and parenting program, and the teenage parent demonstration. *Evaluation Review* 23(2):107-145.

Granovetter, M. 1973. The strength of weak ties. *American Journal of Sociology* 78(6):1360-1380.

Guzzo, K. B. 2011. New fathers' experiences with their own fathers and attitudes toward fathering. *Fathering: A Journal of Theory, Research, and Practice about Men as Fathers* 9(3):268-290.

Guzzo, K. B., and F. F. Furstenberg. 2007. Multipartnered fertility among young women with a nonmarital first birth: Prevalence and risk factors. *Perspectives on Sexual and Reproductive Health* 39(1):29-38.

Haas, S. A. 2006. Health selection and the process of social stratification: The effect of childhood health on socioeconomic attainment. *Journal of Health and Social Behavior* 47(4):339-354.

Hairston, C. F. 2009. *Kinship care when parents are incarcerated: What we know, what we can do*. Baltimore, MD: Annie E. Casey Foundation.

Hampton, K. N., C.-J. Lee, and E. J. Her. 2011. How new media affords network diversity: Direct and mediated access to social capital through participation in local social settings. *New Media & Society* 13(7):1031-1049.

Haveman, R., B. Wolfe, and K. Pence. 2001. Intergenerational effects of nonmarital and early childbearing. In *Out of wedlock: Causes and consequences of nonmarital fertility*, edited by L. L. Wu and B. Wolfe. New York: Russell Sage Foundation. Pp. 287-316.

Hayslip, B., Jr., and P. L. Kaminski. 2005. Grandparents raising their grandchildren: A review of the literature and suggestions for practice. *The Gerontologist* 45:262-269.

Haythornthwaite, C. 2005. Social networks and Internet connectivity effects. *Information, Community & Society* 8(2):125-147.

Haythornthwaite, C., and B. Wellman. 1998. Work, friendship, and media use for information exchange in a networked organization. *Journal of the American Society for Information Science* 49(12):1101-1114.

Henretta, J. C. 2007. Early childbearing, marital status, and women's health and mortality after age 50. *Journal of Health and Social Behavior* 48(3):254-266.

Heuveline, P., and J. M. Timberlake. 2004. The role of cohabitation in family formation: The United States in comparative perspective. *Journal of Marriage and Family* 66(5): 1214-1230.

Hines, A. 2008. Consumer trends in three different worlds. *The Futurist* 42(4).

Hofferth, S. L., and F. Goldscheider. 2010. Family structure and the transition to early parenthood. *Demography* 47(2):415-437.

Hofferth, S. L., J. H. Pleck, and C. K. Vesely. 2012. The transmission of parenting from fathers to sons. *Parenting: Science and Practice* 12(4):282-305.

Horwitz, A. V., and H. R. White. 1998. The relationship of cohabitation and mental health: A study of a young adult cohort. *Journal of Marriage and Family* 60(2):505-514.

House, J., K. Landis, and D. Umberson. 1988. Social relationships and health. *Science* 241(4865):540-545.

Hughes, M. E., and L. J. Waite. 2002. Health in household context: Living arrangements and health in late middle age. *Journal of Health and Social Behavior* 43(1):1.

Humphreys, L. 2005. Cellphones in public: Social interactions in a wireless era. *New Media & Society* 7(6):810-833.

Humphreys, L. 2010. Mobile social networks and urban public space. *New Media & Society* 12(5):763-778.

Hunter, N. 2012. The future impact of same-sex marriage: More questions than answers. *Georgetown Law Journal* 100:1855-1879.

Joung, I., K. Stronks, H. Van de Mheen, and J. Mackenbach. 1995. Health behaviours explain part of the differences in self-reported health associated with partner/marital status in the Netherlands. *Journal of Epidemiology and Community Health* 49(5):482-488.

Kerr, D. C., D. M. Capaldi, K. C. Pears, and L. D. Owen. 2009. A prospective three generational study of fathers' constructive parenting: Influences from family of origin, adolescent adjustment, and offspring temperament. *Developmental Psychology* 45(5):1257.

Kessler, R. C., and P. D. Cleary. 1980. Social class and psychological distress. *American Sociological Review* 45(3):463-478.

Kim, H. K., and P. C. McKenry. 2002. The relationship between marriage and psychological well-being: A longitudinal analysis. *Journal of Family Issues* 23(8):885-911.

King, C. T., R. W. Glover, T. C. Smith, R. Coffey, B. Levy, H. Yoshikawa, W. Beardslee, and M. Kordsmeier. 2009. *The CareerAdvance® pilot project: Recommended jobs strategy for families served by the community action project of Tulsa county*. Austin, TX: Ray Marshall Center for the Study of Human Resources.

Kohn, M. L., Slomczynski, K., and Schoenbach, C. 1986. Social stratification and the transmission of values in the family: A cross-national assessment. *Sociological Forum* 1(1):73-102.

Kreager, D. A., S. E. Cavanagh, J. Yen, and M. Yu. 2014. "Where have all the good men gone?" Gendered interactions in online dating. *Journal of Marriage and Family* 76(2):387-410.

Krieger, J., and D. L. Higgins. 2002. Housing and health: Time again for public health action. *American Journal of Public Health* 92(5):758-768.

Lamb, K. A., G. R. Lee, and A. DeMaris. 2003. Union formation and depression: Selection and relationship effects. *Journal of Marriage and Family* 65(4):953-962.

Lareau, A. 2004. *Unequal childhoods: Class, race, and family life*. Berkeley, CA: University of California Press.

Ledbetter, A. M. 2009. Family communication patterns and relational maintenance behavior: Direct and mediated associations with friendship closeness. *Human Communication Research* 35(1):130-147.

Lee, A. I. 1998. Intergenerational financial support among whites, African Americans, and Latinos. *Journal of Marriage and Family* 60:426-441.

Leonard, K. E., and R. D. Eiden. 2007. Marital and family processes in the context of alcohol use and alcohol disorders. *Annual Review of Clinical Psychology* 3:207-232.

Lerman, R. I. 2002. *How do marriage, cohabitation, and single parenthood affect the material hardships of families with children?* Washington, DC: Urban Institute.

Lerner, R. M. 2006. Developmental science, developmental systems and contemporary theories of human development. In *Handbook of child psychology*, 6th ed., Vol. 1, edited by W. Damon and R. M. Lerner. Hoboken, NJ: Wiley. Pp. 1-17.

Lewis, C. E., Jr., I. Garfinkel, and Q. Gao. 2007. Incarceration and unwed fathers in fragile families. *Journal of Sociology & Social Welfare* 34:77.

Lichter, D. T., and Z. Qian. 2008. Serial cohabitation and the marital life course. *Journal of Marriage and Family* 70(4):861-878.

Lichter, D. T., D. K. McLaughlin, G. Kephart, and D. J. Landry. 1992. Race and the retreat from marriage: A shortage of marriageable men? *American Sociological Review* 57(6):781-799.

Lichter, D. T., D. R. Graefe, and J. B. Brown. 2003. Is marriage a panacea? Union formation among economically disadvantaged unwed mothers. *Social Problems* 50(1):60-86.

Loper, A. B., and E. H. Tuerk. 2006. Parenting programs for incarcerated parents: Current research and future directions. *Criminal Justice Policy Review* 17(4):407-427.

López Turley, R. N., and M. Desmond. 2011. Contributions to college costs by married, divorced, and remarried parents. *Journal of Family Issues* 32(6):767-790.

Lopoo, L. M., and B. Western. 2005. Incarceration and the formation and stability of marital unions. *Journal of Marriage and Family* 67(3):721-734.

Manlove, J., C. Logan, E. Ikramullah, and E. Holcombe. 2008. Factors associated with multiple-partner fertility among fathers. *Journal of Marriage and Family* 70(2):536-548.

Manning, W. D., P. J. Smock, and D. Majumdar. 2004. The relative stability of cohabiting and marital unions for children. *Population Research and Policy Review* 23(2):135-159.

Martin, J. A., B. E. Hamilton, M. J. K. Osterman, S. C. Curtin, and T. J. Mathews. 2013. Births: Final data for 2012. *National Vital Statistics Report* 62(9).

Martinson, K., and D. Nightingale. 2008. *Ten key findings from responsible fatherhood initiatives*. Washington, DC: Urban Institute.

Marwick, A. 2013. *Status update: Celebrity, publicity, and branding in the social media age*. New Haven, CT: Yale University Press.

Massoglia, M., B. Remster, and R. D. King. 2011. Stigma or separation? Understanding the incarceration-divorce relationship. *Social Forces* 90(1):133-155.

Mastekaasa, A. 1994. The subjective well-being of the previously married: The importance of unmarried cohabitation and time since widowhood or divorce. *Social Forces* 73(2):665-692.

Mathews, T., and B. E. Hamilton. 2009. *Delayed childbearing: More women are having their first child later in life*. Hyattsville, MD: National Center for Health Statistics.

McLanahan, S., and G. Sandefur. 1994. *Growing up with a single parent: What helps, what hurts*. Cambridge, MA: Harvard University Press.

Merline, A. C., J. E. Schulenberg, P. M. O'Malley, J. G. Bachman, and L. D. Johnston. 2008. Substance use in marital dyads: Premarital assortment and change over time. *Journal of Studies on Alcohol and Drugs* 69(3):352-361.

Mincieli, L., J. Manlove, and M. McGarrett. 2007. *The relationship context of births outside of marriage: The rise of cohabitation*. Bethesda, MD: Child Trends.

Moore, M. R., and J. Brooks-Gunn. 2002. Adolescent parenthood. In *Handbook of parenting*, Vol. 3, edited by M. H. Borstein. Mahwah, NJ: Lawrence Erlbaum Associates. Pp. 173-214.

Murrell, K. 2012. *Two generation approaches: Initial observations and reflections*. Baltimore, MD: Annie E. Casey Foundation.

Murry, V. M., and N. Li. 2014. *Are African Americans living the dream 50 years after passage of the Civil Rights Act?* https://contemporaryfamilies.org/tag/african-americans (accessed August 6, 2014).

Murry, V. M., R. L. Simons, L. G. Simons, and F. X. Gibbons. 2013. Contributions of family environment and parenting processes to sexual risk and substance use of rural African American males: A 4-year longitudinal analysis. *The American Journal of Orthopsychiatry* 83(2, Pt. 3):299-309.

Musick, K. 2007. Cohabitation, nonmarital childbearing, and the marriage process. *Demographic Research* 16(9):249-286.

NCSL (National Conference of State Legislatures). 2014a. *Termination of support—age of majority*. http://www.ncsl.org/research/human-services/termination-of-child-support-age-of-majority.aspx (accessed September 16, 2014).

NCSL. 2014b. *Termination of support—college support beyond the age of majority.* http://www.ncsl.org/research/human-services/termination-of-support-college-support.aspx (accessed September 16, 2014).

NCSL. 2014c. *Termination of child support—exception for adult children with disabilities.* http://www.ncsl.org/research/human-services/termination-of-child-support-exception-for-adult.aspx (accessed September 16, 2014).

Nock, S. L. 1995. A comparison of marriages and cohabiting relationships. *Journal of Family Issues* 16(1):53-76.

Nomaguchi, K. M., and M. A. Milkie. 2003. Costs and rewards of children: The effects of becoming a parent on adults' lives. *Journal of Marriage and Family* 65(2):356-374.

O'Connor, M., A. Sanson, M. T. Hawkins, P. Letcher, J. W. Toumbourou, D. Smart, S. Vassallo, and C. A. Olsson. 2011. Predictors of positive development in emerging adulthood. *Journal of Youth and Adolescence* 40(7):860-874.

Oesterle, S. 2013. Background paper: Pathways to young adulthood and preventive interventions targeting young adults. In *Improving the health, safety, and well-being of young adults: Workshop summary*, edited by Institute of Medicine and National Research Council. Washington, DC: The National Academies Press. Pp. 147-176.

Oppenheimer, V. K. 2003. Cohabiting and marriage during young men's career-development process. *Demography* 40(1):127-149.

Papacharissi, Z. 2012. Without you, I'm nothing: Performances of the self on twitter. *International Journal of Communication* 6:18.

Payne, K. K. 2011. *Sequencing of family experiences.* Bowling, OH: National Center for Family & Marriage Research.

Payne, K. K. 2012. *Timing of first marital birth.* Bowling, OH: National Center for Family & Marriage Research.

Pollard, M. S., and K. M. Harris. 2013. *Nonmarital cohabitation, marriage, and health among adolescents and young adults.* Working Paper. Santa Monica, CA: RAND Corporation.

Putnam, R. 2001. Social capital: Measurement and consequences. *Canadian Journal of Policy Research* 2(1):41-51.

Quinn, K., and Z. Papacharissi. 2014. The place where our social networks reside: Social media and sociality. *Media and Social Life* 189.

Rainie, L., and B. Wellman. 2012. *Networked: The new social operating system.* Cambridge, MA: The MIT Press.

Ren, X. S. 1997. Marital status and quality of relationships: The impact on health perception. *Social Science & Medicine* 44(2):241-249.

Rettberg, J. W. 2013. *Blogging.* Cambridge, UK: Polity Press.

Rosenquist, J. N., J. H. Fowler, and N. A. Christakis. 2010a. Social network determinants of depression. *Molecular Psychiatry* 16(3):273-281.

Rosenquist, J. N., J. Murabito, J. H. Fowler, and N. A. Christakis. 2010b. The spread of alcohol consumption behavior in a large social network. *Annals of Internal Medicine* 152(7):426-433.

Ross, C. E. 1995. Reconceptualizing marital status as a continuum of social attachment. *Journal of Marriage and Family* 57(1):129-140.

Rossi, P. P. H. 1990. *Of human bonding: Parent-child relations across the life course.* Piscataway, NJ: Transaction Publishers.

Roulet, M. 2009. *Fatherhood programs and healthy marriage funding.* Madison, WI: Center for Family Policy and Practice.

Rueda, M. R., M. I. Rosner, and M. K. Rothbart. 2011. Attentional control and self-regulation. In *Handbook of self-regulation, second edition: Research, theory, and applications,* edited by K. D. Vohs and R. F. Baumeister. New York: Guilford Press. Pp. 284-299.

Sameroff, A. 2010. A unified theory of development: A dialectic integration of nature and nurture. *Child Development* 81(1):6-22.

Sampson, R. J., J. H. Laub, and C. Wimer. 2006. Does marriage reduce crime? A counterfactual approach to within-individual causal effects. *Criminology* 44(3):465-508.

Sassler, S. 2010. Partnering across the life course: Sex, relationships, and mate selection. *Journal of Marriage and Family* 72(3):557-575.

Sassler, S., and A. Cunningham. 2008. How cohabitors view childbearing. *Sociological Perspectives* 51(1):3-28.

Schoeni, R. F., and K. E. Ross. 2005. Material assistance from families during the transition to adulthood. In *On the frontier of adulthood,* edited by R. A. Settersten, Jr., F. F. Furstenberg, and R. G. Rumbaut. Chicago, IL: University of Chicago Press. Pp. 396-416.

Schulenberg, J. E., and J. L. Maggs. 2002. A developmental perspective on alcohol use and heavy drinking during adolescence and the transition to young adulthood. *Journal of Studies on Alcohol Supplement* (14):54-70.

Scott, M., E. Falkenburger, M. McDaniel, A. Khare, and S. J. Popkin. 2013. *HOST year 2: Implementation and expansion. HOST brief* 2. Washington, DC: Urban Institute. http://www.urban.org/UploadedPDF/412824-HOST-Year-2-Implementation-and-Expansion.pdf (accessed August 4, 2014).

Semyonov, M., and N. Lewin-Epstein. 2001. The impact of parental transfers on living standards of married children. *Social Indicators Research* 54(2):115-137.

Settersten, R., and B. E. Ray. 2010. *Not quite adults: Why 20-somethings are choosing a slower path to adulthood, and why it's good for everyone.* New York: Random House.

Shaffer, A., K. B. Burt, J. Obradovic, J. E. Herbers, and A. S. Masten. 2009. Intergenerational continuity in parenting quality: The mediating role of social competence. *Developmental Psychology* 45(5):1227-1240.

Shanahan, M. J. 2000. Pathways to adulthood in changing societies: Variability and mechanisms in life course perspective. *Annual Review of Sociology* 26(1):667-692.

Shaw, K., S. Goldrick-Rab, C. Mazzeo, and J. A. Jacobs. 2005. *Putting poor people to work: How the work-first ideology eroded college access for the poor.* Unpublished book manuscript. Philadelphia, PA: Temple University.

Shouls, S., M. Whitehead, B. Burstrom, and F. Diderichsen. 1999. The health and socioeconomic circumstances of British lone mothers over the last two decades. *Population Trends-London* 41-46.

Silk, J. S., L. Steinberg, and A. S. Morris. 2003. Adolescents' emotion regulation in daily life: Links to depressive symptoms and problem behavior. *Child Development* 74(6): 1869-1880.

Simmel, G. 1950. *The sociology of Georg Simmel*, edited by K. Wolff. New York: The Free Press.

Simons, R. L., J. Beaman, R. D. Conger, and W. Chao. 1993. Childhood experience, conceptions of parenting, and attitudes of spouse as determinants of parental behavior. *Journal of Marriage and Family* 55(1):91-106.

Small, M. L. 2009. *Unanticipated gains: Origins of network inequality in everyday life*. New York: Oxford University Press.

Smith, S. 1995. *Two generation programs for families in poverty: A new intervention strategy*, Vol. 9. Portsmouth, NH: Greenwood Publishing Group.

Smock, P. J. 2000. Cohabitation in the United States: An appraisal of research themes, findings, and implications. *Annual Review of Sociology* 26:1-20.

Smock, P. J., and F. R. Greenland. 2010. Diversity in pathways to parenthood: Patterns, implications, and emerging research directions. *Journal of Marriage and Family* 72(3):576-593.

Staff, J., J. E. Schulenberg, J. Maslowsky, J. G. Bachman, P. M. O'Malley, J. L. Maggs, and L. D. Johnston. 2010. Substance use changes and social role transitions: Proximal developmental effects on ongoing trajectories from late adolescence through early adulthood. *Development and Psychopathology* 22(4):917-932.

Swartz, T. T. 2009. Intergenerational family relations in adulthood: Patterns, variations, and implications in the contemporary United States. *Annual Review of Sociology* (35): 191-212.

Sweeney, M. M. 2002. Two decades of family change: The shifting economic foundations of marriage. *American Sociological Review* 132-147.

Teachman, J. D., L. M. Tedrow, and K. D. Crowder. 2000. The changing demography of America's families. *Journal of Marriage and Family* 62(4):1234-1246.

Thoits, P. A. 1983. Multiple identities and psychological well-being: A reformulation and test of the social isolation hypothesis. *American Sociological Review* 48(2):174-187.

Thomas, A., and I. V. Sawhill. 2005. For love and money? The impact of family structure on family income. *The Future of Children* 15(2):57-74.

Umberson, D., and J. K. Montez. 2010. Social relationships and health a flashpoint for health policy. *Journal of Health and Social Behavior* 51(Suppl. 1):S54-S66.

Umberson, D., and K. Williams. 1999. Family status and mental health. In *Handbook of the sociology of mental health*. New York: Springer Publishing. Pp. 225-253.

Umberson, D., T. Pudrovska, and C. Reczek. 2010a. Parenthood, childlessness, and well-being: A life course perspective. *Journal of Marriage and Family* 72(3):612-629.

Umberson, D., R. Crosnoe, and C. Reczek. 2010b. Social relationships and health behavior across the life course. *Annual Review of Sociology* 36:139-157.

Upchurch, D. M., L. A. Lillard, and C. W. Panis. 2002. Nonmarital childbearing: Influences of education, marriage, and fertility. *Demography* 39(2):311-329.

U.S. Census Bureau. 2010. *America's families and living arrangements: 2010*. https://www.census.gov/population/www/socdemo/hh-fam/cps2010.html (accessed October 2, 2014).

U.S. Census Bureau. 2013. *Median age at first marriage: 2013 American Community Survey 1-year estimates*. http://factfinder2.census.gov/faces/tableservices/jsf/pages/productview.xhtml?pid=ACS_13_1YR_B12007&prodType=table (accessed September 24, 2014).

Wagner, B., and K. M. Harris. 2014. Health and social stratification in family information pathways. Unpublished paper presented at 2014 Annual Meeting Population Association of American, Boston, MA, May.

Waite, L. J. 1995. Does marriage matter? *Demography* 32(4):483-507.

Wallerstein, J. S., and J. M. Lewis. 2004. The unexpected legacy of divorce. *Psychoanalytic Psychology* 21(3):353-370.

Ward, R. A., and G. D. Spitze. 2007. Nestleaving and coresidence by young adult children: The role of family relations. *Research on Aging* 29(3):257-277.

Ward, R., G. Spitze, and G. Deane. 2009. More the merrier? Multiple parent-adult child relations. *Journal of Marriage and Family* 71(1):161-173.

Wasserman, S., and K. Faust. 1994. *Social network analysis: Methods and applications (structural analysis in the social sciences)*. New York: Cambridge University Press.

Wellman, B., and S. D. Berkowitz. 1997. *Social structures: A network approach*. Greenwich, CT: JAI Press.

Westin, M., and R. Westerling. 2006. Health and healthcare utilization among single mothers and single fathers in Sweden. *Scandinavian Journal of Public Health* 34(2):182-189.

White, L., and N. Lacy. 1997. The effects of age at home leaving and pathways from home on educational attainment. *Journal of Marriage and Family* 59(4):982-995.

Wickrama, K. A., L. G. Simons, and D. Baltimore. 2012. The influence of ethnicity and adverse life experiences during adolescence on young adult socioeconomic attainment: The moderating role of education. *Journal of Youth and Adolescence* 41(11):472-487.

Wildsmith, E., N. R. Steward-Streng, and J. Manlove. 2011. *Childbearing outside of marriage: Estimates and trends in the United States*. Bethesda, MD: Child Trends.

Williams, K., S. Sassler, A. Frech, F. Addo, and E. Cooksey. 2011. Nonmarital childbearing, union history, and women's health at midlife. *American Sociological Review* 76(3): 465-486.

Williams, K., S. Sassler, A. Frech, F. Addo, and E. Cooksey. 2013. Mothers' union histories and the mental and physical health of adolescents born to unmarried mothers. *Journal of Health and Social Behavior* 54(3):278-295.

Wilson, B. 2012. *Coresident grandparents: Caregivers versus non-caregivers (FP-12-18)*. Bowling Green, OH: National Center for Family & Marriage Research. http://ncfmr.bgsu.edu/pdf/family_profiles/file115686.pdf (accessed October 2, 2014).

Wilson, W. 1987. *The truly disadvantaged: The inner city, the underclass, and public policy*. Chicago, IL: University of Chicago Press.

Wood, R. G., B. Goesling, and S. Avellar. 2007. *The effects of marriage on health: A synthesis of recent research evidence*. Washington, DC: Mathematica Policy Research, Inc.

Wood, R. G., Q. Moore, A. Clarkwest, and A. Killewald. 2014. The long-term effects of building strong families: A program for unmarried parents. *Journal of Marriage and Family* 76(2):446-463.

Wu, Z., and R. Hart. 2002. The effects of marital and nonmarital union transition on health. *Journal of Marriage and Family* 64(2):420-432.

Wu, Z., M. J. Penning, M. S. Pollard, and R. Hart. 2003. "In sickness and in health" does cohabitation count? *Journal of Family Issues* 24(6):811-838.

Zaslow, M. J., K. A. Moore, J. L. Brooks, P. A. Morris, K. Tout, Z. A. Redd, and C. A. Emig. 2002. Experimental studies of welfare reform and children. *The Future of Children* 12(1):79-96.

Zhang, Z., and M. D. Hayward. 2006. Gender, the marital life course, and cardiovascular disease in late midlife. *Journal of Marriage and Family* 68(3):639-657.

4

Education and Employment

Key Findings

- While many young adults gain enough education and labor market experience to succeed in life, doing so has always posed some challenges for other young adults, especially those from economically disadvantaged or minority backgrounds. These challenges are greater today than in earlier eras, and not only for those whose families have been disadvantaged.
- The cost of college has grown substantially, and many students have difficulty making the investment, yet prospects for well-paying jobs for high school graduates without some postsecondary credentials are slim. For this and other reasons, many young adults enter college, but dropout rates are high, and the numbers of years needed to complete degree programs have risen.
- Well-compensated entry-level jobs are becoming more difficult to find, even for young college graduates, and especially in the aftermath of the Great Recession. Moreover, many companies do not provide health insurance or other economic benefits, and low earnings plague many young workers because of technological change and globalization, as well as the weakening of institutions and mechanisms (such as unions and government regulations) that have traditionally protected less-educated workers.

- Educational attainment during young adulthood has lifelong implications not only for economic well-being but also for health. Over the long run, the more educated a young adult becomes, the healthier she or he will be in adulthood.
- Given the important linkages among education, employment, and health and safety outcomes for young adults, the very weak education and employment outcomes of two groups of young adults raise particular concern: those who are disconnected and those who have disabilities and chronic health conditions.
- Overall, there is some evidence on successful workforce programs for adults and youth with relatively strong basic skills, and limited evidence on programs designed to improve success rates for disadvantaged students who enroll in college. Integrating useful labor market information or training into developmental efforts appears highly promising. But the ability to replicate and scale up the best programs and to identify successful efforts for those with greater skill deficiencies or disabilities remains limited.

Social scientists view the transition to adulthood as a function of progression in five interrelated domains: completing education, gaining full-time employment, becoming financially independent from parents, entering marriage/romantic partnership, and becoming a parent (IOM and NRC, 2013; Shanahan, 2000). There is agreement that all of these tasks of adulthood are now taking longer to accomplish than in generations past. Among the challenges young people face as they transition to adulthood, two can be considered centrally important: (1) progressing toward and completing their educational attainment, and (2) becoming employed and earning enough to gain independence from their families. From a developmental perspective, the transition to adulthood is a critical period for forging work- and career-related identities, with initial plans and training confronting market realities. Those who cannot gain a foothold in the world of work during this time may continue to lag behind their more successful age-mates. Thus, reflecting one of the major themes of this report, what happens during young adulthood is integral to long-term socioeconomic trajectories.

Not only is working an important aspect of becoming adult, but employment and health, including behavioral health, are highly correlated across individuals:

- Individuals with compromised health have greater difficulty attaining and maintaining employment, and involuntary loss of employment can have a negative impact on physical and behavioral health when it occurs among adults (Fergusson and Horwood, 1997; Montgomery et al., 1999; Paul and Moser, 2009).
- One study found that psychological health in childhood had a greater impact than physical health in childhood on adult earnings (Goodman et al., 2011). Psychological health problems in childhood reduce adult incomes by 14-28 percent compared with controls. Moreover, this study found that the impact of childhood psychological problems on adult income occurred disproportionately in earlier rather than later adulthood, supporting the notion that young adulthood is a critical window for intervention.
- Health care coverage is disrupted by loss of employment, and loss of coverage can contribute to reduced health care seeking, as discussed in Chapter 6.

To some extent, gaining enough education and labor market experience to succeed has always posed some challenges for young people, especially those from disadvantaged or minority backgrounds. In many ways, however, these challenges appear to be greater today than in earlier eras for a variety of reasons, and not only for those whose families have been disadvantaged.

For one thing, the labor market today poses serious challenges for young people. The Great Recession, which began formally at the end of 2007 and ended in mid-2009, reduced employment opportunities for youth and young adults more than for any other age group. Furthermore, the recovery from this recession has been both modest and extremely slow, especially in the job market; in 2011, the rate of employment in the population for young adults was only marginally higher than it was at the recession's trough (Sum et al., 2014).

Gaining early work experience has been difficult for many in this environment, including those with college diplomas, and this sluggishness also limits wage gains for many who are employed. Indeed, the evidence suggests that the average young person entering the job market during a major economic downturn may be "scarred" by this experience in terms of lower average earnings for many years (Dahl et al., 2013; Kahn, 2010). Moreover, it is possible that the job market will remain weak going forward, and for years to come, if the current stagnation is more "secular" than "cyclical" in nature (Ball et al., 2014).

Even before 2007, however, the labor market had changed in a variety of ways that increased the challenges faced by young people. Because of a variety of labor market and institutional forces, the earnings of those with no postsecondary education or training credential in the United States have stagnated or declined over time, and the earnings prospects of young people without this education or training are now very limited (Autor et al., 2008; Card and DiNardo, 2005). Of course, having this background is no guarantee of labor market success, especially for young adults in lower-paying fields or from less prestigious educational institutions. But on average, investments in higher education remain worthwhile for those who can afford to make them and are able to complete a postsecondary program of study (Oreopoulos and Petronijevic, 2013).

"A lot of my friends say, 'you need to get an internship, you need something outside of your education, you need to volunteer' to supplement your degree and stand out more."*

Unfortunately, many young adults do not fit into this category. As discussed below, the rate at which young people graduate from high school remains quite low in the United States, and substitutes (such as passing a General Educational Development [GED] test) are not particularly valued in the job market. Many of those who complete high school only face poor labor market prospects. Noncompletion rates also are quite high among those who enroll in 2- or 4-year colleges. Dropout rates are particularly high at 2-year institutions and among those who are disadvantaged and have weak educational skills and records (Holzer and Dunlop, 2013).

Moreover, many people leave these institutions saddled with the debt incurred while pursuing a degree there, and are challenged to earn enough to pay down their debt while providing for themselves and their families. Failure to complete enough education or obtain a well-paying job also has some negative social consequences, such as reluctance to marry (or an inability to stay married), and incarceration rates for such young adults, especially young men of color, are unacceptably high. For young people who are "disconnected" from school and work or disabled, these challenges can be quite severe.

Below we consider these issues at greater length. First, we look at trends in employment outcomes among young people over time, as well as in enrollment, to distinguish those who are productively engaged in work or school as opposed to being "idle" or disconnected. We distinguish trends

* Quotations are from members of the young adult advisory group during their discussions with the committee.

until 2006 from those occurring more recently, with the former reflecting secular and the latter cyclical factors to a great extent. We also consider relative wages and employment rates across young people who have finished various levels of schooling.

In the next section, we look at differences in educational attainment across racial/gender groups as well as family income, and at the extent to which observed differences in employment outcomes can be accounted for by differences in enrollment or completion rates across groups and at different kinds of schools. Since community colleges are a type of institution particularly relevant for disadvantaged young people as a potential gateway to better-paying jobs, we discuss some of their unique characteristics and a set of potential reforms to financial aid or remediation programs that might render them more effective. We also consider other possible sources of education—such as for-profit colleges or career and technical programs—as alternatives to public 2- or 4-year schools with both advantages and disadvantages in their relative benefits and costs.

Next we discuss the short- and long-term implications of education and employment for health and well-being. We also discuss the social implications of students who are relatively less successful in education or employment. We give particular attention to two groups that struggle with education and employment—"disconnected" youth and those with disabilities.

In the following section, we review the policy landscape affecting education and employment outcomes of young adults. We also consider lessons learned to date from evaluation evidence.

Finally, we conclude with conclusions and recommendations for improving opportunities for young people in both higher education and the labor market.

EMPLOYMENT OUTCOMES OF YOUNG ADULTS

Since many young adults remain enrolled in college until their mid-20s or beyond, most data on those aged 16-24 focus on their rates of engagement in the productive activities of schooling and work. We therefore analyze the fractions of youth who are either enrolled, employed, or neither (usually referred to, as above, as "idle" or "disconnected"). We then offer an analysis of the levels of educational attainment, wages or earnings, and rates of employment for those aged 25-29.

Table 4-1 presents data on employment, labor force participation, and unemployment rates, as well as rates of school enrollment and idleness, for

TABLE 4-1 Percent Changes in Labor Market Measures by Demographic Group, 1980-2010

	Ages 16-19			Ages 20-24		
	1980	2006	2010	1980	2006	2010
Employment-to-Population Ratio						
Male, White	48.5	38.6	29.8	76.5	71.7	65.7
Female, White	43.8	41.8	34.9	65.1	69.7	66.9
Male, Black	27.7	21.9	16.0	60.4	51.8	44.9
Female, Black	21.8	26.3	20.4	50.1	57.8	53.4
Male, Hispanic	42.4	35.0	25.0	74.8	74.5	67.1
Female, Hispanic	32.7	29.6	23.8	52.6	57.5	56.7
Labor Force Participation Rate						
Male, White	55.9	47.9	40.6	84.7	79.6	77.8
Female, White	49.5	49.8	44.0	69.9	76.0	75.4
Male, Black	36.8	37.2	30.7	73.8	68.6	65.8
Female, Black	30.2	40.6	35.1	61.5	72.8	71.9
Male, Hispanic	50.5	45.1	37.6	83.8	82.4	80.5
Female, Hispanic	38.7	38.7	34.2	59.0	65.5	68.0
Unemployment Rate						
Male, White	13.3	19.3	26.6	9.7	9.9	15.5
Female, White	11.5	15.9	20.7	6.9	8.2	11.2
Male, Black	24.7	41.2	48.1	18.2	24.5	31.8
Female, Black	27.9	35.3	41.9	18.6	20.6	25.8
Male, Hispanic	16.1	22.4	33.4	10.8	9.6	16.7
Female, Hispanic	15.3	23.6	30.4	10.9	12.3	16.6
Share Enrolled in School						
Male, White	71.0	84.5	85.1	25.2	40.0	41.3
Female, White	70.5	87.4	88.1	22.3	46.3	48.5
Male, Black	68.8	78.9	79.8	19.1	29.4	31.9
Female, Black	70.8	82.3	83.9	21.7	37.5	42.6
Male, Hispanic	61.8	72.0	77.1	18.5	22.4	26.9
Female, Hispanic	62.1	78.1	81.8	17.8	32.3	36.2
Share Not in School and Not Working						
Male, White	8.8	6.1	7.5	12.0	12.2	15.8
Female, White	12.4	5.7	6.1	25.3	14.4	15.0
Male, Black	17.1	14.5	15.1	28.9	33.1	37.1
Female, Black	20.3	11.1	11.1	37.6	25.8	26.0
Male, Hispanic	15.0	10.7	11.4	17.3	16.6	20.8
Female, Hispanic	22.8	12.9	11.3	39.5	29.9	27.9

SOURCE: Adapted with permission from Dennett and Modestino, 2013.

youth aged 16-19 and young adults aged 20-24.[1] The data cover the years 1980, 2006, and 2010. Changes in the period 1980-2006 reflect mainly secular trends in employment and enrollment, while those in the period 2006-2010 more likely reflect cyclical (or temporary) changes, as they indicate peak-to-trough changes in the labor market. Separate results appear by race and gender.

Table 4-1 shows the following developments for teens and young adults in the period 1980-2006:

- School enrollment rates rose considerably, especially among those aged 20-24.
- Employment rates and labor force activity fell for most groups, while unemployment rose.
- Idleness held steady or declined modestly for most groups of young men and dropped substantially for young women, whose enrollment rates rose more and employment dropped less than was the case for young men.
- Black male young adults showed a substantial increase in idleness during this period, and now have the lowest employment rates (and highest rates of idleness) of any group.

For most groups of young people, especially young women, a rise in school enrollment fully offsets their drop in employment. The larger increases in enrollment for those aged 20-24 almost certainly reflect college enrollments, and likely result in more young people with 2- or 4-year college degrees.[2] Yet, reflecting a recurring theme of this chapter (and the report as a whole), these general patterns subsume a great deal of sociodemographic heterogeneity, as school and work trends vary across diverse segments of the population. For example, the rise in idleness among young black men is disturbing—especially given the fact that these data notoriously undercount less-educated young and disconnected men, especially blacks, so that actual rates of idleness and their increases over time are likely to be significantly higher for this population (Pettit, 2012). We also note the relatively low enrollment rate of Hispanic men in this age group, presumably in higher education, while their employment rate is quite high;

[1] The employment rate is defined as the percentage of the civilian noninstitutional population that is employed; the labor force participation rate is the percentage of the same population that is employed or seeking work; and the unemployment rate is the percentage of that labor force that is not employed but seeking work.

[2] A rise in the average number of years it takes to complete a 2- or 4-year degree also contributes to rising enrollment rates at any point in time for this population (Turner, 2007).

the implication is that their earnings growth as they age may lag behind that of other demographic groups.

The data over the period 2006-2010, on the other hand, show quite dramatic declines in employment, rises in unemployment, and declines in labor force activity for both groups, especially among teens. While some increases are seen in school enrollment (especially among Hispanics and/or those aged 20-24), these increases generally are insufficiently large to fully offset declining employment, so that idleness increased for most groups, especially male young adults.

Although unemployment rates for all groups have declined since 2010, these changes have been driven mainly by declining labor force activity rather than higher employment rates. Thus, youth employment has not rebounded strongly. Evidence has accumulated that young people who enter the job market during periods of high joblessness are scarred with low earnings in the future, and the lengthy period of depressed employment will no doubt reduce their earning capacity for many years to come (Dahl et al., 2013; Kahn, 2010). Furthermore, it is unclear whether or when these employment rates will recover, especially for those young people who have left the job market without enrolling in school.

Given these patterns of school and work activity for young people until their mid-20s, what employment rates and earnings levels do we observe for young people aged 25-29? Figure 4-1 and Table 4-2 present average employment and hourly wage rates for young adults by their level of educational attainment and by race and gender in 2010. The results show large differences in both employment rates and wages across different educational groups, with both outcomes rising quite consistently with educational attainment.

It is particularly noteworthy that, since average employment and hourly wages in combination determine annual earnings, gaps in annual pay between those who do and do not have college diplomas will be substantially larger than the differences that appear in Table 4-2. It is also noteworthy that young college graduates (with BAs) have both employment and wage rates that are roughly 30 percent and 60 percent higher, respectively, than the rates for those with only high school (see Figure 4-1), implying that annual earnings are nearly twice as high for the former as for the latter. The data also show significant racial and gender gaps remaining in employment outcomes, while other data (not included here) show large variations across fields of study within each educational level.[3]

[3] At the sub-BA and BA levels, earnings returns to degrees in science, technology, engineering, and mathematics tend to exceed those to degrees in the social sciences and humanities (and other applied fields), while returns to degrees in business, law, and medicine grow much larger at the post-BA level (Holzer and Dunlop, 2013).

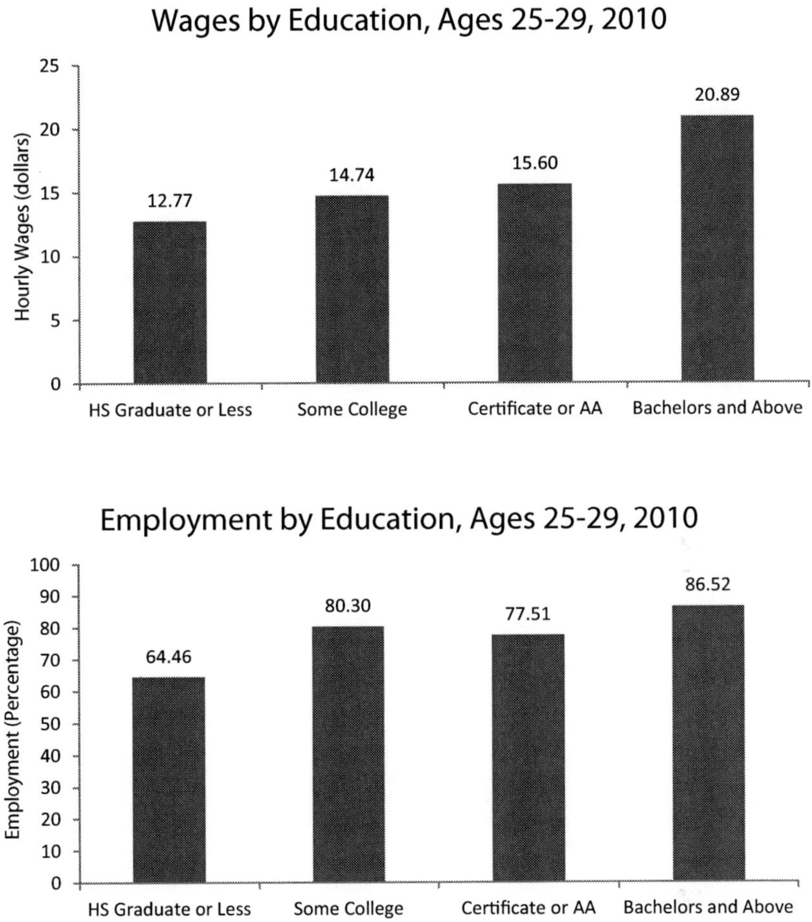

FIGURE 4-1 Wages and employment by education, 2010.
SOURCE: Holzer and Dunlop, 2013, based on data from the Survey of Income and Program Participation (SIPP), reprinted with permission.

A substantial literature now exists that examines the trends over time in the labor market returns to different levels of education, as well as how they vary by race and gender. These studies generally show that

- earnings gaps between those with BAs and with high school only have roughly doubled since 1980 (Autor, 2010; Autor et al., 2008);
- young women have gained ground in employment and earnings relative to young men, although they still lag behind in both (Blau and Kahn, 2006);

TABLE 4-2 Employment Rate and Mean Hourly Wages by Education and by Race/Gender in 2010, Ages 25-29

Education	Race	Gender	Employment Rate	N	Mean Hourly Wage (in 2010 $)
Dropout	Black	Male	0.43	61	$9.58
		Female	0.33	107	$9.69
	Hispanic	Male	0.74	276	$10.93
		Female	0.35	342	$8.14
	White	Male	0.73	302	$12.60
		Female	0.49	250	$10.12
General Educational Development (GED)	Black	Male	0.40	25	$11.08
		Female	0.56	60	$11.32
	Hispanic	Male	0.87	73	$13.08
		Female	0.55	54	$8.33
	White	Male	0.56	214	$15.21
		Female	0.59	192	$12.55
High School	Black	Male	0.73	147	$12.43
		Female	0.57	159	$9.64
	Hispanic	Male	0.76	245	$13.60
		Female	0.47	262	$11.22
	White	Male	0.83	905	$16.29
		Female	0.68	747	$12.14
Some College	Black	Male	0.78	161	$13.59
		Female	0.89	236	$13.47
	Hispanic	Male	0.81	142	$12.55
		Female	0.66	221	$13.77
	White	Male	0.92	840	$16.55
		Female	0.77	858	$14.42
Certificate	Black	Male	0.51	58	$11.45
		Female	0.73	107	$11.93
	Hispanic	Male	0.89	56	$12.17
		Female	0.63	95	$13.81
	White	Male	0.86	283	$16.95
		Female	0.67	354	$13.42
Associate's Degree	Black	Male	0.90	22	$11.90
		Female	0.76	84	$12.35
	Hispanic	Male	1.00	52	$17.03
		Female	0.74	61	$16.32
	White	Male	0.88	355	$17.13
		Female	0.79	450	$17.77
Bachelor's Degree	Black	Male	0.96	36	$20.24
		Female	0.79	107	$16.11
	Hispanic	Male	0.65	52	$14.94
		Female	0.70	84	$15.96
	White	Male	0.93	1,131	$21.40
		Female	0.87	1,359	$18.63

SOURCE: Holzer and Dunlop, 2013, reprinted with permission.

- racial differences in hourly wages among young workers within an educational category are accounted for mainly by gaps in achievement (measured as grades and/or test scores), while gender gaps (in wages and employment) reflect primarily childrearing responsibilities among women and occupational choices (Holzer and Dunlop, 2013);
- very large racial differences in employment (especially among young men) remain and are less fully accounted for by these factors (Holzer et al., 2005); and
- less-educated young white and black men have tended to withdraw from the workforce in response to these trends (Holzer et al., 2005).

Among other factors contributing to differences in employment, discrimination in hiring by race and gender has been clearly documented; "spatial mismatch" (between the locations of jobs and the residences of minorities), along with differences in the strength of informal hiring networks, contribute to employment gaps by race as well (Holzer et al., 2005). Less-educated Hispanic men work at levels above those of their white and black counterparts, reflecting some preference for immigrants in low-wage jobs among employers and also the strength of informal networks in the immigrant community. Even less-educated women have seen rising employment rates in the past two decades as a result of both employment shifts toward the service sector and policy changes. But the gaps in education and achievement across racial groups remain among the most important determinants of observed gaps in earnings (Holzer et al., 2005).

> "Entering the workforce is hard because there's this big debate over getting a job that pays well or experience. In my experience, it was either a job that was convenient, paid well, but it wasn't really what I wanted to be doing or there was a really perfect job in my field, exactly what I wanted to be doing, but it doesn't pay well."

What accounts for the long-term trends in the job market for young adults? Most economists attribute these trends to ongoing technological change, whereby less-educated employees doing routine work are replaced, while demand rises for those with more technical, analytical, and/or communication skills. The forces of globalization also have gained strength in the past decade, resulting in enormous increases in the supply of less-educated workers in international markets that increasingly compete with U.S. workers.

In addition, while the demand for higher education in the U.S. labor market has grown, the supply of workers with higher education has failed to keep pace over the past three decades (Goldin and Katz, 2009). Indeed, employers that offer substantial wage premiums for those with skills gained through higher education often are frustrated by their inability to find appropriately skilled workers in the United States. Thus they often seek such workers abroad (either by offshoring work or by lobbying for fewer limits on immigration of the highly skilled to the United States, such as through the H1-B visa program [e.g., DeLuca, 2014]). At the same time, the effects of these powerful market forces are compounded by the weakening of important institutions that have traditionally protected less-skilled workers from such market forces, such as unions and minimum wage regulation (Autor et al., 2008; Card and DiNardo, 2005).

Furthermore, job losses in the middle of the occupational wage distribution have been larger than those at either the top or the bottom. The resulting polarization of the job market has made it more difficult for less-educated workers to advance, since the production and clerical jobs that used to pay workers with a high school education well are the ones that have diminished most in number (Holzer, 2010). The results of this research do not suggest that the middle of the job market has disappeared, but that its accessibility is limited to those with at least some postsecondary education (Carnevale et al., 2010; Holzer, 2010).[4]

In the future, moreover, even well-educated young workers may see their skills become obsolete in a labor market buffeted by rapid technological changes and growing globalization. The need of workers to adjust their skills and careers by engaging in lifelong learning and mobility in the job market may grow accordingly.

EDUCATIONAL PATTERNS AND OUTCOMES OF YOUNG ADULTS

Because college experience is such a big part of many young adults' lives and because the consequences of educational attainment are so important for the earnings of young adults, it is important to analyze attainment differences and trends in recent years and what accounts for them.

Young adults take many different educational paths, just as they differ widely in paths to family formation, health trajectories, and other dynamic experiences discussed throughout this report. When the type of postsecondary institution (2- versus 4-year colleges) and attendance and graduation

---

[4] In these articles, postsecondary educational attainment can include certificates or significant on-the-job training as well as associate's degrees.

patterns (e.g., stopout, dropout) are taken into account, no one normative pathway describes what most young people do. For example, based on national longitudinal data following high school graduates until age 25 (considering those who graduated from high school between 1977 and 2003), 47 percent graduated from a 4-year college, 12 percent graduated from a 2-year college, 11 percent dropped out, 3 percent were still enrolled, and 28 percent did not attend college at all (Patrick et al., 2013). Of particular importance, extensive variation was seen within each group of college attenders in patterns of late start, stopping out, moving between 2- and 4-year colleges, and so on (see Table 4-3). Although these rates likely will vary by historical period, the fact will remain that whenever education (and work) trajectories across the transition to adulthood are considered, there will be noteworthy heterogeneity in how young people negotiate and experience their educational pathways.

> "I have a lot of friends going into engineering, simply because they think it will give them the highest chance of finding a job—not because they are passionate about it."

Figure 4-2 presents educational attainment trends/outcomes by race/gender as of 2010. The results show that whites still had considerably higher rates of BA attainment relative to blacks or Hispanics, although the attainment of certificates and AA degrees (and some college more generally) among blacks surpassed that among whites. Indeed, whites made substantial strides in attaining BAs during the Great Recession, while for blacks and Hispanics, the observed progress was more limited to sub-BA credentials, implying growing racial gaps in this period among those with postsecondary credentials. At the same time, young women in virtually all racial groups obtained higher education more frequently than young men.

To what extent do ongoing gaps in educational attainment reflect gaps in college enrollment at the 2- and 4-year levels, as opposed to gaps in completion rates among enrollees? Enrollment rates are higher among women than men, among whites than minorities, and among middle- and upper-income families than disadvantaged ones (Holzer and Dunlop, 2013). But even larger gaps can be found in rates of college completion. Figure 4-3 presents data from the National Educational Longitudinal Study (NELS) on completion rates at 2- versus 4-year institutions for all workers and separately by race and gender and by low socioeconomic position of families in 2000. The results show average completion rates (within 6 years of enrolling) of more than 60 percent at 4-year schools, about 35 percent at 2-year schools for achieving AA degrees only, and about 55 percent at 2-year schools for achieving AAs or certificates.

TABLE 4-3 Distribution of College Attendance Patterns Among High School Graduates

Attendance Pattern	Percent	Weighted Sample
4-Year Graduates	46.6	4,668
Stay-in[a] 4-Year Graduate	30.6	3,066
Stay-in Combined[b] 4-Year Graduate	5.8	580
Late-Start[c] 4-Year Graduate	4.4	443
Late-Start Combined 4-Year Graduate	0.9	89
Stopout[d] 4-Year Graduate	4.3	433
Stopout Combined 4-Year Graduate	0.6	57
2-Year Graduates	11.8	1,184
Stay-in 2-Year Graduate	4.6	459
Stay-in Combined 2-Year Graduate	0.9	86
Late-Start 2-Year Graduate	3.9	395
Late-Start Combined 2-Year Graduate	0.2	20
Stopout 2-Year Graduate	1.6	161
Stopout Combined 2-Year Graduate	0.6	63
Still Enrolled at Age 25 (Nongraduates)	3.3	329
Stay-in 4-Year Nongraduate	0.2	21
Stay-in Combined Nongraduate	0.1	12
Late-Start 4-Year Nongraduate	0.9	91
Late-Start 2-Year Nongraduate	0.7	71
Late-Start Combined Nongraduate	0.2	17
Stopout 4-Year Nongraduate	0.7	75
Stopout 2-Year Nongraduate	0.1	13
Stopout Combined Nongraduate	0.3	26
Dropouts	10.8	1,084
Immediate-Start[e] 4-Year Dropout[f]	5.2	522
Late-Start 4-Year Dropout	0.7	74
2-Year Dropout	3.6	357
Late-Start 2-Year Dropout	0.9	87
Combined Dropout	0.4	44
Never Attenders	27.5	2,755

NOTES: Based on national longitudinal data from the Monitoring the Future study, following high school seniors (graduating classes of 1977-2003) into young adulthood; total $N = 10{,}020$.

[a] Stay-in refers to continuous enrollment until graduation.

[b] Combined refers to students who attended both 2-year and 4-year schools across the follow-up waves.

[c] Late-start refers to those who did not attend school until after age 19.

[d] Stopout refers to those who reported dropping out before returning to graduate.

[e] Immediate-start refers to students who enrolled the year following high school.

[f] Dropout refers to those who left school and did not graduate.

SOURCE: Patrick et al., 2013.

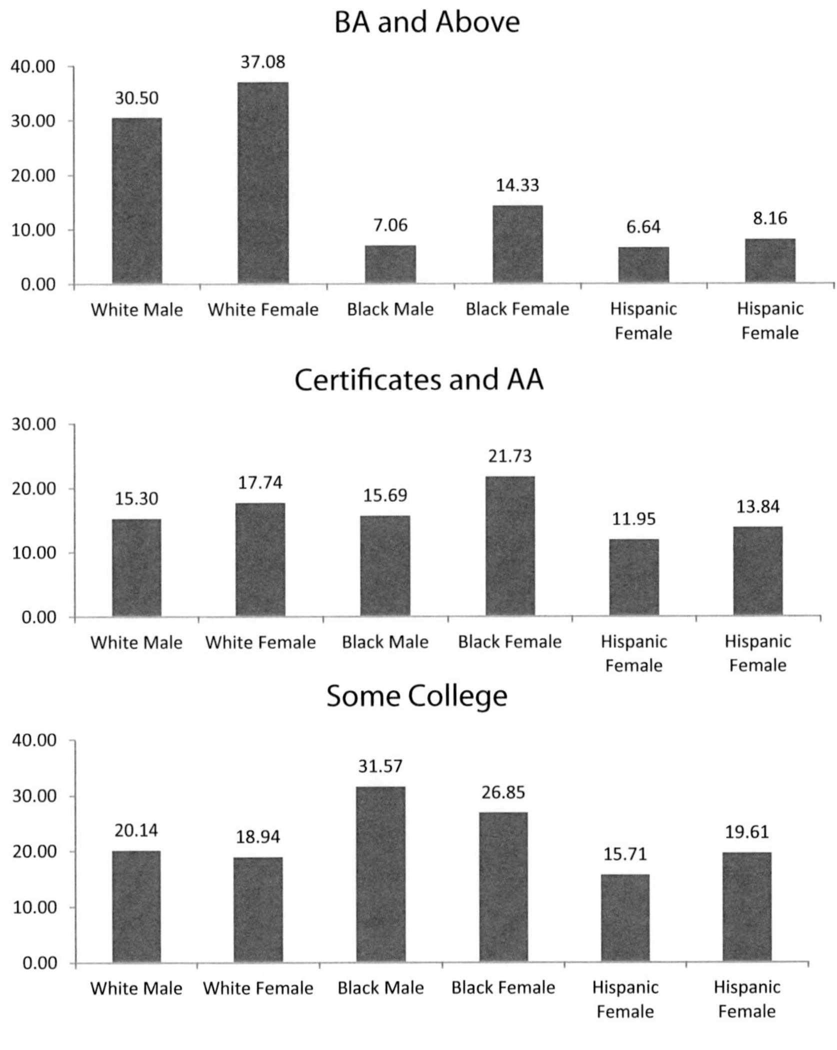

FIGURE 4-2 Educational attainment by race/gender, ages 25-29, 2010.
SOURCE: Holzer and Dunlop, 2013, based on data from the Survey of Income and Program Participation (SIPP), reprinted with permission.

Very large gaps exist in BA completion rates by race and socioeconomic position; more specifically, completion rates for whites exceed those for blacks and Hispanics by about 20-30 percentage points, while those in the bottom quartile of parental socioeconomic position have BA completion rates nearly 40 percentage points lower than those of other students (Holzer

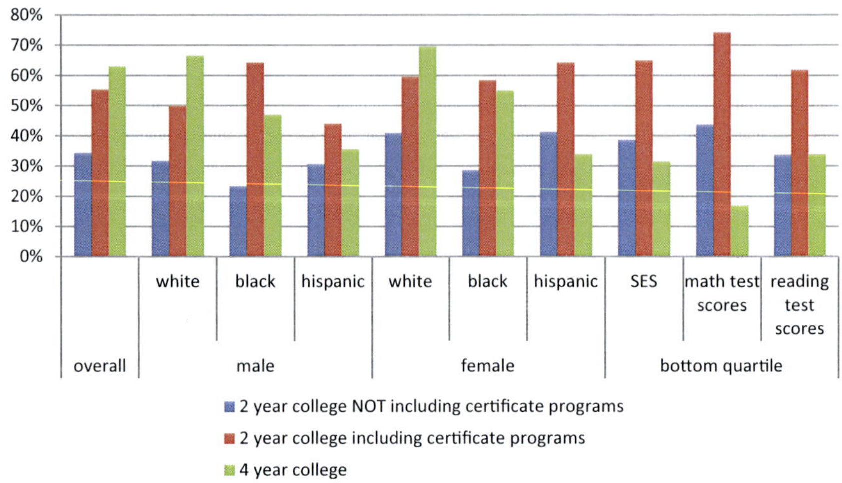

FIGURE 4-3 Completion rates: Total and by demographic/achievement groups, 2000.
NOTE: SES = socioeconomic status.
SOURCE: Holzer and Dunlop, 2013, based on data from the National Educational Longitudinal Study (NELS), 2000, reprinted with permission.

and Dunlop, 2013). Indeed, some recent evidence suggests that differences in educational attainment by socioeconomic position are widening over time (Bailey and Dynarski, 2011). Female completion rates also exceed those of males among both whites and blacks (Bailey and Dynarski, 2011). As for AA (and certificate) attainment, differences in completion by race/gender and socioeconomic position are not as large as they are among BA students, but completion rates at 2-year colleges are quite low across the board (Holzer and Dunlop, 2013). While credits attained even by those who do not finish degree programs generally have some labor market value (Kreisman et al., 2013), in most cases there remains a substantial reward for attaining a degree that the noncompleters do not receive.

What might account for the large observed differences in educational attainment and completion across race/gender and socioeconomic groups? A large body of research attributes these differences to

- cognitive skill gaps reflecting highly uneven academic preparation in the K-12 years (Bound et al., 2010; Holzer and Lerman, 2014),
- rising costs of education and liquidity constraints facing families with lower levels of household wealth (Bound et al., 2010),

- poor information about educational opportunities among lower-income or minority students (Baum and Schwartz, 2014; Hoxby and Turner, 2013), and
- family obligations and pressure to generate income by working full time (Baum and Schwartz, 2014).

It is noteworthy that completion rates vary substantially across institutions as well as demographic groups of students, and are generally higher, even adjusting for student academic preparation, at the more prestigious or elite schools. Some observers have attributed these differences to resource constraints at weaker institutions that limit their ability to provide supports, or even enough key classes to accommodate differences in student needs or schedules (Bound et al., 2010). Thus to the extent that poor information among lower-income young adults leads them to be "undermatched" to colleges and universities in terms of quality, their completion rates (and labor market opportunities thereafter) are lower as well.

Another problem that has recently grown more serious is the accumulation of student debt. The ratio of outstanding debt to income for households with educational debt rose from 0.28 in 1992 to 0.6 in 2010 (Akers and Chingos, 2014). On average, college remains a very good economic investment for those who complete their chosen degree program and gain employment soon after in their chosen fields. For these individuals, the accumulation of debt makes sense, and repayment generally is not burdensome, but for individuals who drop out of college or have difficulty obtaining a job in the current economic environment, debt repayment can be quite difficult.

Of course, the ability of young adults to enroll in college at all will depend on their rates of high school graduation (or attainment of a GED credential). Thus, although most high school dropping out occurs in the earlier teen years, it is clearly relevant to the educational outcomes considered here. Dropout rates in the United States have clearly declined in the past 10-15 years (Murnane, 2013), although they remain somewhat high in comparison with those observed in other industrialized countries, especially among minorities or disadvantaged students.[5]

Low educational attainment also is a particularly serious problem in some geographic locales, such as inner-city neighborhoods with concentrated poverty and many rural areas. Individuals from these areas who attain more education tend to relocate elsewhere and leave behind a more disadvantaged population (Domina, 2006).

Overall, the ongoing (and sometimes growing) gaps in achievement

[5] Murnane (2013) shows that the current high school dropout rate in the United States is about 16 percent, and about 22 percent among blacks and Hispanics.

and educational attainment among young adults from different family backgrounds and between whites and minorities will contribute to ongoing economic inequality in the United States and limited upward mobility for disadvantaged young adults.

Community Colleges: Multiple Roles and Challenges

Community colleges are uniquely positioned to provide both academic and vocational opportunities to young adults, especially those from disadvantaged backgrounds and/or with relatively weaker academic preparation. They can provide a gateway to more traditional higher education in 4-year schools, but also offer AA degrees or certificates (both for credit and noncredit) that have more immediate labor market value. Moreover, these schools are accessible both to young adults directly after high school graduation and to those who decide to return to school after some time away.

The success of community colleges in these different roles appears to vary substantially across institutions. Some see their traditional academic mission as primary, while others focus more on the vocational challenge. And the high rates of program noncompletion at community colleges noted above suggest that there are broad areas in which improvements are needed.

One such area is developmental (or remedial) education. Large numbers of students (perhaps more than half) enter community college academically unprepared for the rigors of postsecondary work, and they often are placed in noncredit remedial classes they must pass before they are allowed to take classes for credit (Aud et al., 2011). But evidence suggests that remedial classes may be unsuccessful in preparing many students, who instead drop out altogether in high numbers (Bettinger et al., 2013; Clotfelter et al., 2013). In some cases, there is even evidence of negative effects of remediation on educational outcomes.

Financial aid is another area in which impacts on student outcomes are not necessarily as positive as they could be. Students often face a bewildering array of federal, state, and institutional programs that provide a mix of grants, loans, and work-study. Application rules tend to be complicated, and complex interactions in eligibility often exist across the many forms of aid. And the Pell grant, the primary federal program for disadvantaged students, is simply a voucher to attend any college, accompanied by few other supports or academic conditions (Dynarski and Scott-Clayton, 2013).

More broadly, the largely unstructured and unassisted experiences of many students in community college (especially those who are disadvantaged and those who are of the first generation in their family to attend college) inhibit their ability to complete programs of study or make successful transitions to 4-year colleges or the labor market. Even the processes of choosing and registering for classes can be chaotic, with many classes not being offered in the needed time slots and much uncertainty about which classes will best lead toward degree completion (Jenkins and Cho, 2012; Rosenbaum et al., 2006; Scott-Clayton, 2011).

Furthermore, students who manage to complete a postsecondary program may not be making the optimal choice of a field of study, given that, as noted earlier, different fields are compensated very differently in the labor market. This suggests the importance of not just academic but also career guidance and information so that students can make better-informed choices. Also important are incentives for academic institutions to be responsive to the job market by expanding instructional capacity in areas of high labor market demand (in which more students might prefer to study) and by ensuring that instructors are fully up to date in their own preparation and the curricula they teach (Holzer, 2014; Jacobson and Mokher, 2009). A lack of well-defined institutional linkages or pathways between higher education and the job market appears to contribute to these difficulties.

The growth of for-profit colleges that compete with traditional community colleges further complicates this picture. Indeed, for-profit schools now receive at least a fourth of Pell grant dollars (Deming et al., 2013). Some observers have noted that the for-profits have greater incentives to be responsive to job market needs, although questions remain about the large debts accrued by students who attend these colleges, especially those who do not complete their degree program, and about quality and marketability more broadly (Deming et al., 2013).

Finally, the growth of massive open online courses (MOOCs) could dramatically change the delivery of higher education over time, in ways that cannot yet be anticipated. Their positive effects could include reductions in the costs of higher education and greater access among minorities and the poor to courses offered at elite colleges and universities. But very little is known to date about the quality of such education, and how credentials thus generated will be valued in the job market. Ongoing experimentation and innovation in this area may provide a clearer picture of the effects of MOOCs over time.

Alternative Routes: High-Quality Career and Technical Education and Work-Based Learning

The ability of students—whether disadvantaged or not—to gain academic credentials, along with work experience, that improve their employment outcomes would likely be stronger if they had the opportunity to choose high-quality career and technical education (CTE) offered in secondary schools. Formerly known as "vocational education," CTE in the United States has languished for several decades, at least in part because of opposition from minority groups and the poor (Holzer et al., 2013). Their opposition stems from the low quality of many earlier programs and the concern that students were being "tracked," often against their will, into a considerably weaker substitute for higher education. This rightfully angered the parents and representatives of minority and disadvantaged students.

However, this is not the only possibility for CTE. In many European Union countries (such as Austria, Germany, and Scandinavia), high-quality CTE enables students to graduate from secondary school and immediately have access to relatively high-paying jobs (Hoffman, 2011; Symonds et al., 2011). In the United States, a range of high-quality models being developed hold great promise for enabling students to achieve both postsecondary and labor market success, rather than one or the other. Under these models, many students would take college preparatory curricula, including rigorous math and science classes. But more of the teaching would be in the context of work- or project-based studies, in which students would gain technical and employability as well as academic skills (Holzer et al., 2013). Very importantly, students would then have a range of high-quality education models from which to choose, all of which should prepare them for both college and careers, and *no students would be tracked away from college against their will.*

Among the models that have been or are being developed for secondary schools in the United States are career academies—schools within broader schools that focus on a particular industry (such as health, information technology, or finance) (Kemple and Willner, 2008). Students take classes and attain work experience in their chosen field while also pursuing more general, college preparatory studies. Career academies clearly improve the employment outcomes of students, especially at-risk young men, for many years after without their having to sacrifice their academic work (see the section Evaluation Evidence in this chapter). Other promising CTE models include High Schools That Work, a model that embeds rigorous math and science instruction in a more vocational setting, and Linked Learning, in which career-oriented studies are provided for all students on a district-wide basis in California (Holzer et al., 2013).

During high school and beyond, career and technical education sometimes comes in the form of work-based learning, whereby students learn while engaging in paid work. The strongest such model is apprenticeship, in which students work for employers (at a somewhat reduced wage) while gaining important training and work experience. The education they receive is strongly contextualized by the work they perform, and they are often highly motivated to persist in and complete the program (because they are being paid to do so). Increasingly, apprenticeships incorporate a postsecondary program of study, usually at a community college. Research evidence (although nonexperimental) suggests strong positive impacts of these programs on subsequent earnings (Reed et al., 2012). Apprenticeships also are popular in many European Union member states, as well as with foreign-based (especially German) companies opening plants in the United States (Schneider, 2013; Schwartz, 2013).

Finally, as discussed further below, a range of "career pathways" are being developed by states around the country. These are usually programs of occupational study in high schools and colleges that combine work experience and academic learning, with students earning a series of specific education credentials along the way. To date there exists no rigorous evaluation evidence as to their impacts on earnings over time. But broadly, work-based learning models that combine strong academic learning with paid work can help young adults attain both the postsecondary education and work experience needed by so many young people today.

HEALTH AND SOCIAL CAUSES AND CONSEQUENCES

Education and Health in the Short and Long Terms

As demonstrated by the evidence reviewed thus far on the long-term economic benefits of educational attainment, the high stakes of young adulthood discussed throughout this report are clearly evident in the educational system. Those high stakes are not strictly economic, as an educational gradient is seen in many other domains of functioning. For example, persistent educational disparities in health are well documented (Baker et al., 2011; Mirowsky and Ross, 2003). In short, more-educated Americans tend to experience significantly less morbidity and fewer functional limitations than their less-educated counterparts, and they report better levels of health overall. Perhaps most strikingly, they have substantially longer life expectancy. These disparities by level of education—typified by comparisons between 4-year college graduates and those who have not entered or graduated from such colleges—tend to become more pronounced across the life course, and on a population level have become more pronounced over time. Of course, some portion of these observed effects of educational attainment on health, including mortality, simply reflects selection effects—preexisting differences in who obtains a college degree and who does not—but not all of it does. Completing higher education—and obtaining more education in general—does appear to support and enhance health (Lauderdale, 2001; Lynch, 2003).

Why might going to college and obtaining more education lead to better health across the life course? Sociologists Mirowsky and Ross (2003) offer some general explanations. First, education leads to greater job stability, higher earnings, and access to work with better benefits, all of which support health and the avoidance of health problems. Second, education cultivates the development of psychological resources, including feelings of personal control and analytical skills that enable people to better manage their health and make more informed health decisions, as well as networks of social support that protect people from health risks and stressors. Third, reflecting the first two mechanisms, education tends to facilitate healthier lifestyles, so that the behavioral profiles of more-educated individuals keep them in good health for longer periods of time. For example, college graduates are more likely to exercise and eat nutritiously, and consequently are less likely to be obese (see Yu, 2012). Similar trends extend to mental health, with lower depression and higher life satisfaction being seen among the more educated (Mirowsky and Ross, 2003). The correlation between education and health may not be completely causal, although no doubt part of it is. There are also other associations between education and long-term health. For example, those with lower educational attainment also had more adverse childhoods; this childhood experience leads to an increased stress response (allostatic load), which leads in turn to long-term health problems (Shonkoff et al., 2012).

The large literature on this subject suggests that education and health are positively related over the long run such that the more educated a young adult becomes, the healthier she or he will be in later life. Yet these long-term patterns may also subsume shorter-term risks associated with obtaining more education. In particular, attending college can be associated with poorer health behaviors relative to individuals of the same age who do not go to college. In recent years, for example, college students have used illicit drugs at slightly higher rates than their noncollege age-mates; in 2012, annual prevalence rates in these two groups were 37 percent and 35 percent, respectively, a disparity driven mainly by marijuana use but also capturing enrollment-related differences in amphetamine use (Johnston et al., 2013). This pattern does not extend to many of the more dangerous drugs, such as cocaine and heroin, nor does it apply to cigarette smoking (in 2012, 13 percent of college students were current smokers, compared with about 26 percent of noncollege young adults) (Johnston et al., 2013). Still, given the consistency of the link between educational attainment and health across the life course, these exceptions to the general rule during young adulthood are notable.

Perhaps no health risk among young adults on college campuses receives more attention than alcohol consumption. In 2012, more than two-thirds of college students (68 percent) reported drinking in the past month, compared with just over half (54 percent) of noncollege youth (Johnston et al., 2013). More troublesome is binge drinking (having five or more drinks on a single occasion in the past 2 weeks), which has for decades been consistently higher among college students than among their noncollege age-mates; in 2012, the respective rates were 37 percent and 30 percent

(Johnston et al., 2013). Drinking is widely viewed as a major part of college campus life in the United States, one that runs counter to the general pattern of higher education being conducive to health (Schulenberg and Maggs, 2002; Wechsler and Wuethrich, 2002). Evidence that the college years are a time of steady weight gain as well as a period in which many students have suicidal ideation also suggests that young adults on college campuses (and not just their peers who are not attending college) may need attention with respect to countering health risks (IOM and NRC, 2013; Nelson et al., 2007; Zagorsky and Smith, 2011).

Employment and Health in the Short and Long Terms

The employment and health outcomes of young adults are correlated, although the direction of causation is not always clear. Poor health appears clearly to generate low employment outcomes (Currie and Madrian, 1999). Whether low employment generally causes poor health, especially among young adults, is less clear. Very poor employment opportunities do appear to drive disconnected youth into crime and incarceration, as discussed below, and these outcomes are associated with poor long-term health outcomes, such as HIV infection (Johnson and Raphael, 2009). Research also has shown that sudden involuntary job loss can raise health and mortality risks, especially among older adults (Sullivan and von Wachter, 2009), although it is unclear whether this is true for more sporadic episodes of joblessness among young adults.

> "It is very important for workplaces to have opportunities for guidance, professional and personal development, whether the young adult works as cashier or a manager."

Another potential link between employment and health for young adults involves workplace safety. Young adults are a subset of the workforce with traits that create important requirements for safety, health, and well-being in the workplace. They have behavioral and cognitive attributes and less well-developed work skills, experience, and training that increase their risk for injury compared with older adults. Young adults' vulnerability to occupational injury and illness also may result from their overestimation of their skill level; greater risk taking in their desire to meet their employer's expectations; and greater tendencies to be distracted as a result of performing multiple activities, such as texting and driving motor vehicles, simultaneously. Shorter employment histories and fewer cumulative encounters with workplace safety training also tend to make young adults less familiar with health and safety protections, such as state or federal occupational safety and health standards, hazard or injury reporting systems, and rights under workers' compensation statutes in the event of on-the-job injury (CDC, 2013).

Data on nonfatal occupational injuries are provided by the U.S. Bureau of Labor Statistics for young adults according to the age groups 16-19, 20-24, and 25-34. It is generally believed that these data understate the actual incidence of work-related injuries among young adults because of their reticence to report such injuries to their employer or their lack of awareness of reporting systems. Compared with older workers, young adult workers have higher nonfatal injury rates in the private sector but lower injury rates in the public sector, where work hazards differ (BLS, 2013). In 2012, nonfatal work injuries involving days away from work in private industry were 111 per 10,000 full-time workers for those aged 16-19, 109 per 10,000 full-time workers for those aged 20-24, and 100 per 10,000 full-time workers for those aged 25-34, compared with 102 per 10,000 full-time workers for all workers (BLS, 2013). Industries contributing the most to work injuries among young adults are the leisure and hospitality industry, the food and beverage industry, grocery stores, and the motor vehicle and parts industry. The major type of injury among young adult workers is musculoskeletal, particularly strains and sprains of tendons and ligaments (BLS, 2013). Cuts, lacerations, and burns are common injury types in the food preparation and restaurant industries. Data on injuries requiring emergency department (ED) visits, drawn from a surveillance sample of hospitals, have shown that work-related injuries are seen twice as often among workers under age 25 as among workers above this age, and that the leisure, hospitality, and retail industries account for slightly more than three-quarters of ED visits by young adult workers (CDC, 2013).

Compared with older workers, young adults have lower overall rates of fatal work injuries. Fatality rates for occupational injuries rise progressively from age 20 onward. In 2012, rates of fatal injuries were below 3.0 per 100,000 full-time equivalent workers among workers less than age 34 and above that level for all older age groups. Rates of fatal work injuries are higher for those aged 18-19 than for those aged 20-24 and 25-34, at 2.9, 2.4, and 2.4, respectively, per 100,000 full-time equivalent workers (BLS, 2014).

Fatal occupational injuries among young adults share some important epidemiological characteristics with those among older adults. Men are overwhelmingly affected compared with women, and the same events or exposures cause fatal work injuries in both young and older adults. Most work-related fatal injuries result from transportation collisions in mining, agriculture, and waste management, often with the young adult as driver; gun shootings and other assaults; being struck by objects or equipment; and falls from heights (BLS, 2014). The service and construction industries account for the largest *number* of fatal injuries to young adults, but mining and agriculture have the highest *rates* of such injuries (BLS, 2014).

Disconnected Youth and Youth with Disabilities and Chronic Health Conditions

Given the important linkages among education, employment, and health and safety outcomes for young adults, the very weak education and employment outcomes of two groups raise particular concern: youth who are disconnected and those who have disabilities and chronic health conditions.

Disconnected Youth

As noted earlier, young adults who are out of school and out of work (or idle) for significant periods of time are often called *disconnected youth*.[6] While disconnection can occur at any level of education, it is for those with no postsecondary credential that concern is highest.

The numbers of disconnected youth have almost certainly grown considerably since the beginning of the Great Recession. One very credible recent estimate puts the number at 6.7 million, which constitutes about 17 percent of the population aged 16-24 (Belfield and Levin, 2012). The rates are highest among African Americans and those aged 20-24, almost all of whom have left high school. About half of these youth, and no doubt even more among those who are high school dropouts rather than graduates, appear to be "chronically" disconnected and perhaps have never entered the formal labor market.

Many of these youth have low education (often no high school diploma) and poor basic skills. Disconnected youth also are likely to be scarred by their lack of work experience when they do try to enter the job market, in the form of either low employment rates or low wages (Belfield and Levin, 2012). Young women who are disconnected are frequently single mothers (and often became mothers as teens), while disconnected young men tend to be noncustodial fathers in one or more families.[7] Disconnected young men, especially African Americans, also tend to have disproportionately high rates of incarceration and ex-offender status (Pager, 2003).

The combination of having a criminal record and a child support or-

[6] They are also sometimes referred to as *opportunity* youth (see Chapter 1).

[7] Despite the high correlations between teen motherhood (or unwed motherhood more generally) and poor education and employment outcomes, researchers continue to debate the extent to which the former causes the latter. See Hill et al. (2009), Kearney and Levine (2014), and Thomas (2012). The difficult experiences of young noncustodial fathers, especially in multiple families, are documented by Edin and Nelson (2013).

der can substantially reduce future employment prospects for these young men, even when they age out of crime. Employers tend to avoid hiring those with a criminal record (except in economic sectors where there is little contact with customers, children and the elderly, or cash), while those in arrears on their child support payments face high taxes in the form of wage garnishing and thus reduced incentives to work (Edelman et al., 2006; Holzer et al., 2004; Pager, 2003).

> "I was released from the juvenile justice system in June 2012 and I applied to all these large stores, such as Sears and Home Depot, which you think would hire for the manpower. But I was denied. Most often when I got to the question of the criminal conviction, that's what automatically changed the whole conversation."

Any approach designed to help this population therefore requires policies that address a range of difficult personal circumstances and barriers, including low levels of education, basic skills, and work experience, along with the stigma and disincentives associated with a criminal record and child support debt.

Youth with Disabilities and Chronic Health Conditions

High school students receiving special education services (those identified as having a disability that interferes with their educational performance) do not do as well in school as the general population of high school students and are less likely to complete high school. Most youth with disabilities (72 percent) graduate from or complete certification for secondary school, but completion rates vary greatly with the type of disability (U.S. Department of Education, 2005). The highest rates of completion are among those with visual (95 percent) and hearing (90 percent) impairments, while the lowest rates are among those with emotional disturbance (56 percent). On average, students with disabilities who receive grades earn a lower grade point average and have much higher course failure rates than the general population of students (Newman et al., 2011a). The rate of ever failing a course in high school is highest among those with emotional disturbance (77 percent) and lowest among those with autism (27 percent). As in the general population, students with disabilities from households with lower incomes or of minority race have lower secondary school academic performance and attainment.

One study found that at ages 21-25, 60 percent of former special education students had had some postsecondary education, compared with 67 percent of their age-mates in the general population (Newman et al.,

2011b). Postsecondary school enrollment was highest among those with visual (71 percent) or hearing (75 percent) impairments and lowest among those with an intellectual disability (29 percent) (Newman et al., 2011b). Among those enrolling in postsecondary schooling, former special education students are twice as likely to enroll in 2-year colleges and almost twice as likely to complete that education compared with those in the general population. However, they are only half as likely to enroll in 4-year colleges and much less likely to complete 4-year college (34 percent versus 51 percent) compared with the general population (Newman et al., 2011b). Race or ethnicity and household income are not associated with different rates of postsecondary school enrollment or completion among former special education students. These findings highlight the central role of 2-year colleges for vulnerable young adults.

Not all students with disabilities or chronic health conditions are served in special education. Fewer than 10 percent of students with mental illness, for example, are enrolled in special education (Forness et al., 2012). Studies that reflect the broad spectrum of youth with mental illness confirm their low high school performance and completion rates (Davis and Vander Stoep, 1997). Epidemiological work suggests that these low rates of high school performance and attainment are due largely to the direct impact of childhood adversity and the presence of conduct and attention-deficit disorders (Breslau et al., 2011). Although colleges are seeing increased rates of students with mental health conditions on campus (Eisenberg et al., 2007), those with a mental illness that predates college entry are less likely to finish college than those without such a condition (Bachrach and Read, 2012; Kessler et al., 1995). Development of a mental health condition while in college also compromises school functioning and completion (Bachrach and Read, 2012). Other mental health issues, such as suicidal ideation or attempts, also are seen among college students. Survey results show that 1 in 10 college students contemplated suicide during the previous year, and 1-2 percent made an attempt (Brener et al., 1999; Kisch et al., 2005). One of the challenges faced by college students with mental illness is the particular social stigma of these conditions, which plays a role in reducing their willingness to request educational accommodations (Salzer et al., 2008) and to seek help for their condition (Eisenberg et al., 2007).

> "My college work suffered due to mental health issues. My university didn't understand what I was going through. I had to pay back $10,000 of scholarship money. They weren't recognizing the mental health issue as an issue."

Ongoing substance use in high school also contributes to educational difficulties—including dropping out of college—during the transition to adulthood (e.g., Patrick et al., 2013). Tobacco use during high school has stronger effects than alcohol and illegal drug use on school struggles (Breslau et al., 2011).

Employment rates at ages 21-25 are comparable among former special education students and their age-mates in the general population (Newman et al., 2011b). However, employment rates among those with learning disabilities or speech/language disabilities are more than 20 points higher than among those with deafness/blindness, orthopedic impairments, autism, multiple disabilities, or mental retardation. Those in the latter disability categories also are more likely to work part time than those in the former categories. It is notable that those with hearing impairments are among former special education students with the highest educational attainment, yet the lowest employment rates. Hourly wages among those who are employed are lower among former special education students than among their age-mates in the general population (Newman et al., 2011b). These findings indicate that for many students, special education services help them achieve employment on par with their same-age peers in the general population. However, numerous subgroups experience employment and income disparities.

Twelve percent of individuals under age 65 receiving Supplemental Security Income (SSI) are young adults aged 18-25 (Social Security Administration, 2012). Receiving these benefits is a strong deterrent to work (e.g., Bond et al., 2007; Burns et al., 2007; Frey et al., 2011). Further, despite some encouraging findings among former special education students described above, studies of employment among young adults with disabilities reveal that many challenges remain for this population. Major barriers to accessing good and satisfying employment include (1) a lack of work experience and restricted aspirations, (2) sporadic patterns of early employment, (3) limited access to postsecondary education and training, and (4) discrimination and prejudice (Lindstrom et al., 2013).

EDUCATION AND EMPLOYMENT POLICY FOR YOUNG ADULTS

The United States currently has a wide array of policies designed to support higher education and workforce development services, for both young and older adults, at the federal, state, and local levels, as well as laws protecting those with disabilities. We first describe the current policy landscape, and then review what can be learned from the research and evaluation literature about the effectiveness of these policies and related programs.

Workforce Programs

The greatest single source of funding for workforce development programs in the United States is the Workforce Innovation and Opportunity Act (WIOA), which succeeded earlier programs and is administered by the U.S. Department of Labor.[8] Title I of WIOA distributes three primary funding streams—for adults, dislocated workers, and youth (up to age 21)—that are allocated by state and local workforce boards. It also funds the Job Corps, one of the original "War on Poverty" programs, which provides job training for youth in residential settings nationwide. Young adults can potentially participate in programs funded by any of these streams, depending on their exact ages and circumstances.

Other titles of WIOA fund adult basic education, the labor market information and job search assistance provided at the roughly 3,000 American Job Centers around the country (formerly known as "One Stop" offices), and other services and access to income support through unemployment insurance that are available at these centers. The workforce services provided to adults and youth at these centers include basic job matching and counseling or testing, with limited availability of vouchers for training that is mainly short term (Besharov and Cottingham, 2011).

It appears that authorized spending on WIOA will be about $6 billion (CBO, 2014), although the actual appropriated amount may be different. This funding has declined dramatically over time in real terms, especially relative to the size of the U.S. workforce or the economy. But workforce funds also are provided by the U.S. Departments of Education, Health and Human Services, and Agriculture through such programs as Vocational Rehabilitation, Temporary Assistance for Needy Families, the Supplemental Nutrition Assistance Program, and a variety of block grant programs.

According to Government Accountability Office estimates (GAO, 2011), 47 such federal workforce programs were disbursing some $18 billion in funding as of 2010, although most of these programs are quite limited in size. Expenditures by these programs total 0.1 percent of national gross domestic product, which is a relatively small sum compared with similar expenditures in other industrial countries. Still, there is likely some scope for savings through consolidation and more effective operation of some of these programs.

At the state and local levels, workforce training and services are administered through WIOA funding and other sources. In recent years, most states have begun to design programs that link economic and workforce development to train workers for the states' high-growth and high-wage

[8] Earlier versions of this legislation included the Comprehensive Employment and Training Act, the Job Training Partnership Act, and the Workforce Investment Act.

industries, although data indicating just how far these programs have come are sparse (Choitz and Harmon, 2014). "Sectoral" efforts, in which providers of training work directly in partnership with employers or industry associations to train workers for existing jobs in high-growth or high-wage industries are beginning to play major roles, as are the "career pathway" models alluded to earlier (Choitz and Harmon, 2014; National Governors Association Center of Best Practices, 2012). Many localities also have developed such partnerships, with some scale (National Fund for Workforce Solutions, 2014).

Finally, a wide range of small programs and pilots have been developed over the years, often with a mix of public and foundation funding, to test a variety of approaches to workforce development. The many small grant programs administered in the past decade by the Bush and Obama administrations have helped support this trend.[9]

Disability Law and Programs

Two federal laws—the Americans with Disabilities Act (ADA)[10] and the Rehabilitation Act of 1973[11]—and their amendments are designed to help individuals with disabilities participate fully in society, including employment and education. Both provide protection from disability-based discrimination and mandate that employers offer reasonable accommodations for employees or applicants with disabilities.

The ADA, a civil rights law, provides protection against discrimination in private, state, and local government employment. None of its elements or amendments are specific to young adults. It provides protections primarily when individuals seek them, such as in requesting reasonable accommodations in the workplace. Thus, for young adults to receive many of the ADA's protections, they must know about the law and pursue their rights.

The protections under the Rehabilitation Act prohibit discrimination in federal agencies, federal employment, the employment of federal contractors, and programs receiving federal financial assistance. The Rehabilitation Act currently is contained within the WIOA, and funds services and programs that include state vocational rehabilitation services, supported employment, independent living, and programs in training and research. Several sections of the current Rehabilitation Act mandate that federal and

---

[9] These competitive grant programs from the U.S. Department of Labor include the High Growth Job Training Initiative, the Workforce Innovation in Regional Economic Development grants, the Trade Adjustment Assistance Community College and Career Training grants, and the Workforce Innovation Funds.

[10] Americans with Disabilities Act of 1990, Public Law 101-336, 101st Cong. (July 26, 1990).

[11] Rehabilitation Act of 1973, Public Law 93-112, 93rd Cong. (September 26, 1973).

state vocational rehabilitation programs engage in activities that support the transition from school to work for individuals with disabilities. These mandates are designed to prevent interruptions in services after individuals leave secondary school, to ensure that secondary students covered by either the Individuals with Disabilities Education Act or the ADA are provided transition services, and that vocational rehabilitation agencies and institutions of higher education have interagency agreements (or other such mechanisms) outlining various aspects of coordination. The services provided by state vocational rehabilitation agencies to those aged 16-24 under these mandates are called transition-age youth services. About 8 percent of transition-age youth with disabilities apply for state vocational rehabilitation services, and 56 percent of them eventually receive those services (Honeycutt et al., 2013). Little research has examined the impact of state vocational rehabilitation transition services (Davis et al., 2013; Honeycutt et al., 2013).

Higher Education

Most public expenditures on higher education—which nationally total more than $160 billion per year—occur at the state level in the form of aid to state colleges and universities as well as community colleges that helps keep tuition well below cost (Barrow et al., 2013). Many analyses of these expenditures suggest that these programs are relatively regressive, with the largest benefits being gained by higher-income families that send their children primarily to the flagship schools in state college and university systems (Barrow et al., 2013; Hansen and Weisbrod, 1969; Johnson, 2005).

Various federal programs also make important contributions to higher education, both public and private. For example, the Pell grant program (part of the Higher Education Act) finances tuition payments for low-income youth and adults aimed at breaking the intergenerational cycle of poverty and socioeconomic disadvantage (reflecting the generational theme of this report). This program has expanded dramatically in recent years, and its expenditures now total roughly $35 billion (Crandall-Hollick, 2012; Dynarski and Scott-Clayton, 2013). Since many students go to college—especially 2-year and for-profit institutions—to obtain a vocational degree or certificate, the Pell grant has effectively become the largest financer of vocational training in the United States. The federal government also operates direct loan and work-study programs, as well as a range of federal tax credits for tuition payments (Dynarski and Scott-Clayton, 2013).

Although much vocational education occurs in colleges and is funded by U.S. Department of Education programs, a wide gulf remains between these colleges and the job centers funded by the U.S. Department of Labor through the WIOA that provide workforce services in many localities. This gulf appears to be beginning to break down, however, with an increasing number of job centers being located on community college campuses and with representatives of colleges sitting on local workforce boards. But a good deal more needs to be done in this regard.

The transition from secondary to postsecondary education involves vast changes in disability policy and practice as students move from a system of entitlement (Individuals with Disabilities Education Act) to one of eligibility (GAO, 2009). Section 504 of the Rehabilitation Act, the ADA, and their amendments provide guidelines regarding students with disabilities in colleges, but the main focus is on providing equal access and preventing discrimination rather than promoting student success in college (GAO, 2009). According to the ADA, any college that receives federal funding must provide equal access through the use of reasonable accommodations and auxiliary aids (e.g., sign language interpreters). One of the greatest changes from high school to college is that school districts are obligated to identify and serve students with disabilities in high school, whereas colleges have reduced obligations to provide the array of services and supports required of high schools for their students with disabilities. Essentially, responsibility shifts from the school to the student; students themselves must disclose their disability to access accommodations in college. The result is practices that vary greatly across colleges (Cory, 2011; GAO, 2009) and may impose a greater burden on those with stigmatized disabling conditions (e.g., Yang et al., 2013).

Finally, it is important to mention the role of CTE, discussed earlier, much of which begins in secondary school but continues into higher education at the 2-year college level. The Carl D. Perkins Act provides roughly $1 billion per year to fund CTE programs at the secondary and postsecondary levels. This funding constitutes less than 10 percent of public funds expended on CTE (Holzer et al., 2013). In recent years, however, the Perkins Act has required states to develop a range of "career clusters" and "programs of study" (also known as the aforementioned "career pathways") that often begin in high school or community college and continue thereafter through a series of well-defined steps by which students gain educational credentials and work experience on their way toward specific well-paying careers. These programs are increasingly playing a role in state-level economic and workforce development efforts (Holzer et al., 2013).

Evaluation Evidence

A large literature evaluating the impacts of job training programs on worker outcomes has been generated over the past few decades. A smaller literature on the impacts of programs in higher education is developing as well (Heckman et al., 1999; Holzer, 2009, 2013; LaLonde, 1996).

The results of the literature on job training can be summarized as follows:

- Training for adults through the WIA or its predecessor (the Job Training Partnership Act of 1982) has had modest positive impacts on the future earnings of disadvantaged adults (including young adults).
- The best sectoral programs—such as Per Scholas and the Wisconsin Regional Training Partnership for adults or Year Up for youth (Maguire et al., 2010; Roder and Elliott, 2011)—as well as apprenticeships can have large positive impacts on the earnings of disadvantaged adults and youth, although these impacts are limited to individuals with fairly strong basic skills (and how long they persist is unknown, especially if the trained workers ultimately switch jobs and industries).
- It is difficult to find programs that have persistent positive impacts on the education or earnings of youth and young adults, especially teens and those in their early 20s, although there is evidence of shorter-term impacts. For instance, the positive impacts of the Job Corps fade after a few years, but more for teens than for young adults (Bloom, 2010; LaLonde, 1996; Schochet et al., 2008). Some recent summer employment programs for those enrolled in school also show promising impacts (Schwartz et al., 2014).
- It is also quite difficult to find training programs that raise the earnings of young or older adults who are "difficult to employ" and have a range of barriers to employment (Bloom and Butler, 2007).
- Limited research supports current practices designed to assist high school students with disabilities in transitioning to postsecondary education or employment. No practices with strong evidence of efficacy have emerged in this age group.

In terms of higher education, it is known that on average, completing a BA or AA degree has strong positive earnings impacts for disadvantaged young adults, and even certificate programs have some modest positive effects, especially in particular fields (Carnevale et al., 2010; Holzer and Dunlop, 2013). But noncompletion rates are extremely high for low-income students at 4-year schools and for almost all students at 2-year schools, as noted above. Indeed, there is even some question as to whether Pell grants actually increase college attainment for poor young adults at all, because so few recipients tend to finish the courses of study they be-

> "Sometimes work gets in the way of finishing my degree and sometimes my degree gets in the way of finishing my work. One thing I found useful was having a job that tied into my degree."

gin (Long, 2013). As observed earlier, many of these students must complete developmental (or remedial) education classes to make up for deficiencies in their earlier academic preparation before they can take courses for credit in their chosen field, and dropouts rates from these remedial programs are extremely high.

Still, a growing evaluation literature is beginning to generate more evidence on programs and practices that improve completion rates for young adults in high school as well as college. These studies have yielded the following findings:

- Among other "whole school" reforms, success in high school can be enhanced by allowing students to choose among smaller high schools with clear themes.
- Preparation for GED tests (which are themselves becoming more rigorous) for young adults is best offered in highly structured environments or combined with information of interest, such as on labor markets in sectors with high employment growth.
- Developmental programs are more successful when they are accelerated or when they integrate remediation into academic or applied vocational teaching.
- Younger students are more successful at completing full-time programs with a range of supports than part-time programs.
- Providing individual-specific and straightforward information about selective colleges and financial aid prospects to high-achieving high school students from low-income families can greatly improve the quality of the colleges they attend and thus their completion rates.
- Learning communities, mandatory participation in certain counseling activities, coaching, and financial aid conditioned at least partly on student performance can all have positive impacts on completion rates among disadvantaged young adults.
- Programs to "reengage" disconnected youth in school have a mixed track record and are very challenging, although a few (like the National Guard ChalleNGe program) have clearly been successful.[12]

---

[12] Programs that have been rigorously evaluated and have led to these inferences include Small Schools of Choice in New York City and the Talent Development model at the high school level; and the National Guard ChalleNGe program, GED Bridge at LaGuardia Com-

A range of public programs are currently using rigorous evaluation methods to extend the base of knowledge on what is cost-effective in this realm. Various experimental efforts also have been funded by private foundations, although these efforts are more sporadic and include limited formal evaluation.[13] In addition, while rigorous evidence on how to reconnect young adults who have "disconnected" remains thin, at least a few programs (such as Roca and the Crittenden Women's Union in Boston and the Gateways to College program in Portland, Oregon, and other sites) have shown promising outcomes and need rigorous evaluation. "Two-generation" models, aimed at improving both the employment and parenting skills of young adults while providing early education to their young children, are becoming more popular as well and require further study.[14] These models are discussed further in Chapter 3.

High-quality career and technical programs, such as the career academies in high school discussed above and later efforts for young adults, can have positive impacts on employment and earnings prospects (Kemple and Willner, 2008). Some support is growing for the notion that math and science can be taught successfully in applied project-based contexts. And apprenticeships and other forms of work-based learning, also discussed earlier, appear to have positive impacts on earnings as well (Reed et al., 2012).

There currently are no large-scale approaches with the demonstrated capacity to improve the educational and vocational outcomes of young adults with disabilities. Only two pilot programs to this end have been funded (the Youth Transition Demonstration [Social Security Administration, 2014] and the Promoting Readiness of Minors in Supplemental Security Income [PROMISE] program of the Social Security Administration and the U.S. Department of Education [U.S. Department of Education, 2013, 2014]). Both programs focus on youth receiving SSI, which is a subset of youth under age 18 with disabilities. The Transition Youth Demonstration program, which targeted youth aged 14-25, did not yield models with

munity College, I-BEST in Washington State, and Accelerated Studies to Associate Programs at the City University of New York at the college level. See Bloom and Unterman (2012); Brock (2010); Kemple et al. (2005); Martin and Broadus (2013); Millenky et al. (2011); Scrivener and Weiss (2013); and Zeidenberg et al. (2010).

[13] Efforts to systematically evaluate the impacts of educational programs include Innovation Strategies for Increasing Self-Sufficiency at the U.S. Department of Health and Human Services and the Center for Economic Opportunity in New York City.

[14] These programs often address the difficulties experienced by poor parents with "executive functioning"—in other words, planning ahead, making sensible choices, showing self-restraint, and staying focused. Researchers increasingly believe that parents with executive functioning difficulties create highly stressful environments for their children, which then impedes the children's cognitive and noncognitive skill development. See, for example, Chase-Lansdale and Brooks-Gunn (2014).

positive outcomes that could be scaled up to the state level. The PROMISE grants, initiated in 2013, target youth aged 14-16 who receive SSI. The grants will test five states' and one state consortium's efforts to prevent SSI dependence by improving employment outcomes through the provision of services and improved coordination of services designed to support school success and career launches. Each state's approach will share broad guidelines for service coordination, and possibly some important policy waivers, but no single approach is used across the different sites, and none of the approaches have been rigorously tested.

Some innovative policies and programs in Europe use approaches that have not been tried in the United States (Moreno et al., 2014). These include national youth employment strategies that benefit youth both with and without disabilities and balance youth preparation and employer incentives (Norway); youth-specific programs that partner private enterprise with vocational rehabilitation services that provide the wages and training for the youth (Germany); and disability benefit programs specifically for young adults, with associated vocational services (Norway and Sweden). These approaches have not been evaluated, but offer suggestive directions for innovation.

Overall, there is some evidence on successful workforce programs for adults and youth with relatively strong basic skills, and limited evidence on programs designed to improve success rates for disadvantaged students who enroll in college. Integrating useful labor market information or training into developmental efforts appears promising. But the ability to replicate and scale up the best programs and to identify successful approaches for those with greater skill deficiencies or disabilities remains limited.

CONCLUSIONS AND RECOMMENDATIONS

The transition to adulthood is a critical time during which individuals need to accomplish a number of important tasks, including the completion of their education and the beginning of their career. In recent years, however, young adults in the United States have experienced unusual difficulty obtaining higher education credentials and early work experience. To improve opportunities for young adults, and especially to provide pathways for upward mobility for those from disadvantaged backgrounds, it will be necessary to raise success rates in education and the workforce for a wide range of young Americans. Doing so will also improve young Americans' health and social well-being.

To achieve greater opportunity and success will require accomplishing two major goals: (1) raising completion rates in high school and among those who enroll in postsecondary institutions, and (2) ensuring that the skills and credentials they attain are those the labor market actually rewards. Accomplishing these goals will in turn require better integrating institutions of secondary and higher education with workforce agencies and ensuring that both are more responsive to labor market needs than is the case today. Instead of siloed agencies in each realm, the two need to work together more effectively to prepare young Americans for available and well-paying jobs (Holzer, 2011).

Interventions with positive impacts on completion rates and on the alignment of education and employment have been developed and rigorously evaluated, as discussed in the previous section. However, efforts to replicate and scale up these programs need to be undertaken. Accordingly, we make the following policy recommendations.

Recommendation 4-1: State governments, with support from the U.S. Department of Education, should experiment with and evaluate a range of interventions designed to improve graduation rates at high schools and colleges, as well as the rates at which high school dropouts receive their General Educational Development (GED) credential and enroll in college or job training. These experiments should be primarily attempts to scale up interventions that have already been rigorously evaluated and generated positive impacts, such as (1) GED preparation or accelerated developmental education programs in college that integrate training (or at least labor market information) with remediation, (2) financial assistance that is more closely tied to individual performance as well as family income, (3) the provision of more information about college quality to high school students, and (4) mandated academic and career counseling for college students.

To encourage experimentation and evaluation of these interventions, the committee recommends the following specific actions:

- The U.S. Department of Education should continue to provide competitive grants for states that implement such interventions state- or county-wide and rigorously evaluate them, as it has done recently through its High School Graduation Initiative.
- The U.S. Department of Education should provide technical assistance for any states that undertake such interventions.
- State governments should encourage local school systems and the 2- and 4-year colleges in their state to implement such interventions, including by providing resources and assistance, and should rigorously evaluate them.
- State and local school systems should particularly experiment with and evaluate programs designed to reduce the enormous dispari-

ties in high school and college completion that now exist by race, family income, and geographic location (urban versus rural).

- State governments should promote the adoption by colleges of health and social supports that appear to encourage academic success among young adult enrollees.

Recommendation 4-2: State governments, with support from the U.S. Departments of Education and Labor, should implement and evaluate education and workforce development approaches that are more closely tied to high-demand economic sectors. These approaches should include sectoral models and partnerships (e.g., among employers, community colleges, and intermediaries), career pathways, high-quality career and technical education in high school, apprenticeships, and other forms of work-based learning.

To facilitate the implementation of these education and workforce development approaches, the committee recommends the following specific actions:

- The U.S. Departments of Education and Labor should provide competitive grants—perhaps modeled on the Race to the Top program for K-12 education, which had large impacts on state policy and practice—for states that implement such interventions at a medium or large scale and rigorously evaluate them.
- The U.S. Departments of Education and Labor should provide technical assistance for any states that undertake such interventions.
- State governments should encourage local colleges and workforce boards to implement such interventions, including by providing resources and assistance, and should rigorously evaluate them.

Because public resources can be expected to be highly limited in future years, it is necessary to make better use of the public resources being spent today—which include at least $160 billion for higher education (Barrow et al., 2013). Although a much smaller amount is spent on workforce development, even here there is room for improvement: the 47 different federal programs in this area no doubt could benefit from some consolidation, as well as from review of which programs are cost-effective and which are not.

To improve both the education and employment outcomes of young adults and the efficiency of resources spent on higher education and workforce development will require improving both the *information* available to students and workers and the *incentives* for education institutions to improve the outcomes of their students, as discussed in the section on community colleges above. Students and workers need better information about programs of study in different institutions, about completion rates (among students like themselves), and about labor market rewards so they can make better-informed choices regarding where and what to study. Students need not only access to more data, which are potentially available in administrative records at the state level, but also more and better career counseling from well-trained providers, perhaps in newly improved American Job Centers, that should be much more accessible to college students. Institutions also need to be held more accountable for the outcomes they generate in terms of degree completion and earnings of their graduates. Instead of receiving flat subsidies from their states regardless of whether students succeed along these dimensions, some part of these subsidies should be based on the success of the institutions' students. A number of states around the country are beginning to implement performance-based subsidies for higher education, although we believe more needs to be done to encourage this process. Careful design of these incentives is important so as not to generate perverse incentives for colleges to be more selective in admissions (e.g., by excluding more disadvantaged students) or lower their academic standards in high-demand fields. Accordingly, we make the following policy recommendation.

Recommendation 4-3: State governments should experiment with and evaluate providing performance-based subsidies to their public colleges and universities, with performance being measured by credits earned, time to degree, and graduation rates. Weight also should be given to the subsequent labor market employment and earnings of graduates. States should ensure as well that college students have access to up-to-date labor market information and career counseling based on that information.

To facilitate state governments' implementation of these education and workforce development incentives, the committee recommends the following specific actions:

- The U.S. Departments of Education and Labor should provide competitive grants for states' use of performance-based subsidies for public colleges and universities. These grants should be targeted at states that implement such incentives state-wide and rigorously evaluate them.
- The U.S. Departments of Education and Labor should provide technical assistance for any states that undertake such incentives.
- States should give substantial weight to performance measures for specifically disadvantaged populations to help ensure that colleges meet performance requirements by applying improved practices to

populations similar to those they have been serving, rather than by raising admission requirements to exclude more-disadvantaged students.

Implementing the above recommendations will be even more challenging as the labor market continually evolves in the 21st century and requires ever-higher levels of skills (NRC, 2012). One cannot necessarily extrapolate from recent trends in labor demand and supply to predict just what skills will be needed.[15] Many young Americans will likely need to engage in lifelong learning to ensure that their skills remain competitive and they are able to secure new jobs and careers, as many of those gained in the past will likely become obsolete.

Key Areas for Research

Given existing knowledge gaps, research is needed in two overarching areas to help improve young adults' education and employment outcomes:

- **How to improve success rates in higher education and the labor market for young people at all levels of skill and success.** In considering policies to improve success rates in higher education and the labor market, it is important to make improved opportunities available to young people at all levels of skill and success, including those who are currently disconnected from school and work and those currently or formerly incarcerated. High-quality options for serving these populations and preventing more students from dropping out and disconnecting need to be expanded. However, knowledge of what works cost-effectively for the most difficult-to-serve populations who are already disconnected is quite limited.[16] Accordingly, besides better policies and better data from the states, as recommended above, it will be necessary to engage in an ongoing process of experimentation with new approaches in this area and to undertake a robust research and evaluation agenda to identify what works. For example, research is needed on the efficacy of a variety of new models of higher education made possible by the Internet, such as distance learning and MOOCs, as well as new

[15] Brynjolffson and McAfee (2014) and Cowen (2013) suggest that dramatic labor market changes and growing turbulence will occur in the coming decades as a result of technological change, although Levy and Murnane (2013) predict a continuation of recent trends, with growing opportunities for those with complex analytical and communication skills and declining opportunities for those whose work is more routine.

[16] The newly announced federal government initiative My Brother's Keeper should provide some opportunity to gain this knowledge.

modes of job search and work for youth that rely more heavily on social media. Also important is to continue to monitor and evaluate trends in for-profit colleges and universities, and consider whether any further regulations are needed in this area. Needed as well is a better understanding of the long-term life trajectories of those who fail to succeed in education and employment and thus have difficulty making the transitions that are so crucial for young adults.

- **How to improve success rates in higher education and the labor market for young adults with disabilities.** An important concern is improving opportunities for young adults with disabilities and ensuring that policies and programs target their specific challenges. As described above, research on practices designed to assist high school students with disabilities in transitioning to postsecondary education or employment is limited. Two lines of research would be valuable. First, it would potentially be fruitful to test the extent to which young adults with disabilities are assisted by programs and policies that have shown positive outcomes in the general population, such as those mentioned in Recommendation 4-1 and described in greater detail above. Second, because young adults with disabilities likely will not be fully served by programs for the general population, new or modified programs for these young adults will need to be developed and rigorously evaluated. The programs described earlier that showed promise in Europe may serve as a basis for innovation. Once interventions with positive outcomes have been identified, they will need to be scaled up through mechanisms such as those described in Recommendations 4-1 and 4-2.

REFERENCES

Akers, B., and M. M. Chingos. 2014. *Is a student loan crisis on the horizon?* Washington, DC: The Brookings Institute.

Aud, S., W. Hussar, G. Kena, K. Bianco, L. Frohlich, J. Kemp, and K. Tahan. 2011. *The condition of education 2011.* NCES 2011-033. U.S. Department of Education, National Center for Education Statistics. Washington, DC: U.S. Government Printing Office.

Autor, D. 2010. *The polarization of job opportunities in the U.S. labor market: Implications for employment and earnings.* Washington, DC: Center for American Progress and The Hamilton Project.

Autor, D. H., L. F. Katz, and M. S. Kearney. 2008. Trends in U.S. wage inequality: Revising the revisionists. *Review of Economics and Statistics* 90(2):300-323.

Bachrach, R. L., and J. P. Read. 2012. The role of posttraumatic stress and problem alcohol involvement in university academic performance. *Journal of Clinical Psychology* 68(7):843-859.

Bailey, M., and S. Dynarski. 2011. Inequality in postsecondary education. In *Whither opportunity:? Rising inequality, schools, and children's life chances*, edited by G. J. Duncan and R. Murane. New York: Russell Sage Foundation. Pp. 117-132.

Baker, D. P., J. Leon, E. G. S. Greenaway, J. Collins, and M. Movit. 2011. The education effect on population health: A reassessment. *Population and Development Review* 37(2):307-332.

Ball, L., B. DeLong, and L. Summers. 2014. *Fiscal policy and full employment.* Washington, DC: Center on Budget and Policy Priorities.

Barrow, L., T. Brock, and C. E. Rouse. 2013. Postsecondary education in the United States: Introducing the issue. *The Future of Children* 23(1):3-16.

Baum, S., and S. Schwartz. 2014. *Student aid, student behavior, and educational attainment.* http://umdcipe.org/conferences/DecliningMiddleClassesSpain/Papers/Schwartz.pdf (accessed October 17, 2014).

Belfield, C., and H. Levin. 2012. *The economics of investing in opportunity youth.* New York: Civic Enterprises.

Besharov, D. J., and P. H. Cottingham. 2011. *The Workforce Investment Act: Implementation experiences and evaluation findings.* Kalamazoo, MI: WE Upjohn Institute.

Bettinger, E. P., A. Boatman, and B. T. Long. 2013. Student supports: Developmental education and other academic programs. *The Future of Children* 23(1):93-115.

Blau, F. D., and L. M. Kahn. 2006. The U.S. gender pay gap in the 1990s: Slowing convergence. *Industrial and Labor Relations Review* 60(1):45-66.

Bloom, D. 2010. Programs and policies to assist high school dropouts in the transition to adulthood. *The Future of Children* 20(1):89-108.

Bloom, D., and D. Butler. 2007. Overcoming employment barriers: Strategies to help the "hard-to-employ." In *Reshaping the American workforce in a changing economy*, edited by H. J. Holzer and D. S. Nightingale. Washington, DC: Urban Institute. Pp. 155-180.

Bloom, H. S., and R. Unterman. 2012. *Sustained positive effects on graduation rates produced by New York City's small public high schools of choice.* Policy brief. New York: MDRC.

BLS (Bureau of Labor Statistics). 2013. *Nonfatal occupational injuries and illnesses requiring days away from work, 2012.* http://www.bls.gov/news.release/osh2.toc.htm (accessed July 3, 2014).

BLS. 2014. *Revisions to the 2012 Census of Fatal Occupational Injuries (CFOI) counts.* http://www.bls.gov/iif/oshwc/cfoi/cfoi_revised12.pdf (accessed August 4, 2014).

Bond, G., H. Xie, and R. Drake. 2007. Can SSDI and SSI beneficiaries with mental illness benefit from evidence-based supported employment? *Psychiatric Services* 58(11):1412-1420.

Bound, J., M. F. Lovenheim, and S. Turner. 2010. Why have college completion rates declined? An analysis of changing student preparation and collegiate resources. *American Economic Journal-Applied Economics* 2(3):129-157.

Brener, N. D., S. S. Hassan, and L. C. Barrios. 1999. Suicidal ideation among college students in the United States. *Journal of Consulting and Clinical Psychology* 67(6):1004-1008.

Breslau, J., E. Miller, W.-J. J. Chung, and J. B. Schweitzer. 2011. Childhood and adolescent onset psychiatric disorders, substance use, and failure to graduate high school on time. *Journal of Psychiatric Research* 45(3):295-301.

Brock, T. 2010. Young adults and higher education: Barriers and breakthroughs to success. *The Future of Children* 20(1):109-132.

Brynjolfsson, E., and A. McAfee. 2014. *The second machine age: Work, progress, and prosperity in a time of brilliant technologies.* New York: W.W. Norton & Company.

Burns, T., J. Catty, T. Becker, R. E. Drake, A. Fioritti, M. Knapp, C. Lauber, W. Rössler, T. Tomov, and J. Van Busschbach. 2007. The effectiveness of supported employment for people with severe mental illness: A randomized controlled trial. *Lancet* 370(9593): 1146-1152.

Card, D., and J. DiNardo. 2005. The impact of technological change on low-wage workers: A review. In *Working and poor: How economic and policy changes are affecting low-wage workers*, edited by R. M. Blank, S. Danziger, and R. F. Schoeni. New York: Russell Sage Foundation. Pp. 113-140.

Carnevale, A. P., N. Smith, and J. Strohl. 2010. *Help wanted: Projections of job and education requirements through 2018*. Indianapolis, IN: Lumina Foundation.

CBO (Congressional Budget Office). 2014. *Congressional Budget Office cost estimate: S. 1356 Workforce Investment Act of 2013*. Washington, DC: CBO.

CDC (Centers for Disease Control and Prevention). 2013. *Health and safety of young workers: Proceedings of a U.S. and Canadian series of symposia*. http://www.cdc.gov/niosh/docs/2013-144/pdfs/2013-144.pdf (accessed July 7, 2014).

Chase-Lansdale, P. L., and J. Brooks-Gunn. 2014. Two-generation programs in the twenty-first century. *The Future of Children* 24:13-40.

Choitz, V., and T. Harmon. 2014. *Strengthening your career pathways systems: The alliance for quality career pathways*. Washington, DC: Center for Law and Social Policy.

Clotfelter, C. T., H. F. Ladd, C. Muschkin, and J. L. Vigdor. 2013. *Developmental education in North Carolina community colleges*. Paper presented at Association for Public Policy Analysis & Management (APPAM) Research Conference, Baltimore, MD, November 8-10, 2012.

Cory, R. C. 2011. Disability services offices for students with disabilities: A campus resource. *New Directions for Higher Education* 2011(154):27-36.

Cowen, T. 2013. *Average is over: Powering America beyond the age of the great stagnation*. New York: Dutton Adult.

Crandall-Hollick, M. 2012. *The American opportunity tax credit: Overview, analysis, and policy options*. Congressional Research Service Report R42561. Washington, DC: U.S. Government Printing Office.

Currie, J., and B. C. Madrian. 1999. Health, health insurance and the labor market. *Handbook of Labor Economics* 3:3309-3416.

Dahl, M., T. DeLeire, and J. Schwabish. 2013. *A lost generation? The impact of high unemployment rates at college graduation on long-term earnings*. Washington, DC: Congressional Budget Office.

Davis, M., and A. Vander Stoep. 1997. The transition to adulthood for youth who have serious emotional disturbance: Developmental transition and young adult outcomes. *The Journal of Mental Health Administration* 24(4):400-427.

Davis, M., J. Delman, and T. Duperoy. 2013. Employment and careers in young adults with psychiatric disabilities. In *Tools for system transformation for young adults with psychiatric disabilities: State of the science papers*, edited by M. Davis. Worcester: University of Massachusetts Medical School, Department of Psychiatry, Center for Mental Health Services Research, Transitions RTC. Pp. 59-95.

DeLuca, M. 2014. *Tech demands more H-1B visas as critics cry foul*. http://www.nbcnews.com/business/business-news/tech-demands-more-h-1b-visas-critics-cry-foul-n77161 (accessed October 14, 2014).

Deming, D., C. Goldin, and L. Katz. 2013. For-profit colleges. *The Future of Children* 23(1):137-163.

Dennett, J., and A. S. Modestino. 2013. *Uncertain futures? Youth attachment to the labor market in the United States and New England*. Boston, MA: Federal Reserve Bank of Boston.

Domina, T. 2006. Brain drain and brain gain: Rising educational segregation in the United States, 1940-2000. *City & Community* 5(4):387-407.

Dynarski, S., and J. Scott-Clayton. 2013. Financial aid policy: Lessons from research. *The Future of Children* 23(1):67-91.

Edelman, P. B., H. J. Holzer, and P. Offner. 2006. *Reconnecting disadvantaged young men.* Washington, DC: Urban Institute.

Edin, K., and T. J. Nelson. 2013. *Doing the best I can: Fatherhood in the inner city.* Oakland: University of California Press.

Eisenberg, D., E. Golberstein, and S. E. Gollust. 2007. Help-seeking and access to mental health care in a university student population. *Medical Care* 45(7):594-601.

Fergusson, D. M., and L. J. Horwood. 1997. Early onset cannabis use and psychosocial adjustment in young adults. *Addiction* 92(3):279-296.

Forness, S. R., S. F. Freeman, T. Paparella, J. M. Kauffman, and H. M. Walker. 2012. Special education implications of point and cumulative prevalence for children with emotional or behavioral disorders. *Journal of Emotional and Behavioral Disorders* 20(1):4-18.

Frey, W. D., R. E. Drake, G. R. Bond, A. L. Miller, H. H. Goldman, and D. S. Salkever. 2011. *Mental health treatment study.* Rockville, MD: Westat.

GAO (Government Accountability Office). 2009. *Higher education and disability: Education needs a coordinated approach to improve its assistance to schools in supporting students.* Washington, DC: Government Accountability Office.

GAO. 2011. *Multiple employment and training programs: Providing information on colocating services and consolidating administrative structures could promote efficiencies.* http://www.gao.gov/new.items/d1192.pdf (accessed August 5, 2014).

Goldin, C. D., and L. F. Katz. 2009. *The race between education and technology.* Cambridge, MA: Harvard University Press.

Goodman, A., R. Joyce, and J. P. Smith. 2011. The long shadow cast by childhood physical and mental problems on adult life. *Proceedings of the National Academy of Sciences of the United States of America* 108(15):6032-6037.

Hansen, W. L., and B. A. Weisbrod. 1969. The distribution of costs and direct benefits of public higher education: The case of California. *Journal of Human Resources* 4(2):176-191.

Heckman, J. J., R. J. LaLonde, and J. A. Smith. 1999. The economics and econometrics of active labor market programs. *Handbook of Labor Economics* 3(A):1865-2097.

Hill, C. J., H. J. Holzer, and H. Chen. 2009. *Against the tide: Household structure, opportunities, and outcomes among white and minority youth.* Kalamazoo, MI: W.E. Upjohn Institute.

Hoffman, N. 2011. *Schooling in the workplace: How six of the world's best vocational education systems prepare young people for jobs and life.* Cambridge, MA: Harvard Education Press.

Holzer, H. J. 2009. *Workforce development as an antipoverty strategy: What do we know? What should we do?* http://hdl.handle.net/10419/35478 (accessed July 7, 2014).

Holzer, H. J. 2010. *Is the middle of the U.S. job market really disappearing? A comment on the "polarization" hypothesis.* Washington, DC: Center for American Progress.

Holzer, H. J. 2011. *Raising job quality and skills for American workers: Creating more-effective education and workforce development systems in the states.* Washington, DC: The Hamilton Project.

Holzer, H. J. 2013. Workforce development programs. In *Legacies of the war on poverty,* edited by M. Bailey and S. Danziger. New York: Russell Sage Foundation. Pp. 121-150.

Holzer, H. J. 2014. Improving employment outcomes of disadvantaged students. In *Policies to address poverty in America,* edited by M. Kearney, B. Harris, and K. Anderson. Washington, DC: The Hamilton Project. Pp. 87-95.

Holzer, H. J., and E. Dunlop. 2013. *Just the facts, ma'am: Postsecondary education and labor market outcomes in the U.S.* Bonn, Germany: IZA (Institute for the Study of Labor).

Holzer, H. J., and R. Lerman. 2014. *Cognitive skills in the U.S. labor market: For whom do they matter?* Unpublished paper. Washington, DC: American Institutes for Research.

Holzer, H. J., S. Raphael, and M. A. Stoll. 2004. Will employers hire former offenders? Employer preferences, background checks, and their determinants. In *The impact of incarceration on families and communities*, edited by M. Patillo-McCoy, D. Weiman, and B. Western. New York: Russell Sage Foundation. Pp. 205-243.

Holzer, H. J., P. Offner, and E. Sorensen. 2005. Declining employment among young black less-educated men: The role of incarceration and child support. *Journal of Policy Analysis and Management* 24(2):329-350.

Holzer, H., D. Linn, and W. Monthey. 2013. *The promise of high-quality career and technical education: Improving outcomes for students, firms, and the economy*. Washington, DC: The College Board and The Georgetown Law Center on Poverty, Inequality, and Public Policy.

Honeycutt, T., A. Thompkins, M. Bardos, and S. Stern. 2013. *State differences in the vocational rehabilitation experiences of transition-age youth with disabilities*. Washington, DC: Mathematica Policy Research.

Hoxby, C., and S. Turner. 2013. *Informing students about their college options: A proposal for broadening the expanding college opportunities project*. www.hamiltonproject.org/files/...and.../THP_HoxbyTurner_FINAL.pdf (accessed July 7, 2014).

IOM (Institute of Medicine) and NRC (National Research Council). 2013. *Improving the health, safety, and well-being of young adults: Workshop summary*. Washington, DC: The National Academies Press.

Jacobson, L., and C. Mokher. 2009. *Pathways to boosting the earnings of low-income students by increasing their educational attainment*. http://files.eric.ed.gov/fulltext/ED504078.pdf (accessed July 7, 2014).

Jenkins, D., and S.-W. Cho. 2012. *Get with the program: Accelerating community college students' entry into and completion of programs of study*. New York: Community College Research Center.

Johnson, R. C., and S. Raphael. 2009. The effects of male incarceration dynamics on acquired immune deficiency syndrome infection rates among African American women and men. *Journal of Law and Economics* 52(2):251-293.

Johnson, W. R. 2005. Are public subsidies to higher education regressive? *Education* 1(3): 288-315.

Johnston, L., P. O'Malley, J. Bachman, and J. Schulenberg. 2013. *Monitoring the future national survey results on drug use, 1975-2012: Volume 2, college students and adults ages 19-50*. Ann Arbor: Institute for Social Research, University of Michigan.

Kahn, L. B. 2010. The long-term labor market consequences of graduating from college in a bad economy. *Labour Economics* 17(2):303-316.

Kearney, M. S., and P. B. Levine. 2014. *Media influences on social outcomes: The impact of MTV's 16 and Pregnant on teen childbearing*. http://www.wellesley.edu/sites/default/files/assets/kearney-levine-16p-nber_submit.pdf (accessed August 4, 2014).

Kemple, J., and C. Willner. 2008. *Career academies: Long-term impacts on labor market outcomes, educational attainment, and transitions to adulthood*. New York: MDRC.

Kemple, J. J., C. Herlihy, and T. J. Smith. 2005. *Making progress toward graduation*. New York: MDRC.

Kessler, R. C., C. L. Foster, W. B. Saunders, and P. E. Stang. 1995. Social consequences of psychiatric disorders, I: Educational attainment. *American Journal of Psychiatry* 152(7):1026-1032.

Kisch, J., E. V. Leino, and M. M. Silverman. 2005. Aspects of suicidal behavior, depression, and treatment in college students: Results from the spring 2000 National College Health Assessment Survey. *Suicide and Life-Threatening Behavior* 35(1):3-13.

Kreisman, D., S. Dynarski, B. Jacob, and P. Bahr. 2013. *The returns to course credits, certificates, and degrees: Evidence from Michigan's community colleges*. Paper presented at Association for Public Policy Analysis & Management (APPAM) Annual Fall Research Conference, Washington, DC.

LaLonde, R. J. 1996. The promise of public sector-sponsored training programs. *The Journal of Economic Perspectives* 9(2):149-168.

Lauderdale, D. S. 2001. Education and survival: Birth cohort, period, and age effects. *Demography* 38(4):551-561.

Levy, F., and R. J. Murnane. 2013. *Dancing with robots: Human skills for computerized work*. Washington, DC: Third Way.

Lindstrom, L., L. G. Kahn, and H. Lindsey. 2013. Navigating the early career years: Barriers and strategies for young adults with disabilities. *Journal of Vocational Rehabilitation* 39(1):1-12.

Long, B. T. 2013. Supporting access to higher education. In *Legacies of the war on poverty*, edited by M. Bailey and S. Danziger. New York: Russell Sage Foundation. Pp. 93-120.

Lynch, S. M. 2003. Cohort and life-course patterns in the relationship between education and health: A hierarchical approach. *Demography* 40(2):309-331.

Maguire, S., J. Freely, C. Clymer, M. Conway, and D. Schwartz. 2010. *Tuning into local labor markets: Findings from the Sectoral Employment Impact Study*. Philadelphia, PA: Public/Private Ventures.

Martin, V., and J. Broadus. 2013. *Enhancing GED instruction to prepare students for college and careers: Early success in LaGuardia Community College's Bridge to Health and Business Program*. Policy brief. New York: MDRC.

Millenky, M., D. Bloom, S. Muller-Ravett, and J. Broadus. 2011. *Three-year results of the National Guard Youth ChalleNGe evaluation*. New York: MDRC.

Mirowsky, J., and C. E. Ross. 2003. *Education, social status, and health*. Piscataway, NJ: Transaction Publishers.

Montgomery, S. M., D. G. Cook, M. J. Bartley, and M. Wadsworth. 1999. Unemployment pre-dates symptoms of depression and anxiety resulting in medical consultation in young men. *International Journal of Epidemiology* 28(1):95-100.

Moreno, L., T. Honeycutt, S. McLeod, and C. Gill. 2014. *Lessons for programs serving transition-age youth: A comparative analysis of the U.S. and 10 other countries in the Organisation for Economic Co-operation and Development (OECD)*. Washington, DC: Mathematica Policy Research.

Murnane, R. J. 2013. *U.S. high school graduation rates: Patterns and explanations*. Washington, DC: National Bureau of Economic Research.

National Fund for Workforce Solutions. 2014. *National fund for workforce solutions*. http://www.nfwsolutions.org (accessed July 2, 2014).

National Governors Association Center of Best Practices. 2012. *State sector strategies coming of age: Implications for state workforce policy makers*. Washington, DC: National Governors Association.

Nelson, T. F., S. L. Gortmaker, S. V. Subramanian, L. Cheung, and H. Wechsler. 2007. Disparities in overweight and obesity among U.S. college students. *American Journal of Health Behavior* 31(4):363-373.

Newman, L., M. Wagner, T. Huang, D. Shaver, A.-M. Knokey, J. Yu, E. Contreras, K. Ferguson, S. Greene, and K. Nagle. 2011a. *Secondary school programs and performance of students with disabilities: A special topic report of findings from the National Longitudinal Transition Study-2 (NLTS2)*. NCSER 2012-3000. Washington, DC: National Center for Special Education Research.

Newman, L., M. Wagner, A.-M. Knokey, C. Marder, K. Nagle, D. Shaver, and X. Wei. 2011b. *The post-high school outcomes of young adults with disabilities up to 8 years after high school: A report From the National Longitudinal Transition Study-2 (NLTS2).* http://www.nlts2.org/reports/2011_09_02/nlts2_report_2011_09_02_complete.pdf (accessed September 19, 2014).

NRC (National Research Council). 2012. *Education for life and work: Developing transferable knowledge and skills in the 21st century.* Washington, DC: The National Academies Press.

Oreopoulos, P., and U. Petronijevic. 2013. Making college worth it: A review of the returns to higher education. *The Future of Children* 23(1):41-65.

Pager, D. 2003. The mark of a criminal record. *American Journal of Sociology* 108(5):937-875.

Patrick, M. E., J. E. Schulenberg, and P. M. O'Malley. 2013. High school substance use as a predictor of college attendance, completion, and dropout: A national multicohort longitudinal study. *Youth & Society* 1-23, http://yas.sagepub.com/content/early/2013/11/11/0044118X13508961 (accessed July 7, 2014).

Paul, K. I., and K. Moser. 2009. Unemployment impairs mental health: Meta-analyses. *Journal of Vocational Behavior* 74(3):264-282.

Pettit, B. 2012. *Invisible men: Mass incarceration and the myth of black progress.* New York: Russell Sage Foundation.

Reed, D., A. Y.-H. Liu, R. Kleinman, A. Mastri, D. Reed, S. Sattar, and J. Ziegler. 2012. *An effectiveness assessment and cost-benefit analysis of registered apprenticeship in 10 states.* Washington, DC: Mathematica Policy Research.

Roder, A., and M. Elliott. 2011. *A promising start: Initial impacts of year up on low-income young adults' careers.* New York: Economic Mobility Corporation.

Rosenbaum, J. E., R. Deil-Amen, and A. E. Person. 2006. *After admission: From college access to college success.* New York: Russell Sage Foundation.

Salzer, M., L. Wick, and J. Rogers. 2008. Familiarity with and use of accommodations and supports among postsecondary students with mental illnesses. *Psychiatric Services* 59(4):370-375.

Schneider, H. 2013. Recasting high school, German firms transplant apprentice model to U.S. *The Washington Post*, November 27.

Schochet, P. Z., J. Burghardt, and S. McConnell. 2008. Does Job Corps work? Impact findings from the national Job Corps study. *The American Economic Review* 98(5):1864-1886.

Schulenberg, J. E., and J. L. Maggs. 2002. A developmental perspective on alcohol use and heavy drinking during adolescence and the transition to young adulthood. *Journal of Studies on Alcohol and Drugs* (14):54-70.

Schwartz, A., J. Leos-Urbel, T. Nicolai, and G. S. Blair. 2014. Expanding summer employment opportunities for low-income youth. In *Policies to address poverty in America*, edited by I. M. Kearney and B. Harris. Washington, DC: The Hamilton Project. Pp. 55-66.

Schwartz, N. D. 2013. Where factory apprenticeship is latest model from Germany. *New York Times*, November 30.

Scott-Clayton, J. E. 2011. *The shapeless river: Does a lack of structure inhibit students' progress at community colleges?* New York: Community College Research Center.

Scrivener, S., and M. J. Weiss. 2013. *More graduates: Two-year results from an evaluation of Accelerated Study in Associate Programs (ASAP) for developmental education students.* New York: MDRC.

Shanahan, M. J. 2000. Pathways to adulthood in changing societies: Variability and mechanisms in life course perspective. *Annual Review of Sociology* 26(1):667-692.

Shonkoff, J. P., A. S. Garner, B. S. Siegel, M. I. Dobbins, M. F. Earls, L. McGuinn, and D. L. Wood. 2012. The lifelong effects of early childhood adversity and toxic stress. *Pediatrics* 129(1):e232-e246.

Social Security Administration. 2012. *SSI annual statistical report, 2012*. Washington, DC: Social Security Administration.

Social Security Administration. 2014. *Youth transition demonstration*. http://www.ssa.gov/disabilityresearch/youth.htm (accessed July 2, 2014).

Sullivan, D., and T. von Wachter. 2009. Job displacement and mortality: An analysis using administrative data. *The Quarterly Journal of Economics* 124(3):1265-1306.

Sum, A., I. Khatiwada, M. Trubskyy, and S. Palma. 2014. *The plummeting labor market fortunes of teens and young adults*. Washington, DC: The Brookings Institution.

Symonds, W. C., R. B. Schwartz, and R. Ferguson. 2011. *Pathways to prosperity: Meeting the challenge of preparing young Americans for the 21st century*. Report issued by the Pathways to Prosperity Project. Cambridge, MA: Harvard Graduate School of Education.

Thomas, A. 2012. Three strategies to prevent unintended pregnancy. *Journal of Policy Analysis and Management* 31(2):280-311.

Turner, S. 2007. Higher education policies generating the 21st century workforce. In *Reshaping the American workforce in a changing economy*, edited by H. J. Holzer and D. S. Nightingale. Washington, DC: Urban Institute. Pp. 91-116.

U.S. Department of Education. 2005. *Facts from NLTS2: High school completion by youth with disabilities*. http://nlts2.org/fact_sheets/nlts2_fact_sheet_2005_11.pdf (accessed October 17, 2014).

U.S. Department of Education. 2013. *Department awards $211 million for the Promoting the Readiness of Minors in Supplemental Security Income (PROMISE) initiative*. http://www.ed.gov/news/press-releases/department-awards-211-million-promoting-readiness-minors-supplemental-security-i (accessed July 2, 2014).

U.S. Department of Education. 2014. *Rehabilitation services and disability research: Fiscal year 2014 budget request*. http://www2.ed.gov/about/overview/budget/budget15/justifications/k-rehab.pdf (accessed October 2, 2014).

Wechsler, H., and B. Wuethrich. 2002. *Dying to drink: Confronting binge drinking on college campuses*. Emmaus, PA: Rodale Books.

Yang, L. H., D. M. Anglin, A. J. Wonpat-Borja, M. G. Opler, M. Greenspoon, and C. M. Corcoran. 2013. Public stigma associated with psychosis risk syndrome in a college population: Implications for peer intervention. *Psychiatric Services* 64(3):284-288.

Yu, Y. 2012. Educational differences in obesity in the United States: A closer look at the trends. *Obesity* 20(4):904-908.

Zagorsky, J. L., and P. K. Smith. 2011. The freshman 15: A critical time for obesity intervention or media myth? *Social Science Quarterly* 92(5):1389-1407.

Zeidenberg, M., S.-W. Cho, and P. D. Jenkins. 2010. *Washington state's integrated basic education and skills training program (I-best): New evidence of effectiveness*. New York: Community College Research Center, Teachers College, Columbia University.

5

Civic Engagement and National Service[1]

Key Findings

- Volunteering during adolescence and young adulthood is associated with improved health and well-being. Civic engagement and national service can contribute to educational and occupational development and continued citizenship.
- Military service has both positive and negative effects on the health, safety, and well-being of young adults, with positive effects relating to educational and occupational development, and negative effects relating to military deployment, as well as to difficulties with postmilitary transition.
- Young adults who are members of racial/ethnic minorities, of lower socioeconomic position, and lacking a college education tend to be underrepresented in many venues of civic engagement and national service, yet there is evidence that these youth might benefit the most from such activities.
- National service programs have become more competitive and community goal oriented; the military also has changed, largely as a result of extensive deployment in the past decade and a half. Among other implications, these changes mean that

[1] This chapter draws heavily on a paper commissioned by the committee titled "Civic Engagement, Volunteerism, and Young Adult Well-Being: Volunteer Work and National Service as Developmental Opportunities for Social Incorporation," by Constance Flanagan and Victoria Faust. Available online at http://www.iom.edu/youngadults.

past understanding of the effects of engagement in these activities needs to be updated.

- In the past, national service programs focused on both member development and community improvement; more recently, especially for programs under the Corporation for National and Community Service umbrella, the emphasis has shifted more to community improvement. Given the likely benefits of national service for members (found in past research when membership development was a main goal), the decreased emphasis on membership development may result in inconsequential national service experiences for the new generation of young adults, thus creating a critical missed institutional opportunity for improving the transition to adulthood.

Civic engagement and national service encompass a broad range of activities including community service (volunteer and mandated), political involvement, environmental service, several teaching programs, and military service. Finding one's connection to the larger world through participation in such activities is an important aspect of the transition from adolescence to adulthood, setting the stage for the next generation to become active and contributing citizens (Youniss et al., 2002); providing new and alternative opportunities to contribute in meaningful ways and explore the larger world and one's identity; and providing experiences beneficial for work, education, and social relationships. Such involvement and contributions offer opportunities to participate and serve in ways not always provided by other contexts and activities, including work, education, and social relationships.

> "My volunteer work gave me a view of another career path: working with kids, particularly on health care."*

In this chapter we discuss the science and practice regarding civic engagement and national service during the transition to adulthood. We first provide an overview of civic engagement and national service during the transition to adulthood, focusing on the heterogeneity of experiences and possible effects. We then consider national service programs for young adults, giving specific attention to Ameri-

* Quotations are from members of the young adult advisory group during their discussions with the committee.

Corps, including the research conducted to examine program effects. Next, we provide a summary of military service and how it relates to the transition to adulthood. We conclude with policy and research recommendations.

OVERVIEW OF CIVIC ENGAGEMENT AND NATIONAL SERVICE

Volunteerism and Well-Being

Although volunteering is aimed at helping those on the receiving end, it is also associated with, and may contribute to, health and well-being among those who volunteer. Extensive research, some of it longitudinal and experimental, supports the association between volunteering and health and well-being across the life course. Volunteering is not always associated with clear benefits (especially among middle-aged adults), but the body of evidence is striking for the absence of contradictory findings, with essentially no findings of negative effects (Piliavin and Siegl, 2014).[2]

Does volunteering contribute to, rather than simply being associated with, improved health and well-being? This is a key question for the research on volunteering (and for all research concerning any possible effects of experiences during the transition to adulthood), and one not easily answered. Panel studies provide consistent evidence of a positive effect. Independently of other kinds of social participation, such as religious attendance, visiting with friends, or other social activities, and with controls for earlier levels of well-being, volunteering uniquely predicts lowered depression and increased psychological well-being (Flanagan and Bundick, 2011; Musick and Wilson, 2003; Piliavin and Siegl, 2007, 2014; Thoits and Hewitt, 2001). Physiological effects also have been documented: the altruistic nature of volunteering and the social contact increase levels of oxytocin, which decreases anxiety and increases positive mood (Piliavin and Siegl, 2014). In addition, longitudinal and experimental studies with youth from diverse racial/ethnic and social class backgrounds find that volunteering is associated with fewer behavioral problems, including lower rates of course failure, suspension, school dropout, and pregnancy (Moore et al., 1994; Schmidt et al., 2007).

Volunteering in adolescence and early adulthood has been found to have long-term effects. Analyses of the National Educational Longitudinal Study of 1988 panel data suggest that, controlling for a host of background factors, engaging in community service in high school increases the odds

[2] The optimal level of time commitment is not clear in the literature; burnout can come from too much volunteering without sufficient social support.

of graduating from college in early adulthood (Dávila and Mora, 2007).[3] Volunteering is the best single predictor of later volunteering. Panel studies show that volunteer service in high school and college is related to multiple measures of well-being in adulthood, effects that are mediated by volunteering in adulthood (Bowman et al., 2010).

Thus, evidence is suggestive that there are positive benefits on health and well-being of volunteering during adolescence and the transition to young adulthood, but the effect sizes are unclear. Possible explanations for the positive effect of volunteering include the value of expanded community connections, involvement with prosocial peers, structured use of time, and a sense of benevolence and individual and collective efficacy—i.e., that the volunteer "matters" to those in the organization and to the lives of others. Compared with other forms of extracurricular activity, community service has been implicated in adolescents' reports of higher levels of bonding, bridging social capital, intergenerational harmony, and social support (Flanagan et al., 2014).

Changes in Civic Engagement During the Transition to Adulthood

Involvement in civic organizations and volunteering is lower among young adults than among high school students and older adults (Flanagan and Levine, 2010), with some studies showing rebounds around age 26 (Jennings and Stoker, 2004; Kinder, 2006). These shifts likely reflect changing roles and commitments, as well as changing institutions in terms of both opportunities and incentives (Kinder, 2006; Oesterle et al., 2004; Rotolo, 2000; Watts, 1999).

Among recent cohorts of young adults, delays in taking up the habit of voting are consistent with the protracted nature of the transition to adulthood and with delays in other markers of adult status discussed elsewhere in this report (Flanagan and Levine, 2010), a trend not unique to the United States. Across advanced industrial countries, younger generations are less likely than their elder compatriots to vote or contact elected officials (Dalton, 2008; Norris, 2011; Spannring et al., 2008). Since 1964, rates of voter turnout for presidential elections among 18- to 24-year-olds have been consistently lower than among all other age groups (File, 2014). Voting rates have varied across recent election cycles, but with 18- to 29-year-olds still having the lowest turnout rates (File, 2014). In both emerging and developed democracies, young people are less likely than older people

[3] Many high schools require a certain number of hours of community service as a prerequisite for graduation, although the students select their service recipient and the service they provide. "Mandated" high school service is included within the term "volunteering," and studies find similar effects regardless of whether the service is mandated.

to register to vote (Pintor and Gratschew, 2002). Over the past several decades, political trust has declined in advanced industrial democracies, and younger generations account for a disproportionate share of that decline as well (Dalton, 2004).

At the same time, youth are inventing and engaging in alternative forms of political action, including lifestyle/consumer politics (boycotting and buycotting), community advocacy and development, social justice– and interest-based campaigns, use of online technology for organizing and information campaigns, and global activism (Dalton, 2008; Keeter et al., 2002; Norris, 2002). A growing body of scholarship and practice on these new forms of engagement points to their potential for promoting the well-being of young people and the organizations and communities where they reside (Calvert et al., 2013). According to panel data from a nationally representative sample, 18- to 35-year-olds who used the Internet to blog, email, or post comments about political candidates or issues were more likely to participate in political campaigns and community volunteering and problem solving 2 years later. But even those young adults who used the Internet for apolitical interest-driven activities (i.e., discussions, or organizing or participating in social, recreational, fan, or special-interest sites) or who took the lead in an online community were more likely to engage in community and political campaigns 2 years later; online activities driven by friendships, however, were not related to later civic or political engagement (Kahne et al., 2013).

Differences by Social Class, Race/Ethnicity, and Gender

Both forms and levels of civic engagement vary by social class, race/ethnicity, and gender. Historical, community, and social forces can shape civic engagement, and research has shown that negative social and economic indicators such as poverty, involvement in the justice system, and school dropout are risk factors for civic disengagement (Beaumont, 2012; Ginwright, 2011). Research also has shown that traditional forms of civic engagement may not be desirable for everyone (Ginwright, 2011). In research on African American adolescents, Ginwright (2011) found that for these youth, civic engagement often occurs outside of traditional forms of such activity. Instead of volunteering at a local club or campaigning for a local politician, for example, these youth may work to obtain free bus passes for students receiving public assistance. Similar findings might plausibly hold true for young adults. Little research to date has focused on what can or should be done to address existing civic inequalities and stratifications for young adults with fewer resources or from disadvantaged backgrounds (Beaumont, 2012).

Civic engagement class divides have long existed in the United States, with political interest and voter turnout being concentrated among the more advantaged segments of society (Pacheco and Plutzer, 2008; Verba et al., 1995). Young African Americans voted at the highest rate of any racial/ethnic group in 2008 and 2012 (Commission on Youth Voting and Civic Knowledge, 2013). Nonetheless, while nearly half (45 percent) of those aged 18-29 voted in the 2012 elections, those who went to college voted at almost twice the rate of their non-college-educated peers (CIRCLE, 2012; Commission on Youth Voting and Civic Knowledge, 2013). In 2012, 71 percent of eligible voters aged 18-29 who had any college experience voted, compared with 24 percent of eligible voters with a high school diploma and only 4 percent of eligible voters without a high school diploma (CIRCLE, 2012). Voters without college experience, compared with those with such experience, are more likely to have children in their household; to have lower income; and to identify as lesbian, gay, or bisexual. They also are less likely to be married and to include mothers who do not hold a full-time job (CIRCLE, 2012). The social class divide in political engagement reflects a larger divide in civic opportunities that begins in childhood (Verba et al., 2003) and is exacerbated by the uneven opportunities for civic practice in middle and high schools (Kahne and Middaugh, 2009). Rates of participation in religious organizations, voluntary associations, grassroots political parties, and unions all have fallen for "non-college youth" (Flanagan et al., 2009; Godsay et al., 2012).

The educational gap in voting has been highly consistent since the voting age was lowered to 18 in 1972 (CIRCLE, 2012). However, analyses of trends in intention to vote among high school seniors point to an increasing divide between those who plan on attending a 4-year college and their peers who do not (Syvertsen et al., 2011). Analyses of voter turnout in the 2012 elections show that policies also matter. Specifically, young people without college experience who lived in states with photo ID requirements were less likely to vote in 2012 than their counterparts in states without such ID laws in place, even when other factors related to voting were accounted for (Commission on Youth Voting and Civic Knowledge, 2013).

Regarding gender differences, college women are less likely than men to aspire to political careers at the local or national level (Lawless and Fox, 2013), to discuss politics on a regular basis, and to believe they have leadership qualities and skills that would qualify them for office (Kawashima-Ginsberg and Thomas, 2013). That being said, with the exception of programs that target particular groups, women are more likely than men to enroll in national service programs.

Summary of Causes and Consequences of Civic Engagement in Youth

In her recent book on the political theories of youth, Flanagan (2013) summarizes convergent findings from research on adolescent and young adult civic engagement and offers the following relevant conclusions:

> "You get that feeling that you're actually making an impact when you get to sit and talk with a 5th grader about what is college, what is higher education, why should you go, and do you have the opportunity. Many high-risk youth don't have the confidence that they can go to college, that it is a door for them to step through."

> First, youth are more likely to be civically active as adults if they have had opportunities during adolescence to work collaboratively with peers and adults on engaging issues and to discuss current events with parents, teachers, and peers. Interest in political issues tends to be generated by controversy, discussion, and the perception that it matters to take a stand. Second, young people's sense of social incorporation (solidarity with others, identification with community institutions, being respected and heard by adults) is a psychological factor that is positively related to youth assuming social responsibility for others in their community and for taking civic actions (voting and volunteering) in young adulthood. These relationships are true for youth from different social class and ethnic minority backgrounds. Third, there is a class and racial divide in the civic opportunities available to young people: cumulative disadvantage built up over the K-12 years (including the lack of opportunities to practice civic skills, the competing demands on attention and time of living in economically stressed communities, and especially events such as dropping out of school or getting arrested) depresses civic incorporation and civic action later in life. Fourth, besides opportunities, there are traits of personality (extraversion, confidence, optimism) that predispose some youth to join organizations and get engaged in civic action. Fifth, youth's engagement in meaningful civic projects is positively associated with their psychosocial well-being and mental health. (Flanagan, 2013, pp. 2-3)

NATIONAL SERVICE PROGRAMS FOR YOUNG ADULTS

Institutions are the venues whereby people are recruited into civic life (Verba et al., 1995), and the nature of these recruitment contexts has changed over the past three decades. Unionized workplaces used to be a venue for the civic recruitment of young adults who did not go on to college; over the past three decades, however, union work and the potential for recruitment for this venue have decreased (Finlay et al., 2011, p. 1729). College has been and continues to be a venue for civic recruitment (Zaff et al., 2009). For college students, many opportunities exist both on and off campus, and a number of organizations and initiatives are devoted to encouraging civic engagement among students. For example, Project Pericles is a not-for-profit organization that "encourages and facilitates commitments by colleges and universities to include social responsibility and participatory citizenship as essential elements of their educational programs."[4] An additional example of an opportunity for civic participation is the Federal Work-Study Program. This program provides part-time jobs for students that need financial assistance (at approximately 3,400 postsecondary institutions), which helps them earn money for their education expenses.[5] The program encourages community service work and work related to the student's course of study. Other opportunities for civic participation can occur through a wide range of institutions such as religious organizations, voluntary associations, unions, and political parties, although young adults, especially those who do not attend college (as noted above), are less likely to be involved in these institutions now than they were in the 1970s (Flanagan et al., 2009).

As a substitute for or in addition to college, national service can offer opportunities for civic engagement, building social connections, exposure to training opportunities, and recruitment into civic life for those from disadvantaged backgrounds. In fact, when youth from disadvantaged families were asked why they had enrolled in AmeriCorps national service programs, they said they wanted to make connections, get job training, and earn a stipend to further their education (Finlay and Flanagan, 2008). Not only does national service provide modest financial support for school, smoothing pathways to educational institutions, but it also may enable participants to gain financial and personal resources, including health benefits; to hone their leadership, organizing, and communication skills; to connect with organizations in the community; and ultimately to be recruited into many forms of civic, social, and economic life.

National Service Programs in the United States

Historically, the enabling legislation for national service programs has invoked two major goals: meeting the needs of communities and developing the capacities and character of volunteer members. Young adulthood has been framed in each piece of legislation as a unique phase in life that is formative of later life trajectories. When Franklin D. Roosevelt proposed

---

[4] See http://www.projectpericles.org/projectpericles/about (accessed October 22, 2014).

[5] See http://www2.ed.gov/programs/fws/index.htmlAs (accessed October 22, 2014).

the Civilian Conservation Corps, he argued that a period of prolonged unemployment would have negative lifelong impacts on the character of a generation. In 1961, when there were ample opportunities for young adults to find remunerative work, it was the assets of young adults that John F. Kennedy invoked when he proposed that the Peace Corps recruit young educated and talented Americans to share their resources with citizens of the developing world and, in the process, serve as ambassadors of the United States (Abt Associates, 2004). Each U.S. president since then has had his signature national service initiative. Lyndon B. Johnson started VISTA (Volunteers in Service to America) as part of the "War on Poverty." George H. W. Bush created the Office of National Service in the White House and the Points of Light Foundation to promote volunteerism, and signed into law the National and Community Service Act of 1990. In 1993, Bill Clinton created the Corporation for National and Community Service (CNCS), which included AmeriCorps, one of the most recognizable current national service programs. And George W. Bush's development of the USA Freedom Corps in 2002 expanded volunteerism and national service partnerships, mainly in the area of homeland security (fire corps, medical reserve corps, disaster preparedness).

The most recent expansion of national service legislation, the 2009 Edward M. Kennedy Serve America Act, signed by President Obama, was intended to reinforce, alter, and in some cases build on a wide variety of service opportunities. In its initial year, fiscal year (FY) 2010, it helped increase federal dollars allocated specifically for AmeriCorps positions (CNCS, 2010); as of FY 2014, funding levels for positions are about $63 million over 2009 levels (CNCS, 2014b). In general, there has been an increase in funding for national service programs, although not to the levels needed given the service opportunities allotted. In short, aside from administrative changes to service opportunities, the recent sweeping support for national service embodied in this act remains largely unrealized.[6]

The current umbrella programs coordinated by CNCS include AmeriCorps, Senior Corps, the Social Innovation Fund,[7] and the Volunteer

[6] In some cases, programs that were initially funded, such as Summer of Service, which supported middle school youth from disadvantaged families for participating in service, were defunded by Congress the following year because of budget cuts. Organizations such as ServiceNation and ServeNext have established a grassroots coalition to hold public officials accountable for the implementation of the Serve America Act.

[7] The Social Innovation Fund (SIF) is a CNCS program and White House initiative, combining public and private resources for people in low-income communities in three areas: economic opportunity, healthy futures, and youth development. Although SIF is not a service program, some of the SIF funding for youth development includes programs that may impact young adults, such as Year Up and YouthBuild. See http://www.nationalservice.gov/programs/social-innovation-fund for more detail (accessed October 22, 2014).

Generation Fund.[8] In accordance with the Serve America Act, CNCS activities are now aligned under priority areas of disaster services, economic opportunity, education, environmental stewardship, healthy futures, and veterans and military families. A major objective of the CNCS 2011-2015 strategic plan is to extend the accessibility of CNCS-supported national service to a more diverse audience. Strategies for achieving this objective include giving funding priority to organizations and programs that engage underrepresented populations. Additional priority measures in the plan include increasing the percentage of CNCS-supported participants who are aware of community needs and community-driven solutions, as well as the percentage of participants reporting a connection to the national service community (CNCS, 2011).

Below is a summary of one of the most popular and recognizable national service programs—AmeriCorps—along with associated research. We also describe other, more youth-focused programs (more detail on these programs and associated research is provided in Appendix C).

AmeriCorps

According to Frumkin and colleagues (2009, p. 395), "AmeriCorps, a national program administered by CNCS, provides grants to public and nonprofit organizations to support community service. AmeriCorps comprises three major programs: AmeriCorps State and National, AmeriCorps VISTA, and AmeriCorps National Civilian Community Corps (NCCC)." AmeriCorps State and National and NCCC programs focus largely on direct service provision. In contrast, VISTA is more decentralized, focused on building capacity in local communities through individuals or small groups. Individuals learn about AmeriCorps programs through various routes, including public service announcements, social media, and formal (e.g., college) and informal networks.

One of the goals of AmeriCorps is to enable those who want to serve to do so. Thus attempts are made to remove barriers and to be inclusive. To counterbalance 1 year of full-time service, AmeriCorps members, often referred to as Corps members, obtain job and life skills training, a yearly living stipend ($10,900 to $21,800, depending on the program), health benefits, child care benefits, training, and forbearance of student loans (the interest for which is forgiven upon the completion of service) (Finlay et al., 2011). Often, they do not receive room and board, but many programs

[8] The Volunteer Generation Fund supports voluntary organizations and state service commissions to increase the impact of volunteers in addressing critical community needs. The fund's investments focus on volunteer management practices that increase volunteer recruitment and retention, which may impact young adults.

have access to resources and networks that can support members in meeting these needs.

Education Award. To counterbalance 1 year of full-time or continual part-time service, AmeriCorps participants obtain an education award that can be used to repay qualified student loans or toward higher education or vocational training. The education award must be used within 7 years of receipt (Abt Associates, 2008). In alignment with policies guiding federal financial aid distribution, however, members with convictions on their records, including a drug charge such as possession, cannot lawfully use their education awards. Corps members are eligible for the education award if they successfully completed their term of service or left for a compelling reason. Opportunities exist for alternative uses of the education award, although currently these alternatives apply only for members over age 55. According to Abt Associates (2011, p. 2), "The 2009 Edward M. Kennedy Serve America Act made changes to the maximum amount of the education award. The amount is now tied to the maximum amount of the U.S. Department of Education's Pell grant. For terms of service that are supported using 2009 (or earlier) funds the award continues to be $4,725 for a year of full-time service, and is prorated for part-time service based on that full-time amount. For terms of service that are supported with 2010 funds, the award value increases to $5,350."

Qualified educational institutions around the country can contribute matching grants (varying in maximum amounts and restrictions) to AmeriCorps members that apply their education award to tuition and qualified expenses, as determined by the school's financial aid department. For example, the University of Arizona offers 2 years of base tuition costs to former AmeriCorps members, but only for those who have served in the University of Arizona Cooperative Extension's AmeriCorps and VISTA projects. The list of schools providing such benefits is available on the AmeriCorps website (CNCS, 2014d).

AmeriCorps State and National Program. As described by Frumkin and colleagues (2009, p. 397), "AmeriCorps State and National is by far the largest of the AmeriCorps programs, supporting participants through a network of local community-based organizations, educational institutions, and other agencies. One-third of AmeriCorps State and National grant funds are distributed according to a population-based formula to governor-appointed state service commissions, which in turn make grants to local nonprofits and public agencies." AmeriCorps State and National members are enlisted by sponsoring agencies such as nonprofits, educational institutions, and other organizations to work toward addressing local community needs (Frumkin et al., 2009). Organizations receiving AmeriCorps funds are required to obtain up to 48 percent matching funds. Some intermediary and sponsoring agencies acquire this money through a site matching contribution, while others use private philanthropic or state-granted dollars.

There are approximately 500,000 applications per year for approximately 80,000 AmeriCorps positions (many of which are part time) (CNCS, 2014a). Because an individual can apply to up to 10 sites, however, these application data include some duplication of cases. Currently, about 15,000 members serve full time, with more than 60,000 more serving in part time or education award-only positions across the country. Note that an increase in part-time positions is a significant change. According to the national longitudinal study summarized below, during the 1999-2000 program year, approximately 75 percent of members served full time (Abt Associates, 2004). This change can be attributed to the development of various models designed to be flexible so as to fit both the interests and needs of members and the community. For example, individuals may be serving "full time," as in 40 hours per week of service that is recognized and supported by AmeriCorps, but only for several months during the summer for national parks maintenance or during the school year for educational support.

AmeriCorps members may opt to serve for a maximum of four terms of service. However, members are eligible only for the total equivalent of two education awards, or $11,290 (as of 2014) (CNCS, 2014c). The minimum requirement for eligibility is that an individual be a U.S. citizen, national, or lawful resident alien aged 17 or older. Although there is no age limit, most participants are young adults. AmeriCorps programs vary in their expectations and requirements for incoming members.

Many, although not all, AmeriCorps members serve in teams and address community needs in collaboration with agencies at the state and local levels and nonprofit organizations (CNCS, 2014a). Examples of AmeriCorps members' work range from providing transportation to medical appointments for elderly residents, to doing house repairs, to assisting teachers in elementary schools. The 2009 Edward M. Kennedy Serve America Act expanded the kinds of service to include areas of the environment, homeland security and first responders, and health.

Participants may have opportunities during their year of service to interact with diverse groups of individuals, to learn and practice civic skills, and to engage with older adult mentors, although the mix of opportunities varies by programs and sites (Abt Associates, 2004). In addition to on-the-job learning, up to 20 percent of a member's time can be used for member development and training. Specific AmeriCorps training opportunities come from individual sites, AmeriCorps program structures, state commissions, and national workshops and conferences. Training typically includes reflective learning, team building, service project development, and professional development. Although mechanisms for accessing such opportunities vary, two common structures that support civic and skill development are strong staff mentorship and team-based training. Team-based programs often consist of 5 to 50 members who train together and collaboratively complete local service projects. In some instances, civic development activities can include inviting a legislator to visit a service day, designing a community project, wrestling with individual differences across a team, developing a network of support, and completing an effective citizenship curriculum. In the past, programs utilized a toolkit for members called Effective Citizenship through AmeriCorps, which included modules on active citizenship, identifying community problems, conducting news searches and policy analyses, discussing rights and freedoms, and considering values in conflict (Constitutional Rights Foundation, 2001). These particular activities, however, became less common as the emphasis on demonstrating community impact eclipsed the goal of member development.

Research on AmeriCorps. In summer and fall 1999, CNCS commissioned Abt Associates to conduct a nationally representative longitudinal study of AmeriCorps members. The initial sample included 2,000 people who were first-time, full-time members either in 108 of the AmeriCorps State and National programs or in 3 of the NCCC programs and who had registered between September 1999 and January 2000 (Abt Associates, 2004). A comparison group of 1,524 people was selected from among individuals who indicated interest in AmeriCorps by contacting CNCS for information but did not enroll. Data were collected at baseline (1999), at the end of the service period (2000), 3 years after baseline (2002), and 8 years after baseline (2007). Of the initial sample of 4,153 who completed a baseline survey, 3,300 completed Wave 2 (in 2000), 2,975 completed Wave 3 (in 2002), and 2,240 finished the final survey (in 2007). Data were analyzed using propensity score matching (based on national and community service interest, demographics, and previous civic engagement). This is a common strategy in nonrandomized experiments to help address selection concerns, thus providing better leverage on potential program effects; nonetheless, given the nonrandomized design, appropriate caution is necessary regarding any program effects.

In examining the AmeriCorp participants and the comparison group over time, both short- and long-term positive program effects were found, especially in terms of civic engagement, members' community connections, knowledge about community problems, and contributions to community-based activities. Participation in AmeriCorps also was found to have positive effects on outcomes that could be considered both civic and work related—i.e., increasing confidence in one's capacity to work with local government and to lead a successful community-based change effort. AmeriCorps participation was found to have other positive effects on employment-related outcomes (public service employment), especially for ethnic minorities. Few statistically significant effects were established for measures of participants' attitudes toward education or educational attainment (measured as confidence in the ability to obtain an education, personal responsibility for success, and actual progress) or for particular life skills measures, although life satisfaction increased more for AmeriCorps participants than for the comparison group over the 8 years. One negative outcome was found for the AmeriCorp NCCC participants (residential model of service): 3 years after baseline, this group was less likely to endorse intergroup contact as an important goal, although that attitude had disappeared at the 8-year follow-up (Abt Associates, 2004, 2008; Frumkin et al., 2009). Overall, despite the need for appropriate caution regarding the extent to which AmeriCorp participation caused the various outcomes, there were many positive effects on civic engagement and some on employment—both priority areas of focus for national service; however, there were few effects for educational outcomes or other life skills, which also are priority areas.

McBride and Lee (2012) found that 30 percent of the AmeriCorps participants did not finish their service term; ethnic minorities, those with lower levels of education, and those with a disability were most likely to be in this group. Reasons given for not completing were personal or health (38 percent), program dissatisfaction (26 percent), financial reasons (15 percent), taking a job (8 percent), and being asked to leave (5 percent). In addition, according to members' reports, the likelihood of completing the service period was increased if the program members were involved in planning service activities, and if the program matched activities to career interests, helped develop mentor relationships, and encouraged members to reflect with others on the service experience.

Concerning reasons for joining AmeriCorps, those with lower family incomes were more likely to report that they were influenced by the education award or social connections (e.g., a peer was a member, AmeriCorps previously helped their family) or by a need for social connections (e.g., desire to make friends). Other reasons endorsed by all groups, regardless of family income, included needing a job, believing they would develop useful skills, and altruism (Finlay and Flanagan, 2009).

Finlay and colleagues (2011, p. 1732) found that, "As expected given their commitment to national service, Corps participants were more likely than the comparison group to endorse community participation (activities, meetings) and involvement in civic organizations (on issues of concern); however, they were less likely to endorse local or national voting." Regardless of the Corps member's socioeconomic position, serving with team members and community members from diverse backgrounds boosted civic commitments and behaviors over the course of the program. In addition, for members of lower socioeconomic position, feelings of belonging to a community and collective efficacy boosted civic commitments and behaviors. For those of higher socioeconomic position, opportunities in the program to lead and manage boosted those outcomes (Flanagan and Kim, 2013).

Concerning the potential of national service as a pathway to employment, the 8-year follow-up found that AmeriCorps participation had impacts on attitudinal and behavioral employment outcomes. Based on self-report measures, Corps State and National program members accepted responsibility for employment success (assessment of the extent to which they were personally responsible for job attainment success) and were more likely to work in the public sector, the arts, religion, or military service compared with the comparison group (Frumkin et al., 2009).

It is worth noting that less intense volunteer experiences also have been linked to employment outcomes. Spera and colleagues (2013) analyzed 10 2-year cohorts (2002/2003-2011/2012) in the Current Population Survey to assess the effect of volunteering on subsequent gainful employment. Based on respondents 16 and older who, in their first survey year, reported that they were either unemployed or not in the labor force but interested in working, the researchers identified a final sample of 70,535 in the 10 cohorts. After controlling for a number of demographic and community-level factors, they found that volunteering was associated with a 27 percent increase in odds of employment in the second survey year. The relationship between volunteering and employment was strongest for those without a high school diploma or General Educational Development credential and for those living in rural areas. The positive relationship between volunteering and employment was stable across gender, race and ethnicity, age, time, and community type/size.

Other National Service Programs

In 2014, the top 10 national direct grantees (national organizations receiving grants) were YouthBuild National, City Year National, Notre Dame Mission Volunteers, Washington Service Corps, Minnesota Reading Corps, Public Allies National, Health Corps, Teach for America, Habitat for Humanity, and Jumpstart. Five of these focus on youth explicitly, while two (YouthBuild and Public Allies) hire almost exclusively disadvantaged youth.[9] Some programs, such as YouthBuild, Public Allies, and PASCO (a regional service corps that engages all of its members in leadership devel-

[9] Note that the Serve America Act defines "disadvantaged youth" as those who have one or more of the following characteristics: are out of school, are unemployed, are aging out of foster care, have limited English proficiency, are homeless or runaway, are at risk to leave secondary school without a diploma, are former juvenile offenders or at risk of delinquency, or have a disability.

opment), intentionally recruit "opportunity youth" and give priority to member development. Other programs, such as Wisconsin's Fresh Start program, that involve youth from marginalized communities in service vary by state. While these programs receive funding from a diverse array of sources, they, often with supplemental support from AmeriCorps, make up the networked community of service programs that engage disadvantaged youth participants in civic opportunities.

New Directions in National Service: Implications for Young Adult Development

Based on changes in the Serve America Act, an increase in service opportunities for young people can be anticipated. While current funding allocations encourage programs to hire disadvantaged youth, one can also expect to see a greater level of professionalization of service in light of the rigorous goals for community impact through the CNCS distribution of resources. Senior AmeriCorps officials have suggested that retention rates for AmeriCorps, which in the aggregate are well over 90 percent, are an indicator of such professionalization, driven by increased competition for and the nature of the positions.[10] The largest number of current positions focus on education, with basic educational attainment being required to achieve benchmarks established by performance measures. In the past, a wide array of activities related to construction work, gang-related or antiviolence work, and other areas established positions for members of various skill levels. Now, however, the roles of the members and the types of projects are driven by performance measurement goals, with, as noted earlier, an emphasis on demonstrating community effects.

Indeed, increasing the national service impact on community needs is the primary objective in the CNCS 2011-2015 strategic plan (CNCS, 2011). To achieve this objective, CNCS is engaging in a rigorous evaluation strategy, including allocating millions of dollars to program evaluation and evaluation capacity building. With respect to member training, funding formulas take into account only how members are trained in best practices for the implementation of interventions. CNCS previously supported longitudinal studies of participants' civic development and has funded evaluations of participant impact alongside rigorous impact evaluations for programs such as Youth Corps (Abt Associates, 2004). Presently, strategic priorities include CNCS-supported participants remaining engaged in their communities and finding opportunities for professional, educational, or civic growth through their service. The present performance measures for funding allocation at

[10] Personal communication, B. Basl, AmeriCorps, May 7, 2014.

the national level, however, do not provide for continual monitoring for civic development of participants.

CNCS's new strategic priorities leave open the possibility that the emphasis will shift toward the development of national service programs that require higher skill levels upon entry. For this reason, it is important for those interested in the civic development of youth, and in particular of disadvantaged youth, to continue monitoring the goals, measures, and strategies of CNCS, as well as the development of other national service programs such as the Civic Justice Corps. It is also important to consider the value and fate of programs that have historically operated in the name of youth development and functioned largely independently of CNCS. Overall, the growing deemphasis on member development represents a lost opportunity to incorporate into national service programs mechanisms that could improve health and well-being during the transition to adulthood, as well as the productivity and citizenship of future generations.

MILITARY SERVICE

Although long compulsory during times of war, military service is now voluntary, and the military is increasingly made up of many diverse groups of Americans, most of whom are young adults. The past decade and a half has been a particularly difficult time for military service, as several ongoing conflicts during the "War on Terror" have led to multiple deployments to war zones for many service members. As a result, recent cohorts of young adults are likely to feel the after-effects of military service for many decades to come (MacLean and Elder, 2007).

In 2012, young adults aged 25 or younger accounted for 42.7 percent of active duty military personnel at any one time and an even larger majority of enlisted servicemen and women (48.8 percent) (DoD, 2013). For most of these young adults, military service is not the start of a long career. Instead, it is a bridge between their adolescent experiences in their communities and secondary schools and their adult experiences in higher education and the labor market. In this way, the military is a context for the transition into adulthood for many Americans (Kelty et al., 2010).

This transitional nature of military service is one reason why many young people in the United States enlist in the military in the first place. In contrast to the growing trend in other forms of national service, the military is viewed as giving attention to the improvement of its young adult members. Thus, young people see this form of public service as a channel for social and economic mobility, the cultivation of important life skills (e.g., responsibility, leadership) and work skills (e.g., technology, trades) that they can carry forward into their adult lives, an exit from problematic or disadvantaged circumstances, and the opportunity to turn their lives around

(Kelty et al., 2010), and therefore worth the risk. Thus, today's military tends to attract young people from somewhat lower socioeconomic backgrounds (especially racial/ethnic minorities from lower-income families), as well as those who face significant risks as they transition into adulthood (e.g., those with a history of problems at school or delinquency) (Kelty et al., 2010; Segal and Segal, 2004; Teachman and Tedrow, 2014). Military service is widely viewed as a potential break in the intergenerational transmission of inequality, although it does not always live up to this potential (Bailey, 2013). It is important to note, however, that the military pathway is not open to all, with ineligibility being due to, for example, overweight, mental health concerns, and substance use (Mission: Readiness Military Leaders for Kids, 2009). Young adults with a criminal record may also be ineligible to join the military, and with few exceptions, a high school diploma is an eligibility requirement (Mission: Readiness Military Leaders for Kids, 2009).

As noted, the introduction of all-volunteer military forces led to far greater diversity both demographically and socioeconomically. For example, African Americans and Latino/as are significantly overrepresented in the military relative to the general population, and immigrants now make up 5 percent of the active duty forces. The military also has seen a large-scale influx of women (who now make up 15 percent of the forces) and the rapid expansion of their roles, including combat in the most recent military engagements in the Middle East. Furthermore, with the repeal of the federal Don't Ask Don't Tell policy in 2010 (which had been in effect since the mid-1990s), the service of gays and lesbians has become more visible (Bailey, 2013; Kelty et al., 2010). Thus, just as young adulthood has changed historically, the experiences of young adults in the military have evolved.

Military service is widely assumed to have profound effects on the life course. Understanding what those effects are, however, is challenging because servicemen and women are what is known as a "selective" population. That is, as is true for any sort of national service, people who join the military are likely to be different from people who do not, and those differences may be related to their general adjustment and functioning in the short and long terms. Consequently, whether the observed outcomes of those in the military reflect the causal influences of military service or the factors that selected people into the military in the first place can be difficult to determine. Still, when studies include controls for these selection biases, results suggest that military service does influence the lives of young men and women. Those effects often are a mix of positive and negative, with the mental stresses and physical risks of deployment undercutting some of the potential social and economic advantages of serving (MacLean and Elder, 2007; Sheppard et al., 2010).

The various social roles and activities discussed in Chapter 3 are a window into how the military can affect the life trajectories of young people who serve. The tendency in the general population for young adults to delay family formation until later in their 20s is less pronounced in the military. Indeed, young adults in the military are more likely than civilians in the same age range to marry, and when they do marry, they tend to do so at younger ages. Among junior military personnel, 36 percent of men and 37 percent of women are married; among their similarly aged civilian counterparts with comparable earnings, only 24 percent of men and 33 percent of women are married (Clever and Segal, 2013).

The same trend can be seen in fertility and parenting. In 2012, 43.9 percent of active duty members had children, and for 42,081 members this was their first child, with 53.1 percent of these first-time parents being aged 20-25 (DoD, 2013). The average age at which active duty members have their first child varies across the different branches of service, with the highest average age occurring among Air Force members (26.2) and the lowest among Marine Corps members (24.0) (DoD, 2013). Many features of military service likely facilitate this earlier family formation, including wage stability, subsidized housing (which often is based on family size and therefore sensitive to fertility), free health care, and a large military child care system. In addition, many military and civilian organizations focus on supporting military families (Huebner et al., 2009). Examples of formal military support include the Family Readiness System[11] and the Yellow Ribbon Reintegration Program[12]; examples of other formal support systems include schools, hospitals, and nonprofit organizations (e.g., YMCA Military Outreach,[13] United Service Organizations, Inc.[14]). These supports and protections may help keep families together when a spouse/parent is actively serving (and even deployed). However, formal networks alone do not ultimately change situations for families. Military families often rely primarily on informal network supports such as other unit members, friends, and family (Martin and McClure, 2000).

After service is complete, however, many of the strains of military life (including deployment) can have effects leading to a postservice divorce rate higher than that among civilians (Kelty et al., 2010; Lundquist, 2004). In general, as discussed in more detail below, the transition to civilian life can be stark and difficult overall.

Two worrisome patterns in the domain of military family life concern

---

[11] See http://www.militaryonesource.mil (accessed October 22, 2014).

[12] See http://www.yellowribbon.mil/index.php?Itemid=0 (accessed October 22, 2014).

[13] See http://www.ymca.net/military-outreach (accessed October 22, 2014).

[14] See http://www.uso.org/About-Us/The-Organization/USO-Military-Family-Programs.aspx (accessed October 22, 2014).

child maltreatment and intimate partner violence. Historically, rates of child maltreatment have been higher in the general population than in the military, reflecting the many supports and resources available to military families. Yet rates of child maltreatment in the military population also tend to spike during times of military conflict and deployment, with nearly 50 percent more cases being seen during times of deployment than at other times (Gibbs et al., 2007; McCaroll et al., 2008). The past decade and a half would then be expected to be a period in which child maltreatment has been a particular problem among members of the military, and some evidence supports that expectation. A study of child maltreatment in Texas, which has a large military population, revealed that the difference in the child maltreatment rate between the military and civilian populations reversed during the 2000s, such that the military rate was higher than the civilian rate (Rentz et al., 2007). Although these statistics are not exclusive to that population, they also are highly relevant to the young adult population. Not only do young adults make up the majority of the military (and the recently deployed), they are more likely than older service members to have young children at home. In addition, rates of intimate partner violence are higher among active duty military members than in the general population, a pattern that extends to veterans as well (Fonseca et al., 2006; Stamm, 2009).

Beyond the family context, young adulthood is when most people are in school or entering the labor market. As a result, young adults enlisting in the military without plans to make it a career are momentarily stepping outside this traditional socioeconomic attainment path. At the same time, however, service in the military is closely related to education and employment outside the military. Given the overrepresentation of young people from historically disadvantaged racial/ethnic groups in the all-volunteer forces, military service has many features that can boost their future prospects. For example, it offers better pay and greater job security than most occupations available to those who enlist, and it offers more equitable treatment than many young adults would find in the broader labor market. Moreover, the GI Bill (which was significantly expanded after September 11, 2001) offers financial support for tuition and related living expenses for veterans who wish to pursue their education (Kelty et al., 2010). This widely used benefit provides an entrée to higher education for many young adults who would otherwise likely bypass college. As a result, although young adults who serve in the military have lower educational attainment than their same-age peers through the mid-20s, they tend to catch up (although not completely) as they move into their late 20s and early 30s. In addition, with the exception of whites, young adults who serve in the military tend to earn as much or even more income than their civilian counterparts through adulthood. One socioeconomic factor to consider is that early military service is related to more migration (i.e., moving from place to place) in adulthood. This pattern is notable given that voluntary migration helps adults achieve a better fit with the labor market, increasing their long-term job prospects and, in the process, their earnings (Bailey, 2013; Kelty et al., 2010).

Young adults serving in the military thus make earlier family role transitions and have more concrete supports for socioeconomic attainment than young adults who bypass the military (especially those of similar socioeconomic and racial/ethnic backgrounds). These family and socioeconomic differences, along with the physical aspects of military training and work, would suggest that young adults in the military are in better health. Yet veterans are in no better physical shape than civilians, and they have a range of physical problems and limitations that are directly related to military service (e.g., disabilities, chronic injuries) (Kelty et al., 2010; Teachman, 2011).

Mental health is even more of a concern. Nearly one-fifth of servicemen and -women involved in the recent deployments in Iraq and Afghanistan have experienced mental disorders, with depression and posttraumatic stress disorder (PTSD) being among the most common and most often discussed (Kelty et al., 2010). For example, Hoge and colleagues (2006) report the results of two studies of large numbers of deployed service members in the Middle East. In the first study, in the early 2000s, they found that exposure to firefights and PTSD symptomatology were strongly associated and that only a small proportion (less than one-quarter) of those affected sought help. In a follow-up several years later, the link between combat exposure and PTSD remained strong, but more of those affected were seeking help, perhaps because of growing awareness of the problem (Hoge et al., 2004, 2006). Suicide also is a significant issue, with rates of suicide attempt and completion being higher among those with service experience than in the general population (Kaplan et al., 2007).

All of these mental and physical health patterns refer to military personnel of all ages, as young adults are rarely singled out in studies. Again, however, most military service members—especially those deployed for combat—are young adults.

It is also worth noting that the transition from military to civilian life, which increasingly occurs during young adulthood, can be problematic. In a short amount of time, young adults exiting the military go from strong daily institutional support and oversight to considerable daily self-direction. The pace and pervasiveness of this transition can overwhelm one's coping capacity. In recognition of this problem, the U.S. Departments of Defense, Labor, and Veterans Affairs offer the Transition Assistance Program (DoD, 2014).

Given the special relevance of military service to the transition from adolescence to adulthood, more attention is warranted to the specific segment of the military consisting of young adults. Young adult servicemen and -women are different from other servicemen and -women, and today's servicemen and -women are different from their counterparts in the past. Those differences need to be understood.

CONCLUSIONS AND RECOMMENDATIONS

For some, national service is a logical next step after college; for those who do not go on to college, it can be a means for social incorporation, skill development, and network building. If national service is to provide such an alternative to college, especially for disadvantaged youth, it must provide at least some of the scaffolds (mentoring, counseling, education and training, communication, guided practice in leadership and teamwork) that are built into curricular and cocurricular college life. Although the primary goal of military service is clearly national security, it does provide this sort of scaffolding and member development, if only as incentives for service and to support its primary goal. In contrast, other forms of national service, particularly those under the CNCS umbrella, are increasingly moving away from an emphasis on member development. No doubt, investing in member development is challenging because national service programs are designed to respond to the needs of communities, and developing the capacities of those who serve can pose competing priorities for funding and allocation of staff. For example, one criticism leveled at national service is that engaging well-meaning but inexperienced people for short-term stints in service and allocating valuable resources to their training may not be particularly helpful to the host sites and communities. In 1999, CNCS invested in an 8-year study of the impact of its programs on members. As discussed in this chapter, however, programs are no longer expected to focus on or assess member development. The committee views this shift as a lost opportunity to optimize the transition to adulthood, especially for disadvantaged youth.

Thus, to help enhance young adults' health, safety, and well-being, it would be beneficial to revive the historical emphasis on member development, including educational benefits as a reward for service (e.g., the GI Bill for World War II veterans, deferred college loans for Peace Corps volunteers). President Clinton invoked these and other precedents when he made the case for the AmeriCorps educational stipend—based on a reciprocal contract between the nation and those who serve it. National service has been promoted as an antidote to youth unemployment (Boteach et al., 2009), and national panel studies have shown that volunteering increases the odds of future gainful employment across racial/ethnic, gender, and age groups, and especially for people with low levels of education (Spera et al., 2013). Overall, although more rigorous experimental and long-term studies clearly are needed, existing evidence indicates that national service programs can have a positive impact on young adults' health, safety, and well-being. Accordingly, we make the following recommendation:

Recommendation 5-1: The Corporation for National and Community Service, the U.S. Department of Labor, and other entities that fund service programs should expand and improve opportunities for service for all young adults. They also should emphasize member development (in addition to community impact) in program evaluations, including the short- and long-term effects of service on participants' health and well-being.

Potential strategies for implementing this recommendation include the following:

- Develop a leadership pipeline into the public and nonprofit sectors, linking skill development in service with these career opportunities.
- Increase diversity in the leadership of service programs because most programs serve low-income communities, and leadership matters in the way community service is framed and provided.
- Increase interest among more federal agencies (the U.S. Departments of Justice, Labor, and Education) in the potential of service for the development of human capital. Examples of funding from sources other than the Corporation for National and Community Service already exist (e.g., U.S. Department of Labor funding for YouthBuild and the Civic Justice Corps). In July 2013, President Obama issued an executive order for a Task Force on the Expansion of National Service, tasking 20 different federal agencies to consider how they could tap into national service to accomplish their missions.
- Expand incentives that encourage service:
  - Encourage more colleges and universities (e.g., those in the Campus Compact) to match the educational stipends earned by AmeriCorps members. Roughly 100 colleges now match the award.
  - Provide more opportunities for college loan forgiveness to encourage individuals to enter national service. Expand loan forgiveness programs to link national service opportunities to areas in which community needs are identified (professional corps, law school legal aid). (Such models are developing in Michigan and Pennsylvania.)
  - Extend local and municipal credit for military service in the civil service employment test to civic service programs.
  - Where feasible, provide opportunities for future assistance in the labor market, such as by having members demonstrate competence that can lead to occupational certification or providing information on jobs and credible references.

Finally, further research is needed on national service among young adults and its role in improving their health, safety, and well-being. The following three areas are priorities for research on national service, including military service, to better inform salient policy and programs, with particular emphasis on reaching and involving disadvantaged youth:

- Identify factors that contribute to and enhance civic engagement and increase involvement in national service among young adults.
- Conduct more rigorous experimental studies to determine how civic engagement and national service impact trajectories of the health, safety, and well-being of young adult participants.
- Give specific attention to institutional supports and individual characteristics that facilitate successful transitions from national service to education, employment, social relationships, and citizenship.

REFERENCES

Abt Associates. 2004. *Serving country and community: A longitudinal study of service in AmeriCorps. Early findings.* Washington, DC: CNCS.

Abt Associates. 2008. *Still serving: Measuring the eight-year impact of AmeriCorps on alumni.* Washington, DC: CNCS.

Abt Associates. 2011. *National evaluation of youth corps: Findings at follow-up.* Washington, DC: CNCS.

Bailey, A. K. 2013. Veteran status and spatial mobility across the life course. In *Life course perspectives on military service*, edited by J. M. Wilmoth and A. S. London. New York: Routledge. Pp. 185-199.

Beaumont, E. 2012. *What does recent research suggest about civic learning and civic action in young adults 18-30?: Some insights and foundations for further work.* http://www.spencer.org/resources/content/3/9/2/documents/ElizabethBeaumont.pdf (accessed August 25, 2014).

Boteach, M., J. Moses, and S. Sagawa. 2009. *National service and youth unemployment: Strategies for job creation amid economic recovery.* http://cdn.americanprogress.org/wp-content/uploads/issues/2009/11/pdf/nation_service.pdf (accessed August 18, 2014).

Bowman, N., J. Brandenberger, D. Lapsley, P. Hill, and J. Quaranto. 2010. Serving in college, flourishing in adulthood: Does community engagement during the college years predict adult well-being? *Applied Psychology: Health and Well-Being* 2(1):14-34.

Calvert, M., M. Emery, and S. Kinsey. 2013. *Youth programs as builders of social capital.* Hoboken, NJ: Jossey-Bass.

CIRCLE (The Center for Information and Research on Civic Learning and Engagement). 2012. *Young voters in the 2012 presidential election: The educational gap remains.* Medford, MA: CIRCLE.

Clever, M., and D. R. Segal. 2013. The demographics of military children and families. *The Future of Children* 23(2):13-39.

CNCS (Corporation for National and Community Service). 2010. *Helping all Americans serve their country: Progress on the Obama Administration's service vision.* http://www.nationalservice.gov/sites/default/files/documents/10_0421_wh_serviceagenda.pdf (accessed August 15, 2014).

CNCS. 2011. *Corporation for National and Community Service strategic plan 2011-2015.* http://www.nationalservice.gov/newsroom/marketing/fact-sheets/2011-2015-strategic-plan (accessed August 18, 2014).

CNCS. 2014a. *AmeriCorps NCCC.* http://www.nationalservice.gov/programs/americorps/americorps-nccc (accessed August 18, 2014).

CNCS. 2014b. *Fiscal Year 2014.* http://www.nationalservice.gov/about/budget-and-performance/budget/fiscal-year-2014 (accessed August 21, 2014).

CNCS. 2014c. *Segal AmeriCorps education award frequently asked questions.* http://www.nationalservice.gov/documents/education-award-faqs (accessed August 21, 2014).

CNCS. 2014d. *University of Arizona.* http://www.nationalservice.gov/programs/americorps/segal-americorps-education-award/matching-institutions/University-of-Arizona (accessed August 14, 2014).

Commission on Youth Voting and Civic Knowledge. 2013. *All together now: Collaboration and innovation for youth engagement.* Medford, MA: CIRCLE.

Constitutional Rights Foundation. 2001. *A guide to effective citizenship through AmeriCorps.* Los Angeles, CA: Constitutional Rights Foundation.

Dalton, R. J. 2004. *Democratic challenges, democratic choices: The erosion of political support in advanced industrial democracies.* Oxford, UK: Oxford University Press.

Dalton, R. J. 2008. *Citizen politics: Public opinion and political parties in advanced industrial democracies.* Washington, DC: Congressional Quarterly Press.

Dávila, A., and M. T. Mora. 2007. *Do gender and ethnicity affect civic engagement and academic progress.* Medford, MA: CIRCLE.

DoD (U.S. Department of Defense). 2013. *2012 demographics: Profile of the military community.* Washington, DC: Office of the Deputy Undersecretary of Defense.

DoD. 2014. *Transition Assistance Program.* http://prhome.defense.gov/Portals/52/Documents/RFM/TVPO/files/TVPO%20101%20(FINAL).pdf (accessed July 23, 2014).

File, T. 2014. *Young-adult voting: An analysis of presidential elections, 1964-2012.* Washington, DC: U.S. Census Bureau.

Finlay, A. K., and C. Flanagan. 2008. *Institutional impacts of AmeriCorps service work for vulnerable and nonvulnerable populations.* Paper presented at the biennial meeting of the Society for Research on Adolescence Conference, Chicago, IL.

Finlay, A. K., and C. Flanagan. 2009. *Making educational progress: Links to civic engagement during the transition to adulthood.* http://www.civicyouth.org/PopUps/WorkingPapers/WP_67_Finley_Flanagan.pdf (accessed August 18, 2014).

Finlay, A. K., C. Flanagan, and L. Wray-Lake. 2011. Civic engagement patterns and transitions over 8 years: The AmeriCorps National Study. *Developmental Psychology* 47(6):1728.

Flanagan, C. 2013. *Teenage citizens: The political theories of the young.* Cambridge, MA: Harvard University Press.

Flanagan, C., and M. Bundick. 2011. Civic engagement and psychosocial well-being in college students. *Liberal Education* 97(2):15-25.

Flanagan, C., and T. Kim. 2013. *Boosting civic engagement: A longitudinal study of AmeriCorps.* Paper presented at Community Engagement: Applying What We Know, Annual Meetings of the American Psychological Association, Honolulu, HI.

Flanagan, C., and P. Levine. 2010. Civic engagement and the transition to adulthood. *The Future of Children* 20(1):159-179.

Flanagan, C., P. Levine, and R. Settersten. 2009. *Civic engagement and the changing transition to adulthood.* Medford, MA: CIRCLE.

Flanagan, C. A., T. Kim, J. Collura, and M. A. Kopish. 2014. Community service and adolescents' social capital. *Journal of Research on Adolescence.* doi: 10.1111/jora.12137 (epub ahead of print).

Fonseca, C. A., K. B. Schmaling, C. Stoever, C. Gutierrez, A. W. Blume, and M. L. Russell. 2006. Variables associated with intimate partner violence in a deploying military sample. *Military Medicine* 171(7):627-631.

Frumkin, P., J. Jastrzab, M. Vaaler, A. Greeney, R. T. Grimm, K. Cramer, and N. Dietz. 2009. Inside national service: AmeriCorps' impact on participants. *Journal of Policy Analysis and Management* 28(3):394-416.

Gibbs, D. A., S. L. Martin, L. L. Kupper, and R. E. Johnson. 2007. Child maltreatment in enlisted soldiers' families during combat-related deployments. *Journal of the American Medical Association* 298(5):528-535.

Ginwright, S. 2011. Hope, healing, and care: Pushing the boundaries of civic engagement for African American youth. *Liberal Education* 97(2):34-39.

Godsay, S., K. Kawashima-Ginsberg, A. Kiesa, and P. Levine. 2012. *That's not democracy: How out-of-school youth engage in civic life and what stands in their way.* Medford, MA: CIRCLE.

Hoge, C. W., C. A. Castro, S. C. Messer, D. McGurk, D. I. Cotting, and R. L. Koffman. 2004. Combat duty in Iraq and Afghanistan, mental health problems, and barriers to care. *New England Journal of Medicine* 351(1):13-22.

Hoge, C. W., J. L. Auchterlonie, and C. S. Milliken. 2006. Mental health problems, use of mental health services, and attrition from military service after returning from deployment to Iraq or Afghanistan. *Journal of the American Medical Association* 295(9):1023-1032.

Huebner, A. J., J. A. Mancini, G. L. Bowen, and D. K. Orthner. 2009. Shadowed by war: Building community capacity to support military families. *Family Relations* 58(2):216-228.

Jennings, M. K., and L. Stoker. 2004. Social trust and civic engagement across time and generations. *Acta Politica* 39(4):342-379.

Kahne, J., and E. Middaugh. 2009. Democracy for some: The civic opportunity gap in high school. In *Policies for youth civic engagement*, edited by J. Youniss and P. Levine. Nashville, TN: Vanderbilt University Press. Pp. 29-58.

Kahne, J., N.-J. Lee, and J. T. Feezell. 2013. The civic and political significance of online participatory cultures among youth transitioning to adulthood. *Journal of Information Technology & Politics* 10(1):1-20.

Kaplan, M. S., N. Huguet, B. H. McFarland, and J. T. Newsom. 2007. Suicide among male veterans: A prospective population-based study. *Journal of Epidemiology and Community Health* 61(7):619-624.

Kawashima-Ginsberg, K., and N. Thomas. 2013. *Civic engagement and political leadership among women: A call for solutions.* Medford, MA: CIRCLE.

Keeter, S., C. Zukin, M. Andolina, and K. Jenkins. 2002. *The civic and political health of the nation: A generational portrait.* Medford, MA: CIRCLE.

Kelty, R., M. Kleykamp, and D. R. Segal. 2010. The military and the transition to adulthood. *The Future of Children* 20(1):181-207.

Kinder, D. R. 2006. Politics and the life cycle. *Science* 312:1905-1908.

Lawless, J. L., and R. L. Fox. 2013. *Girls just wanna not run: The gender gap in young Americans' political ambition.* Washington, DC: Women and Politics Institute, American University.

Lundquist, J. H. 2004. When race makes no difference: Marriage and the military. *Social Forces* 83(2):731-757.

MacLean, A., and G. H. Elder, Jr. 2007. Military service in the life course. *Sociology* 33(1): 175-196.

Martin, J. A., and P. McClure. 2000. Today's active duty military family: The evolving challenges of military family life. In *The military family: A practice guide for human service providers*, edited by J. A. Martin, L. N. Rosen, and L. R. Sparacino. Westport, CT: Praeger. Pp. 3-24.

McBride, A. M., and Y. Lee. 2012. Institutional predictors of volunteer retention: The case of AmeriCorps national service. *Administration & Society* 44(3):343-366.

McCarroll, J. E., Z. Fan, J. H. Newby, and R. J. Ursano. 2008. Trends in U.S. army child maltreatment reports: 1990-2004. *Child Abuse Review* 17(2):108-118.

Mission: Readiness Military Leaders for Kids. 2009. *Ready, willing, and unable to serve.* Washington, DC: Mission: Readiness Military Leaders for Kids.

Moore, C., J. P. Allen, K. H. Herre, S. Philliber, and G. Kuperminc. 1994. Teen outreach: A successful program preventing school failure, school dropout, and teen pregnancy. In *Using what we know about at-risk youth: Lessons from the field*, edited by R. C. Morris. Lancaster, PA: Technomic Publishing. Pp. 117-128.

Musick, M. A., and J. Wilson. 2003. Volunteering and depression: The role of psychological and social resources in different age groups. *Social Science & Medicine* 56(2):259-269.

Norris, P. 2002. *Democratic Phoenix: Reinventing political activism.* Cambridge, UK: Cambridge University Press.

Norris, P. 2011. *Democratic deficit: Critical citizens revisited.* Cambridge, UK: Cambridge University Press.

Oesterle, S., M. K. Johnson, and J. T. Mortimer. 2004. Volunteerism during the transition to adulthood: A life course perspective. *Social Forces* 82(3):1123-1149.

Pacheco, J. S., and E. Plutzer. 2008. Political participation and cumulative disadvantage: The impact of economic and social hardship on young citizens. *Journal of Social Issues* 64(3):571-593.

Piliavin, J. A., and E. Siegl. 2007. Health benefits of volunteering in the Wisconsin Longitudinal Study. *Journal of Health and Social Behavior* 48(4):450-464.

Piliavin, J. A., and E. Siegl. 2014. Health and well-being consequences of formal volunteering. In *Handbook of prosocial behavior*, edited by D. Schroeder and W. G. Graziano. Oxford, UK: Oxford University Press.

Pintor, R. L., and M. Gratschew. 2002. *Voter turnout since 1945: A global report.* Stockholm, Sweden: International Institute for Democracy and Electoral Assistance.

Rentz, E. D., S. W. Marshall, D. Loomis, C. Casteel, S. L. Martin, and D. A. Gibbs. 2007. Effect of deployment on the occurrence of child maltreatment in military and nonmilitary families. *American Journal of Epidemiology* 165(10):1199-1206.

Rotolo, T. 2000. A time to join, a time to quit: The influence of life cycle transitions on voluntary association membership. *Social Forces* 78(3):1133-1161.

Schmidt, J. A., L. Shumow, and H. Kackar. 2007. Adolescents' participation in service activities and its impact on academic, behavioral, and civic outcomes. *Journal of Youth and Adolescence* 36(2):127-140.

Segal, D. R., and M. W. Segal. 2004. America's military population. *Population Bulletin* 59(4).

Sheppard, S. C., J. W. Malatras, and A. C. Israel. 2010. The impact of deployment on U.S. military families. *American Psychologist* 65(6):599.

Spannring, R., G. Ogris, and W. Gaiser. 2008. *Youth and political participation in Europe: Results of the comparative study EUYOPART.* Germany: Barbara Budrich Publishers.

Spera, C., R. Ghertner, A. Nerino, and A. DiTommaso. 2013. *Volunteering as a pathway to employment: Does volunteering increase odds of finding a job for the out of work.* Washington, DC: Office of Research and Evaluation, CNCS.

Stamm, S. 2009. Intimate partner violence in the military: Securing our country, starting with the home. *Family Court Review* 47(2):321-339.

Syvertsen, A. K., L. Wray-Lake, C. A. Flanagan, D. Wayne Osgood, and L. Briddell. 2011. Thirty-year trends in U.S. adolescents' civic engagement: A story of changing participation and educational differences. *Journal of Research on Adolescence* 21(3):586-594.

Teachman, J. 2011. Are veterans healthier? Military service and health at age 40 in the all-volunteer era. *Social Science Research* 40(1):326-335.

Teachman, J., and L. Tedrow. 2014. Delinquent behavior, the transition to adulthood, and the likelihood of military enlistment. *Social Science Research* 45:46-55.

Thoits, P. A., and L. N. Hewitt. 2001. Volunteer work and well-being. *Journal of Health and Social Behavior* 42(2):115-131.

Verba, S., K. L. Schlozman, and H. E. Brady. 1995. *Voice and equality: Civic voluntarism in American politics.* Cambridge, UK: Cambridge University Press.

Verba, S., N. Burns, and K. L. Schlozman. 2003. Unequal at the starting line: Creating participatory inequalities across generations and among groups. *The American Sociologist* 34(1-2):45-69.

Watts, M. W. 1999. Are there typical age curves in political behavior? The "age invariance" hypothesis and political socialization. *Political Psychology* 20(3):477-499.

Youniss, J., S. Bales, V. Christmas-Best, M. Diversi, M. McLaughlin, and R. Silbereisen. 2002. Youth civic engagement in the twenty-first century. *Journal of Research on Adolescence* 12(1):121-148.

Zaff, J. F., J. Youniss, and C. M. Gibson. 2009. *An inequitable invitation to citizenship: Non-college-bound youth and civic engagement.* Washington, DC: Philanthropy for Active Civic Engagement.

6

Public Health

Key Findings

- Young adults are at elevated risk of morbidity and mortality in a surprising variety of ways compared with adolescents and older adults.
- Policies and programs aimed at reducing the incidence and prevalence of disease and injury among young adults can be improved by taking a developmental perspective.
- The differential effects of public health interventions on subpopulations of young adults have not been adequately explored. Efforts to address health inequities will have to account for the transitional experiences of young adults, given that the effects of interventions during this period of life are likely to last for several decades.
- Mobile digital media and social networking have the potential to play a pivotal role as vehicles for public health interventions, and research on the effectiveness of these technologies is a high priority.
- The most successful public health interventions for young adults have been those that involve comprehensive, multilevel strategies using ecological approaches in multiple channels and venues to influence changes at the individual, organizational, and societal levels that can be sustained over time.

- The heightened vulnerability of young adults to a variety of health and safety risks supports an extension of some protective health policies beyond the legal definition of adulthood.
- An effective approach to public health policy and practice focused on young adults requires better integration and coordination of federal and state public health programs and effective use of the preventive services component of the Patient Protection and Affordable Care Act.

When their health, safety, and well-being are viewed from a developmental life-course perspective, young adults are at elevated risk of morbidity and mortality in a surprising variety of ways compared with adolescents and older adults. What makes this surprising is that conventional wisdom suggests young adults ought to be in peak physical condition, given that they are beyond the pitfalls of adolescence and not yet experiencing the declines of aging. The vulnerability is even greater among those of lower socioeconomic position and from racial and ethnic minorities, who are exposed to greater risks and dangers than their more advantaged peers and lack safety nets to protect them (NIHCM, 2007). Policy makers and practitioners have recognized that the health, safety, and well-being of adolescents can be enhanced—during adolescence and thereafter—by basing policy and practice on an integrated understanding of this distinct period of development. A key conclusion of this report is that the health, safety, and well-being of young adults can similarly benefit from bringing a life-course perspective to bear on public health policies and programs and on the delivery of health care.

As chronic health conditions become the key health challenge for the 21st century, community-based prevention efforts will increasingly become an important focus for both the public health and health care delivery systems. It is important to recognize the mutually reinforcing connection between effective population-level and individual-level interventions. At the same time needs for treatment are reduced through prevention, public health activities can help increase the effectiveness of health interventions. In fact, Milstein and colleagues (2011) estimate that if protective public health interventions were integrated with coverage and care approaches, in 10 years they could save 90 percent more lives in the United States and in 25 years 140 percent more lives than could be saved through coverage and care approaches without such interventions (Milstein et al., 2011).

This chapter addresses policies and programs undertaken by the public health system (public agencies and their partners at the national, state, and community levels) aimed at reducing the incidence and prevalence of disease and injury among young adults. The next chapter addresses the delivery of health care services for young adults, including both preventive services and treatment delivered by primary care physicians and other health care providers. The chapter begins with a brief overview of public health perspectives and activities. After highlighting the public health issues associated with young adulthood, we then review the literature on the effectiveness of public health initiatives, particularly those targeting health and safety problems with elevated prevalence among young adults, and summarize features of public health interventions that have been successful in reducing the risk of morbidity and mortality among young adults. Next we give special attention to the potentially pivotal role of mobile digital media and social networking as vehicles for public health interventions. We then turn to the role of public health policies, such as those related to the purchase of alcohol and tobacco, in protecting the health, safety, and well-being of young adults. In the next section, we look at the extent to which state and federal public health programs focus on those issues most salient to young adults, and on how these programs can be improved and better coordinated to best address these issues. The final section presents conclusions and recommendations.

OVERVIEW OF PUBLIC HEALTH PERSPECTIVES AND ACTIVITIES

The mission of public health has been defined as "organized community efforts aimed at the prevention of disease and promotion of health. It links many disciplines and rests upon the scientific core of epidemiology" (IOM, 1988, p. 41). Figure 6-1 shows how the different sectors involved, while acting individually, also work together as a public health system in pursuing health goals. Moreover, contemporary public health activities are grounded in an ecological approach that takes account of cross-level influences on individual health behaviors and conditions, including the natural, social, and built environments and the contributions of other government agencies or sectors—such as transportation, environment, economic development, and education—that influence population health (IOM, 2011, 2012b; Sallis et al., 2008). Similarly, public health interventions encompass a wide array of policies and programs, ranging from tax policies to media campaigns.

Although broad action on multiple determinants involving diverse public and private actors is needed to achieve the greatest effects on population health, the governmental public health infrastructure serves an essential coordinating role and, in many contexts, service delivery and regulatory roles (IOM, 2011). In the context of ensuring the health, safety, and well-being of young adults, we focus here on the 10 essential activities of state and local public health agencies listed in Box 6-1, which have become widely accepted in the field (IOM, 2011).

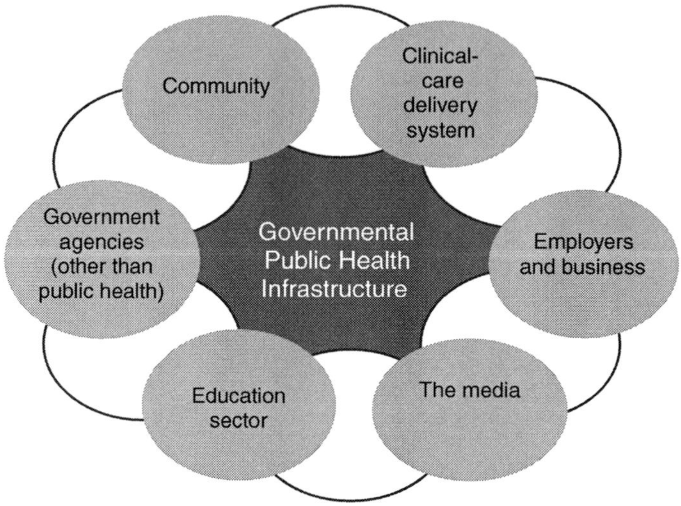

FIGURE 6-1 The intersectoral public health system.
SOURCE: IOM, 2011.

BOX 6-1
10 Essential Public Health Services

1. Monitor health status to identify and solve community health problems.
2. Diagnose and investigate health problems and health hazards in the community.
3. Inform, educate, and empower people about health issues.
4. Mobilize community partnerships and action to identify and solve health problems.
5. Develop policies and plans that support individual and community health efforts.
6. Enforce laws and regulations that protect health and ensure safety.
7. Link people to needed personal health services and ensure the provision of health care when otherwise unavailable.
8. Ensure a competent public and personal health care workforce.
9. Evaluate the effectiveness, accessibility, and quality of personal and population-based health services.
10. Conduct research to attain new insights and innovative solutions to health problems.

SOURCE: IOM, 2011.

The leadership role of public health agencies should not be regarded as synonymous with a directive role. When public health was focused primarily on infectious disease control, its activities often were based on coercive legal authority. However, as the scope of public health has broadened to include preventing chronic disease, promoting healthy communities, and reducing or even eliminating health disparities, collaborative and facilitative approaches have become predominant. Greater attention is being paid to mobilizing and engaging important stakeholders, including community-based organizations, in promoting public health. This multisectoral approach is based on the premise that local agencies and organizations have a better understanding of the local context in which public problems can be studied and solutions can be developed, executed, and sustained (Israel et al., 2008; Minkler and Wallerstein, 2008; Ramanadhan et al., 2012).

It must be noted that the list of essential public health services today would also include ensuring equity within and across different population groups. Despite tremendous investments in research, planning, and deployment of public health strategies and their success, it has become clear that the benefits of these programs are accruing unequally across socioeconomic and racial/ethnic groups (Spalter-Roth et al., 2005). The challenge of erasing persistent health disparities has been the subject of extensive attention in recent years (IOM, 2002, 2012c), and the contributing social and individual factors are now better understood. These factors—which include social class, race and ethnicity, social and economic policies, racism, geography, housing, and communication inequalities, among many others—appear to explain why certain groups experience greater adversity due to risk conditions and also are often unable to take advantage of programs and policies that should ameliorate such conditions (IOM, 2011). A great deal of this work has focused on either childhood poverty or the experience of adults, with much less attention to young adults. But it is clear that any efforts to address health disparities will have to account for the experience of this important age group, as the effects they experience are likely to last for several decades.

PRIORITY PUBLIC HEALTH ISSUES FOR YOUNG ADULTS

Some recent reviews of young adult health have pointed to encouraging trends, such as decreases in rates of suicide, gonorrhea, and cigarette use[1] (Mulye et al., 2009; Park et al., 2006, 2014). However, the mortality rate for young adults aged 20-24 is 93.5 per 100,000, compared with

---

[1] Although use of cigarettes is declining, the use of other tobacco products, such as electronic cigarettes, may be increasing (King et al., 2013).

60.8 among older adolescents (aged 15-19) and 17.4 among younger adolescents (aged 10-14), showing a substantial increase with age (CDC, 2014a). Young adults are at greater risk for short- and long-term impacts on health and have worse health outcomes than adolescents in many areas (Park et al., 2014). Overall, as compared with other age groups, young adults have the highest rate of death and injury from motor vehicles, homicides, mental health problems, sexually transmitted infections (STIs), and substance abuse (Neinstein, 2013). Yet in general, most of the leading causes of illness and death among young adults are largely preventable (Mulye et al., 2009).

Important developmental changes occurring during young adulthood can promote or compromise health and well-being (Harris et al., 2006; Mulye et al., 2009; Neinstein, 2013). Most young adults are transitioning from direct parental supervision to living on their own, which can create a period of vulnerability to unsafe and unhealthy behaviors. Many young adults need help coping with stressful circumstances in school or on the job, and a significant subset are at risk of experiencing acute emotional distress and the onset of major mental disorders (Garcia, 2010). These conditions can, in turn, impact education and workplace achievement in the short term as well as throughout life. There are also profound health and well-being consequences for young adults who have children (as discussed in Chapter 3). Moroever, risk-taking behaviors associated with morbidity and mortality across the life span tend to emerge or peak during young adulthood, with important immediate and long-term health consequences (Park et al., 2006, 2014). For example, use of tobacco and low levels of fitness and poor nutrition increase the probability of developing diseases such as cardiovascular and pulmonary disease and cancer later in life (Santelli et al., 2013). The collective impact of these problems is noticeable at the public health level, where little change in risky behavior has occurred over the past decade. And while in some ways, young adults appear relatively healthy, many public health concerns for young adults remain inadequately and ineffectively unaddressed (Park et al., 2006, 2014).

> "Many people think, 'you just have the blues, and you will get over it.' Many people don't recognize the long-term effects in terms of employment, general quality of life, et cetera."*

For the past 30 years, *Healthy People* has set the national objectives for improving public health. *Healthy People 2020* focuses more on adolescents and young adults as compared with previous decades (Koh et al.,

* Quotations are from members of the young adult advisory group during their discussions with the committee.

2011). Based on guidance from national experts, *Healthy People 2020* identifies 41 "core indicators for adolescent and young adult health," which concentrate on individual outcomes, as well as systems that influence health for these populations.[2] The indicators span seven domains: health care (health insurance coverage, well care, immunizations), healthy development (adult connection, graduation, sleep, transition planning[3]), injury/violence prevention (motor vehicle crashes, riding with a drinking driver, graduated driver licensing laws, homicide, exposure to violence, physical fighting), mental health (suicide rate and attempts, depression, treatment), substance abuse (marijuana use, binge drinking, treatment), sexual and reproductive health (pregnancy prevention, STIs, HIV, reproductive health services), and prevention of chronic disease (oral health, hearing, obesity, physical activity, tobacco) (HHS, 2012a). Although all of the indicators are important for the health, safety, and well-being of young adults, this chapter focuses on an illustrative selection of public health challenges that are related most specifically to the health, safety, and long-term well-being of young adults and that pose substantial public health burdens—motor vehicle injuries; homicide and nonfatal assaultive injuries; sexual assault and intimate partner violence; mental health disorders and suicide; substance abuse; sexual and reproductive health; and chronic disease prevention, including decreasing obesity, reducing tobacco use, and increasing immunizations. Box 6-2 presents key findings on the public health challenges for young adults.

In addition, race, ethnicity, sex, sexual identity, age, disability, education, socioeconomic position, and geographic location all are associated with the health and safety of young adults (Mulye et al., 2009). Among both adolescents and young adults, certain populations have higher rates of risky behaviors, such as unhealthy eating, lack of physical activity, unprotected sexual activity, substance use, and unsafe driving (Park et al., 2014). Some examples are presented in Box 6-3. Major gender differences exist, as well as considerable ethnic and racial disparities, with non-Hispanic black and American Indian/Alaska Native young adults faring worse in many areas (Park et al., 2014). As Box 6-3 shows, many statistics are worse for certain populations than for others, but it is important to note that the differences go both ways. For instance, black males have a higher homicide rate than white males in this age group (100.3 versus 11.4 homicides per 100,000), but the reverse is true for the use of marijuana between early adolescence and young adulthood (Chen and Jacobson, 2012; Smith and Cooper, 2013).

---

[2] See http://www.healthypeople.gov/2020/learn/Draft_Core_Indicators_Web.pdf (accessed October 22, 2014) for a full list of indicators.

[3] Transition planning refers to individuals with special health care needs whose health care provider has discussed transition planning from pediatric to adult health care.

BOX 6-2
Illustrative Public Health Challenges for Young Adults

Below are some of the public health challenges that impose the greatest burdens on the health, safety, and well-being of young adults. They are presented using the *Healthy People 2020* adolescent and young adult domains as a guide.

Injury and Violence Prevention

Reducing Motor Vehicle Injuries

- Motor vehicle crashes account for the largest percentage (approximately 20 per 100,000) of unintentional injury fatalities for 18- to 25-year-olds in the United States (Neinstein, 2013).
- Nonfatal injury rates also are higher among 18- to 25-year-olds than among 12- to 17-year-olds and 26- to 34-year-olds (Neinstein, 2013).
- In 2010, motor vehicle–related hospitalization and treatment of young adults in emergency departments cost the health care system $9 billion (Neinstein, 2013).
- In 2012, 32 percent of 21- to 24-year-olds involved in fatal motor vehicle crashes had blood alcohol levels of .08 or higher, followed by those aged 25-34 (29 percent) (versus 18 percent for those aged 16-20) (NHTSA, 2013).
- Drivers in their 20s accounted for 23 percent of drivers involved in fatal crashes and 27 percent of distracted driving fatalities, 34 percent of which involved use of cell phones (NHTSA, 2014).

Reducing Homicide

- Homicide is the second leading cause of mortality for 18- to 25-year-olds (Neinstein, 2013).
- Young adults aged 18-24 had the highest homicide rate of any age group but also experienced the greatest rate (22 percent) of decline from 2002 (15.2 per 100,000) to 2011 (11.9 per 100,000) (Smith and Cooper, 2013).
- Between 1981 and 2010, firearms accounted for nearly 80 percent of all homicides among 10- to 24-year-olds, and on average, firearms homicides occurred at 3.7 times the annual rate of nonfirearms homicides (CDC, 2013b).

Reducing Nonfatal Assault

- Males aged 18-25 are 70 percent more likely to be assaulted than 12- to 17-year-old males and 50 percent more likely than 26- to 34-year-old males (Neinstein, 2013).
- Young adults aged 18-25 are 220 percent more likely than 12- to 17-year-olds and 75 percent more likely than 26- to 34-year-olds to be injured by firearms (Neinstein, 2013).
- In 2011, more than 700,000 10- to 24-year-olds were treated in emergency departments for physical assault injuries (CDC, 2012).
- In 2011, the nonfatal assault-related injury rate was highest for those aged 20-24, with a rate of 1,867.5 per 100,000 for males and 1,215.1 per 100,000 for females (CDC, 2013d).

***Reducing Sexual Assault and Intimate Partner Violence*[a]**

- Females aged 18-34 are more likely to experience sexual violence (about 4 victimizations per 1,000) than 35- to 64-year-olds (approximately 1.5 per 1,000) (Planty et al., 2013).
- Between 2004 and 2006, more than 100,000 females and 3,500 males aged 10-24 received emergency medical care for nonfatal sexual assault injuries (Gavin et al., 2009).
- The majority of female victims (79.6 percent) experienced their first completed rape before age 25—42.2 percent before age 18 (Black et al., 2011).
- In a study of undergraduate females, almost 20 percent reported experiencing completed sexual assault since entering college (Krebs et al., 2009).
- Almost one-third of female veterans were raped or sexually assaulted while serving in the military (Natelson, 2009), and in fiscal year 2013, among the 3,337 sexual assault investigations in the military, 65 percent of victims were under 25 (DoD, 2014).
- Intimate partner rape, physical violence, and/or stalking has been experienced by 35.6 percent of women and 28.5 percent of men (Black et al., 2011).
- Almost half of women (47.1 percent) and 38.6 percent of men who ever experienced intimate partner rape, physical violence, and/or stalking were aged 18-24 (Black et al., 2011).
- Intimate partner violence can lead to negative physical and mental health outcomes, ranging from gastrointestinal problems, migraines, and depression to posttraumatic stress disorder and suicidal thoughts and behavior (Randle and Graham, 2011; Stewart and Robinson, 1998).

Mental Health Conditions

Preventing Mental Health Disorders

- Approximately 75 percent of lifelong mental health disorders are manifest by age 24 (Kessler et al., 2005), and many conditions, such as depression, anxiety disorders, psychoses, and eating and personality disorders, start before age 24 and persist into adulthood (IOM and NRC, 2013; Patel et al., 2007; Paus et al., 2008).
- Data from the National Study of Drug Use and Health (NSDUH) from 2010 to 2012 indicate that 18.7 percent of 18- to 25-year-olds had had any mental illness in the past year, and 3.9 percent had had a serious mental illness (SAMHSA, 2014). In the past year, among those with any mental illness, 66.6 percent had not received mental health services, and 47 percent with a serious mental illness had not received treatment (SAMHSA, 2014).

continued

BOX 6-2 Continued

Preventing Suicide

- Suicide is the third leading cause of mortality in young adults aged 18-25 (Neinstein, 2013).
- Current young adult suicide rates are almost twice as high as those for adolescents (CDC, 2014d).

Substance Abuse

Reducing Substance Use Disorders

- Compared with adolescents, young adults have a higher rate of drug-related causes of death: 16.7 percent of all deaths among 20- to 29-year-olds have drug-related causes versus 2.2 percent among 10- to 19-year-olds (Mack, 2013).
- NSDUH data from 2012 indicate that 18.9 percent of young adults had substance dependence or abuse disorders, a rate markedly higher than that among 12- to 17-year-olds (6.1 percent) and adults 26 and over (7.0 percent) (SAMHSA, 2013).
- From adolescence to young adulthood, alcohol use increases fourfold, binge drinking (five or more alcoholic drinks on a single occasion in the past 2 weeks) fivefold, and heavy alcohol use (five or more binge drinking episodes in the past month) 10fold (SAMHSA, 2013).
- Among 16- to 34-year-olds, 21- to 25-year-olds are most likely to drive under the influence of alcohol (Neinstein, 2013).
- In 2012, 39.5 percent of 18- to 25-year-olds participated in binge drinking and 12.7 percent in heavy drinking, rates similar to those in 2011 (39.8 percent and 12.1 percent, respectively) (SAMHSA, 2013).
- Among young adults aged 18-22, full-time college students have higher binge drinking rates than non-full-time students (Neinstein, 2013).
- Rates of past-month marijuana use double from adolescence (7.6 percent) to young adulthood (18.8 percent); after age 26, rates of use drop to approximately 5 percent (SAMHSA, 2012).
- About 1.1 percent of 18- to 25-year-olds reported using cocaine in the past month, which is similar to the rate for hallucinogens (SAMHSA, 2013).
- Young adults aged 18-25 have the highest rates of abuse of prescription opioid pain relievers, attention-deficit hyperactivity disorder stimulants, and antianxiety drugs (NIH, 2014).
- Approximately 3,000 young adults died from prescription drug (mainly opioid) overdoses in 2010, which is more than the number who died from heroin and cocaine overdoses; many more needed emergency treatment (NIH, 2014).

Sexual and Reproductive Health

Reducing Unintended Pregnancies and Promoting Healthy Birth Spacing

- In 2012, the mean age of mother at first birth was 25.8, an increase from 25.6 in 2011 and from 21.4 in 1970 (Martin et al., 2013).

- The highest rates of unintended pregnancy occur in 20- to 24-year-olds (50 percent, compared with 25 percent in 25- to 44-year-olds) (Mosher et al., 2012; Neinstein, 2013). This means that about 2.6 million births between 2002 and 2006 among 20- to 24-year-olds were unintended, and these percentages have remained relatively steady since 2002 (Mosher et al., 2012).
- The percentage of unintended pregnancies ending in abortion is 37 percent among 15- to 19-year-olds and 41 percent among 20- to 24-year-olds (Neinstein, 2013).

Sexually Transmitted Infections (STIs)/HIV Prevention

- The Centers for Disease Control and Prevention (CDC) estimates that almost 20 million[b] new STIs occur yearly in the United States; 15- to 24-year-olds account for 50 percent of all new STIs, although they represent just 25 percent of the sexually experienced population (CDC, 2013c).
- Cervical and human papillomavirus (HPV) infections are the most common STIs, with 74 percent of new infections (6.2 million) each year occurring in 15- to 24-year-olds (Neinstein, 2013).
- Between 2008 and 2010, HIV rates increased (CDC, 2013e), with the highest rate of new cases occurring in 20- to 24-year-olds.

Preventing Chronic Diseases

Decreasing Obesity

- Overweight and obesity rates increase from adolescence to young adulthood. Rates are almost 50 percent in male and female 18- to 25-year-olds and are nearly 60 percent in female and more than 70 percent in male 26- to 34-year-olds (Neinstein, 2013).
- Even though young adults are doing better at meeting the recommended physical activity guidelines, about 40 percent still do not do so (Neinstein, 2013).
- In the National Health and Nutrition Examination Survey, males aged 18-24 reported about 5.4 hours a day of sedentary activity versus 7.4 hours for 12- to 17-year-old males; the corresponding figures for females were 5.7 and 8.0 hours (Neinstein, 2013).

Reducing Tobacco Use

- Approximately 90 percent of smokers start smoking by age 18, and 99 percent start by age 26 (HHS, 2012b).
- Of all age groups, young adults have the highest rate of current cigarette smoking, with approximately one of every three young adults under 26 being a smoker (HHS, 2012b).
- Among 18- to 22-year-olds, 21.3 percent of full-time college students reported smoking cigarettes in the NSDUH, compared with 37.2 percent among those not enrolled in college full time (SAMHSA, 2013).
- In 2012, among 18- to 25-year-olds, 10.7 percent had smoked cigars and 5.5 percent had used smokeless tobacco (the highest prevalence of any age group) in the past month (SAMHSA, 2013).

continued

BOX 6-2 Continued

Increasing Immunizations

- Currently, 30 percent of 19- to 26-year-old females, 2.8 percent of 19- to 21-year-old males, and 1.7 percent of 22- to 26-year-old males are initiating HPV vaccination (Kester et al., 2014).
- In 2010, 25 percent of 18- to 25-year-olds received the influenza vaccine, versus 31 percent of 26- to 34-year-olds, and only 12-16 percent of 18- to 25-year-olds received the pertussis vaccine[c] (Neinstein, 2013).

---

[a] Intimate partner violence, as defined by the National Crime Victimization Survey, includes rape or sexual assault, robbery, aggravated assault, and simple assault committed by the victim's current or former spouse, boyfriend, or girlfriend (Catalano, 2013).

[b] This estimate is based on eight common STIs: chlamydia, gonorrhea, hepatitis B virus, herpes simplex virus type 2, HIV, human papillomavirus, syphilis, and trichomoniasis.

[c] The pertussis vaccine prevents against a respiratory disease, commonly known as "whooping cough," that is highly contagious.

BOX 6-3
Illustrative Health Disparities

Below are some of the public health disparities (presented in alphabetical order) that impact the health, safety, and well-being of young adults.

Chronic Disease Prevention

- Among females over 18, the overall prevalence of obesity in 1999-2010 was 51 percent among non-Hispanic blacks, compared with 41 percent among Mexican Americans and 31 percent among non-Hispanic whites (May et al., 2013).

Homicide

- The peak rate of homicide victimization for black males occurs at the age of 23 (100.3 homicides per 100,000 population). This is almost 9 times higher than the peak rate for white males, which occurs at the age of 20 (11.4 homicides per 100,000 population) (Smith and Cooper, 2013).
- Homicide rates among black females peak at age 22 (11.8 homicides per 100,000), compared with white females, whose homicide rate is highest before the age of 2 (4.5 per 100,000) (Smith and Cooper, 2013).

Immunizations

- In females aged 18-26, there were significant increases in uptake of HPV vaccination (≥1 dose) from 2008 to 2012 (11.6 to 34.1 percent). However,

BOX 6-3 Continued

Hispanics and women with limited access to care continued to have lower rates of vaccination (Schmidt and Parsons, 2014).

Intimate Partner Violence

- The rate of intimate partner violence for females of all ages (5.9 per 1,000) is nearly six times that for men of all ages (1.1 per 1,000) (Catalano, 2013).

Mental Health Conditions

- Studies have found that 15- to 24-year-old males are more reluctant to try to find professional care for mental health problems than their female counterparts, and young indigenous and ethnic minorities may be even less likely to do so than whites (Rickwood et al., 2007). Black young adults aged 18-26 are less likely than other racial/ethnic groups to receive mental health services (Broman, 2012).
- A study of 21- to 25-year-olds found that rates of mental disorders and suicidal behavior among those with a predominantly homosexual orientation were 1.5 to 12 times higher than the rates among those with an exclusively heterosexual orientation (Fergusson et al., 2005).

Motor Vehicle Injuries

- Among 20- to 24-year-olds, rates of mortality due to motor vehicle crashes are significantly higher for males (25.8 per 100,000 population) than for females (4.2 per 100,000). The highest rates are among African American males (106.1), followed by non-Hispanic American Indian/Alaska Native males (20.6 per 100,000) (CDC, 2014a).[a]

Nonfatal Assault

- Males aged 18-25 are more than 8 times as likely as their female counterparts to be nonfatally shot (Neinstein, 2013).
- In 2012, among 20- to 24-year-olds, the unadjusted violent victimization rate was 100.6 per 1,000 for persons with disabilities and 36.6 for those without disabilities (Harrell, 2014).
- In 2012, 35.8 percent of overall hate violence survivors and victims were aged 19-29, a slight increase from 2011 (33 percent) (NCAVP, 2013).

Reproductive Health

- In 2012, among unmarried females aged 20-24, birth rates were highest among African Americans (103.5 per 1,000) and Hispanics (96.5 per 1,000), while the birth rate for non-Hispanic whites of the same age was 46.6 per 1,000 (Martin et al., 2013).

Sexual Assault

- Among 18- to 25-year-olds, females are 18 times more likely to be sexually assaulted than males (Neinstein, 2013).

continued

BOX 6-3 Continued

- Among 12- to 34-year-olds, African Americans have the highest rates of sexual assault; among 18- to 25-year-olds, they are 63 percent more likely than whites and 216 percent more likely than Hispanics to be sexually assaulted (Neinstein, 2013).

Sexually Transmitted Infections (STIs)/HIV Prevention

- The rate of HIV diagnosis per 100,000 African American 20- to 24-year-olds (146.9) is more than 4 times the rate for Hispanics (33.3) and almost 12 times that for whites (12.3) in the same age group (CDC, 2013e).
- Among all gay and bisexual males aged 13-24, there was an increase of 22 percent in the incidence of HIV infection from 2008 to 2010 (7,200 to 8,800). The highest incidence within this age group was among African American males, accounting for 4,800 cases (CDC, 2012).

Substance Use

- Past-month alcohol use rates are similar among females (58 percent) and males (63 percent) aged 18-25, with the highest rates being among whites (67 percent) and Hispanics (54 percent) and the lowest among Native Hawaiians/Other Pacific Islanders (43 percent). Binge drinking is higher among males (46 percent) than females (33 percent) of the same age group, and lowest among African Americans (27 percent) and highest among whites (46 percent) and non-Hispanic Native Americans/Alaska Natives (41 percent) (SAMSHA, 2013).
- Past-month marijuana use is higher among males (23 percent) than females (14 percent) aged 18-25, with the highest rates being among African Americans (22 percent) and whites (20 percent), followed by Native Americans/Alaska Natives (16 percent) (SAMSHA, 2013).
- Between early/middle adolescence and young adulthood, whites generally exhibit the highest levels of alcohol use and heavy drinking, while African Americans exhibit the lowest levels, although levels of alcohol use and heavy drinking do not show significant variation across different racial and ethnic groups after age 30 (Chen and Jacobson, 2012).

PUBLIC HEALTH INTERVENTIONS FOR YOUNG ADULTS

Public health interventions include a broad array of activities, such as informing or educating the targeted population about risks, persuading them to reduce risk, creating incentives or disincentives to encourage them to adopt healthy or safe behaviors, and modifying the environment to reduce exposure to risks or to promote or facilitate safe or healthy behaviors. Exposures include not only environmental toxins and dangerous products but also adverse social experiences, such as racism, violence, and social threats or health risks resulting from poor living and working con-

- Even though their levels of marijuana use start to decline after age 29, African Americans have the highest rates of marijuana use after their late 20s compared with whites, Hispanics, and Asians (Chen and Jacobson, 2012).

Suicide

- In the 18-25 age group, non-Hispanic blacks are 1.3 times, Asians 1.7 times, Native Americans/Alaska Natives 1.6 times, and Native Hawaiians/Other Pacific Islanders 7.1 times more likely to have suicidal ideation than whites (Han et al., 2014).
- Among those aged 20-24, suicide is approximately three times higher in males (13.8 per 10,000) than in females (4.7 per 10,000) (CDC, 2014a).
- High school graduates aged 18-25 are 1.3 times more likely than college graduates to have suicidal ideation; unemployment also is associated with a higher risk of suicidal ideation in 18- to 25-year-olds (Han et al., 2014).
- The lifetime prevalence of suicide attempts in gay and bisexual male adolescents and adults was four times that in comparable heterosexual males, and the prevalence among lesbian and bisexual females was almost twice that among heterosexual females. This is the opposite of the gender pattern found in the general population (HHS, 2012c; King et al., 2008).

Tobacco Use

- Past-month cigarette use rates among 18- to 25-year-olds are highest among non-Hispanic Native Americans/Alaska Natives (62 percent), followed by whites (44 percent) and African Americans (32 percent); the rates are lowest among Asians (19 percent) (SAMSHA, 2013).
- Cigarette use is highest for whites through adolescence and young adulthood, while use among African Americans is higher after age 30 than for other racial and ethnic groups (Chen and Jacobson, 2012).

---

[a] These rates do not include those classified as "undetermined intent." If those are added, the rates rise to 42 per 100,000 for males and 13.7 for females, and the highest rate is 58.2 for American Indian/Alaska Native males.

ditions. To the extent that individual behaviors play a causal role, recent public health approaches go beyond changing those behaviors to focus on mobilizing and engaging different sectors to create an environment that facilitates and sustains behavior change, as well as on changing public health practice and policies. These interventions can target the whole population of a community or specific subpopulations thought to be at elevated risk. They can be deployed separately or used in combination, creating synergy. Tools may also include legal requirements or prohibitions. All of these approaches have been used, with varying degrees of success, to address the significant problems identified above that threaten the health, safety, and well-being of young adults, although previously, the focus was primarily on changing individual behavior rather than altering the broader context and environment.

When a multilayer approach is implemented—for example, to reduce the incidence of unsafe driving due to either alcohol use or distracted driving—the likelihood of success is greater (Park et al., 2006). The ecological model or approach assumes that individual behaviors are products of influence at multiple levels, including intrapersonal, interpersonal, organizational, community/built environment, and public policy (Bronfenbrenner, 1979; Sallis et al., 2008). Moreover, a critical assumption is that behaviors are outcomes stemming from interactions across levels and that the context in which behaviors occur can exert significant influence on individuals (Bronfenbrenner, 1979; Sallis et al., 2008). With respect to risky behaviors, for instance, young adults working in the construction industry are likely to be socialized to a different set of norms and practices than those attending 4-year colleges. As an example, the greater use of tobacco among blue-collar workers may be attributable to a lack of knowledge and social supports at the individual level and perhaps to fewer restrictions on smoking in the workplace (Sorensen et al., 2004). Ecological approaches draw on a variety of theories and are robust when applied to specific behaviors. While these approaches have been used for some time, rigorous research has just begun to explore the mechanisms explaining the outcomes of multilevel interventions. In this section, we summarize the evidence base on public health interventions in selected priority areas to illustrate what is known.

Goals of Public Health Interventions

Promoting change in public health is a complex endeavor in terms of both the outcomes expected to result from a campaign and the context in which campaign messages are disseminated and received (Randolph and Viswanath, 2004). Health outcomes vary considerably, including changes in cognition, attitudes, beliefs, affect, salience, preferences, behavioral intentions, and behaviors at the individual level. A campaign may focus on the *initiation* of new behaviors, such as beginning to eat healthfully or engaging in physical activity (Snyder et al., 2004). In the case of risky behaviors, such as unsafe sex and use of tobacco, alcohol, or illicit drugs, one goal is to deter initiation, but a second stage can be directed at those who may not have been deterred or preventing relapse in the case of tobacco or drug use. Other campaigns may reinforce positive health messages, promoting *maintenance,* whether of healthy eating or physical activity (Atkin and Rice, 2012). The temporality of campaign effects is another critical consideration, ranging from short-term effects (e.g., influenza vaccination) to longer-term effects, such as maintaining healthy lifestyles in youth, the effects of which may last well into adulthood (Marcus et al., 2006). The idea of *deferring immediate rewards* to reap future well-being, such as by stopping smoking in youth to protect oneself from cardiovascular diseases or cancer in adulthood, is a challenging message to communicate, particularly to adolescents and young adults (Hoek et al., 2013). Finally, aside from the effects of an intervention on individual behavior, public health campaigns may aim to shape social norms and to promote, advocate, and instill changes at the institutional and community levels (Holder and Treno, 1997; Hornik, 2002; Hornik and Yanovitzky, 2003; Viswanath and Finnegan, 2002).

In the following sections, we briefly review public health campaigns and other interventions in some of the priority areas discussed earlier.[4] We then offer a distillation of lessons learned from these campaigns.

Tobacco Use

Using tobacco can cause cancer and heart and lung disease and can affect fetal well-being (Viswanath et al., 2010b). Tobacco use is estimated to cost 480,000 lives per year as a result of cancer in at least 18 different organ sites and other chronic diseases, such as cardiovascular and chronic obstructive pulmonary diseases (HHS, 2014c; Viswanath et al., 2010b), yet it is one of the most preventable causes of mortality and disease in the United States. Not surprisingly, public health interventions attempting to dissuade people from initiating tobacco use, as well as promoting cessation among users, have received considerable attention.

Tobacco control interventions are an outstanding example of multilevel approaches whereby interventions at one level have been aided by interventions at other levels (NCI, 2008). At the societal and community levels,

[4] To review the interventions focused on young adults that are discussed, we conducted an extensive search of the literature using PubMed and a number of search terms derived from the priority areas specified in Chapter 5, including the combined terms "young adult," and "intervention." Additional search terms included "African American," "Latino," and "low income" to capture a more diverse sample. A secondary search was conducted using "young adult" and "intervention" in the Cochrane Review Database. Searches were restricted to articles published between 2009 and 2014, although reviews that included individual articles before this date were included. Other inclusion criteria were (1) reported findings of an intervention (those reporting only protocols or cost analyses were excluded); (2) inclusion of samples of healthy individuals that were not pregnant or diagnosed with cancer, diabetes, or another chronic condition; and (3) inclusion of samples of young adults aged 18-25 (articles including ages above or below this range were considered only if they were review articles or studies in which the mean age was within this range). The search was not exhaustive; reference lists were not searched for other relevant articles, and other search terms could have been used to identify additional articles. Priority was given to articles that were systematic reviews or emphasized population-level strategies.

evidence shows that comprehensive tobacco control programs, including tax increases, public smoking bans, media campaigns, youth access restrictions, and cessation programs, have reduced the prevalence and intensity of tobacco use (HHS, 2012b; IOM, 2007). At the individual level, media campaigns have focused on promoting knowledge of risks resulting from tobacco use and denormalizing tobacco use behaviors. The focus on individual behaviors is complemented by drawing attention to the deceptive practices of the tobacco industry; offering cessation supports in different institutional settings; promoting support for increased taxes on tobacco; and at the policy level, placing restrictions on marketing, advertising, and using tobacco in different localities, such as the workplace and restaurants (HHS, 2012b; IOM, 2007).

> "I am not sure many people quit smoking because they see an ad from an anti-smoking campaign. I think it is more likely that smoking has negative health effects for them or someone they know and they decide at that point to make a change."

While a large body of work addresses tobacco control interventions among teens and adults (NCI, 2008), interventions focused specifically on young adults have been somewhat limited. A Cochrane review examined the impact of mass media campaigns on smoking prevention among young people (under age 25) (Brinn et al., 2012). Media were defined broadly to include television, radio, newspapers, billboards, posters, leaflets, and booklets. The review examined 7 of 84 studies that met the inclusion criteria and found that they were conducted systematically, drew on sound theories and research-informed interventions, and used extended campaigns to ensure exposure. Brinn and colleagues (2012) report modest evidence that mass media interventions could be successful in the prevention of smoking among young people. In a review of 25 studies examining the effectiveness of multicomponent interventions in reducing smoking uptake among young people, Carson and colleagues (2011) report that one intervention generally was successful in reducing smoking in the short term, and nine showed significant long-term effects. Improvements also were seen in changes in intentions to smoke (six of eight interventions), improved attitudes (five of nine), risk perceptions (two of six), and knowledge of tobacco use (three of six).

In contrast, short-term and/or single-component interventions are less likely to be successful. Villanti and colleagues (2010) conducted a systematic review of 14 studies of interventions promoting smoking cessation among young adults in the United States. The interventions focused on young adults aged 18-24 and were conducted in multiple settings, including universities, a community college, an airforce basic training unit, a quitline, and a rural community. Interventions were delivered either through interpersonal channels, such as peer coaches, counselors, and health educators, or a computer website. The authors report limited support for the efficacy of the interventions, although brief interventions with an extended dose via telephone or electronic media were somewhat effective. Villanti and colleagues (2010) recommend using standardized measures and interventions that take the smoking trajectories among young adults into account and are conducted among diverse population groups.

The use of electronic media, such as telephone quitlines and text messaging, to promote cessation of tobacco use has drawn the attention of several researchers. The Internet and social media hold considerable promise in promoting cessation. Sims and colleagues (2013) compared the effectiveness of cessation counseling through quitlines with a group receiving only mailed self-help material. They report only short-term effects among the group receiving counseling on the telephone. On the other hand, Brown (2013) reviewed eight studies assessing the impact of technology-based interventions that included tailored texts, emails, counseling, and a discussion board on tobacco use among participants aged 18-30 and found that in at least four studies, there was significant 7-day abstinence in the intervention group.

Similarly, Skov-Ettrup and colleagues (2014) report on a randomized controlled trial involving 2,030 daily smokers aged 15-25. The intervention arm received tailored text messages on self-efficacy, beliefs about smoking, and topics chosen by the user, whereas the control group received only generic messages. While there were no significant differences between the two groups in self-reported cessation, the researchers report higher rates of quitting among those in the tailored messaging group who used the text messages. That is, when the participants actually used the messages, the desired effects were much more likely to occur.

This review highlights four points when it comes to tobacco control interventions among young adults. First, comprehensive tobacco control strategies have had a demonstrable effect in reducing the prevalence and intensity of consumption at the population level (HHS, 2012b; IOM, 2007). Second, more focus is needed on developing and testing effective interventions targeting young adults, especially at a time when new tobacco products are being introduced at a rapid pace. Third, most of the interventions appear to have been carried out in colleges or white collar settings, and more effort needs to be made to include population groups of diverse racial, ethnic, and socioeconomic backgrounds. Last, the new information and communication technologies hold considerable promise in promoting tobacco control, but remain underexplored.

Alcohol Use

Alcohol consumption carries a risk of adverse health and social consequences and is the third leading cause of death in the United States (CDC, 2010). It can have a major impact on individuals, families, and communities that can have cumulative effects, contributing significantly to costly social, physical, mental, and public health problems. Alcohol use is associated with both short- and long-term health risks. Short-term risks, most often caused by binge drinking, include injuries, violence, risky sexual behaviors, miscarriages, and alcohol poisoning (CDC, 2014b). Long-term risks include neurological, cardiovascular, psychiatric, and social problems; cancer; liver diseases; and gastrointestinal problems (CDC, 2014b).

Most public health interventions targeting alcohol use by young adults have focused on college students. Paschall and colleagues (2011a,b) conducted a randomized controlled trial in 30 universities where freshmen were delivered an intervention designed to reduce alcohol use and binge drinking. The intervention was delivered over the Internet in two doses and covered such topics as alcohol laws, policies, and risks; setting personal goals; and dealing with friends with alcohol problems. A booster session was delivered 30-45 days later. Limited reductions in alcohol use and binge drinking occurred immediately following the intervention, but the effects did not persist until the second assessment, in the spring semester (Paschall et al., 2011a,b). In another Web-based screening and intervention program targeting college students aged 17-24, Kypri and colleagues (2014) found that intervention group students receiving personalized feedback and information correcting misperceptions of alcohol use among their peers reported only minimal effect. Both of these Internet-based studies show that use of the Internet alone may not be the most effective intervention strategy with respect to outcomes.

> "When I was in college, we had a rule that if you saw somebody who was sick from too much alcohol or from using drugs, you wouldn't get in trouble if you got them the help that they needed. People shouldn't be punished for bad behavior; we should make sure they are getting access to health care."

Similar modest effects were found by Moore and colleagues (2013) in a cluster randomized trial of students in residence halls in Wales, United Kingdom. The intervention focused on correcting misperceptions about the drinking behaviors of peers in order to reduce alcohol consumption. Messages were delivered through nonmedia channels such as posters, coasters, meal planners, and stickers. There were no significant effects on perceived norms or alcohol consumption between the groups, although there were some other modest effects.

On the other hand, a more broad-based community organizing approach focused on changing the environment with respect to high-risk drinking behavior among college students in North Carolina showed positive outcomes (Wolfson et al., 2012). The intervention encompassed campus-community coalitions; action plans; community organizers in each school; and promotion of environmental strategies, including awareness, enforcement, and policy. It also involved correcting misperceptions about alcohol use and limiting exposure to pro-alcohol messages. The intervention had a significant impact on decreasing consequences due to students' own drinking, such as requiring medical treatment, getting a driving under the influence/driving while intoxicated ticket, and being taken advantage of sexually, as well as on alcohol-related injuries caused to others. No differences, however, were seen in actual drinking behavior.

Many environmental policy interventions have been effective in decreasing drinking and driving and motor vehicle crashes that involve alcohol among young adults (Hingson, 2010). However, it has been found that for policies to be effective, they need to be put into action and enforced at the local level (Hingson, 2010). It also has been found that multicomponent college-community approaches among college students that incorporate a legal component can decrease alcohol use and drinking and driving (Hingson, 2010).

Three main lessons can be drawn from this review. First, most interventions addressing alcohol use problems among young adults appear to have been conducted among college students, with virtually little or no focus on noncollege youth. Second, single-component approaches (e.g., only promotion or policy) or those using a single channel (e.g., television) are not effective, while a multipronged approach focusing on both the environment and individual behaviors may be more effective. Schulenberg and Maggs (2002) point out that binge drinking at college campuses is multiply determined and held at high rates by a number of pillars ranging from community standards to students' assumptions about their rights to party. Addressing just one of these pillars is insufficient because the others will pick up the slack and keep the rates high. Third, multimodal community-wide interventions, including legal enforcement, have been shown to reduce drunk driving and alcohol-involved crashes among young adults.

Chronic Disease Prevention

Many interventions for chronic disease prevention center on maintaining a healthy lifestyle and focus on prevention of weight gain, weight loss, healthy eating, and physical activity. Obesity increases the risk of chronic illness and is associated with reduced quality of life and adult success, as well as substantial human and societal costs (IOM, 2012a). Individual effects include illness (e.g., cardiovascular disease, diabetes, hypertension), disability, social ostracism, discrimination, depression, and poor quality of life (IOM, 2012a). Moderate amounts of daily physical activity are recommended for people of all ages both to remain healthy and to improve health. A decline in physical activity is one of the lifestyle changes that can occur during young adulthood.

Many studies have targeted the transition to college, most often using the college setting to recruit participants and deliver intervention components. In one example, undergraduate health classes were used to administer a goal-setting intervention. Participants who wrote if-then statements about healthy eating goals significantly increased their fruit and vegetable consumption relative to participants assigned to a general goal-related task (Chapman et al., 2009). Likewise, over a 15-week period, a college class-based intervention involving 80 students that met three times per week, emphasizing healthy choices and in-class activities, also significantly increased the consumption of fruits and vegetables among participants (Ha and Caine-Bish, 2009). And a sample of college freshmen who were administered an alternative-reality game during a college health education course significantly increased their physical activity compared with controls, although both groups gained a significant amount of weight over the study period, suggesting that other factors in the college experience were impacting weight changes (Johnston et al., 2012).

Online sources also have been used to influence healthy behaviors and weight loss, again in a college setting. For example, Gow and colleagues (2010) administered an intervention using an Internet classroom tool, finding that participants who received the intensive 6-week intervention with feedback on their weight had significantly lower body mass index than controls. The authors note that the combination of monitoring, feedback, and education had a stronger effect on behavior than each component separately. In another study, an Internet-based curriculum that provided 10 online lessons focused on healthy eating and physical activity to students across eight universities significantly increased fruit and vegetable intake and physical activity, with positive, lasting effects being seen over the course of 15-month follow-up (Greene et al., 2012). In another study, however, although an intervention using texts, emails, and a smartphone application led to decreases in body weight and increases in physical activity and healthy eating among the intervention group, no significant differences were observed relative to the control group (Hebden et al., 2014).

Reviews of weight loss interventions among young adults have shown mixed results. Interventions combining diet, exercise, and motivation consistently show weight loss among young adults, although because of the varied components of these interventions, determining what elements are the most effective is problematic (Poobalan et al., 2010). Another review of 37 studies found that university course-based interventions often resulted in weight loss, with many self-monitoring interventions showing positive results as well (Laska et al., 2012). However, both reviews highlight the need to develop and evaluate rigorous weight gain prevention interventions focused on young adults that fully reflect the rapidly shifting life circumstances of this age group and incorporate more diverse populations.

Studies in this area have shown varying degrees of success. Many of the researchers acknowledge that an environmental approach is necessary to fully address the range of issues faced by young adults as they transition into making their own health-related choices, including pressure to engage in certain harmful behaviors.

Prevention of Sexually Transmitted Infections/HIV

STIs are infections that are transmitted primarily through sexual contact. Although they are largely preventable, they remain a significant public health concern, and some have the potential to cause serious health problems, especially if not diagnosed and treated early. The consequences of untreated STIs often are worse for young women than for young men, even though the yearly number of new infections is roughly equal among them (51 percent and 49 percent, respectively) (CDC, 2013c). Although HIV transmission is generally preventable, there is no vaccine or cure. As a result, HIV continues to be a major public health concern.

Several strategies have addressed STI and HIV prevention among diverse samples of young adults across a number of settings, often focusing on increasing condom use and decreasing risky sexual practices. In their sample of U.S. university students aged 18 and older, Norton and colleagues (2012) found that participants exposed to a 60-minute DVD addressing motivation, information, and behavioral skills with respect to increasing condom use and decreasing risky sexual practices changed these behaviors more when the topic was prevention of STIs or unplanned pregnancy than when it was HIV prevention.

Community-based participatory research was used to create a culturally congruent HIV prevention intervention, AMIGAS (Amigas, Mujeres Latinas, Inform andonos, Gui andonos, y Apoy andonos contra el SIDA [friends, Latina women, informing each other, guiding each other, and supporting each other against AIDS]), for young Latina women living in Miami, Florida, modeled after the evidence-based SiSTA (Sistas Informing Sistas about Topics on AIDS) program for African American women (DiClemente and Wingood, 1995; Wingood et al., 2011a). Within the

AMIGAS intervention, Latina health educators delivered four interactive group sessions emphasizing cultural and gender pride, the importance of healthy relationships, HIV knowledge, and how experiences unique to Latina women may increase HIV risk (Wingood et al., 2011a). At the 6-month follow-up, program participants reported significantly more consistent condom use, greater self-efficacy for negotiating safe sex, greater HIV knowledge, and fewer perceived barriers to using condoms compared with controls.

Several studies have targeted African American young adults in various community- and technology-based settings for the reduction of HIV risk behaviors. Aronson and colleagues (2013) developed a pilot intervention with 57 participants that used community-based participatory research partnerships among students, university faculty, and community partners to create a retreat for young adult African American men in which to discuss safe sex, followed by reinforcement messages via electronic media over the course of 3 months. Average number of sex partners and condom errors decreased significantly among participants, with the authors attributing much of this success to the high level of engagement with community partners. In a pilot study by Kennedy and colleagues (2013), a theory-driven, single-session condom promotion program delivered to 18- to 24-year-old African American men recruited from neighborhoods bordering urban community centers significantly increased condom use, perceived condom availability, and positive reasons to use condoms compared with a comparison group that received a general health curriculum. Results suggest that this brief, culturally appropriate prevention program may reduce risky sexual behaviors among high-risk youth from urban communities.

An HIV intervention for young African American women at Planned Parenthood in Atlanta, Georgia, used two computer-based 60-minute interactive sessions also modeled after the SiSTA program (DiClemente and Wingood, 1995; Wingood et al., 2011b). The intervention significantly increased knowledge of HIV prevention, condom self-efficacy, and condom use in participants compared with a control group that received a small-group session on general health topics (Wingood et al., 2011b). Another intervention with low-income African American young women at high risk for HIV used smartphones to stream a soap opera highlighting HIV risk reduction (Jones et al., 2013). Although no statistically significant differences were seen between the intervention and control groups, participants who viewed the videos found them engaging and wished to continue receiving them, prompting further research on how to reach this population on a popular messaging platform.

International studies also have shown success. A Dutch Web-based study involved a tailored intervention for young adults that used a virtual clinic with motivational interviewing, participant-specific feedback, and educational models. Significantly higher condom use and maintenance resulted from the intervention compared with general feedback or treatment as usual (Mevissen et al., 2011). A study in India found that a workplace-based PowerPoint, video, and training session significantly increased positive perceptions of condoms and knowledge of proper wearing techniques among males aged 18-30 (Ray et al., 2012). The authors emphasize that simply providing knowledge may not be sufficient, and that a range of education on behavior, perception, and skill may be needed with this group.

In sum, many interventions targeting STI or HIV prevention saw success when they focused on topics most relevant to young adults; included culturally competent, tailored materials; and introduced skill components along with this tailored feedback.

Human Papillomavirus (HPV) Vaccination

HPV vaccination, recommended for females under 26 and males under 21, entails a series of three shots that protect against HPV infection and HPV's associated health problems, such as cancer and genital warts (CDC, 2014c). Brief intervention techniques highlighting the benefits of HPV vaccination have been shown to increase positive perceptions of the vaccine and increase vaccination intention and reception. For example, Kester and colleagues (2014) recruited a sample of 18- to 26-year-olds at a minority health fair. Intervention group participants received a 5- to 10-minute small-group presentation on HPV infection, detection, and treatment; additional information sources; and a list of locations where the vaccine could be received. Participants had higher HPV knowledge scores and vaccination intention compared with controls.

HPV education also has been delivered to university populations in school computer labs. Intentions to be vaccinated increased significantly among women viewing an HPV website that provided information tailored to their specific perceived barriers to vaccination compared with women who viewed standard information (Gerend et al., 2013). Short videos also were used by Hopfer (2012), with intervention groups watching videos narrated by peers, medical experts, or both, while another arm reviewed a generic video or HPV website or received no message. HPV vaccination nearly doubled among the participants who watched the combined peer-expert video compared with controls; however, these results were not found for the peer- or expert-only videos, highlighting the importance of the communication source and suggesting that peer messages that normalize medical expert messages may play a crucial role in vaccination.

Direct provision of information about HPV and HPV vaccination may be a simple and effective way to motivate young adults to initiate HPV vaccination (Kester et al., 2014). Tailoring this information to ameliorating or removing specific barriers may enhance the effectiveness of this approach (Gerend et al., 2013).

Sexual Assault and Intimate Partner Violence

Black and colleagues (2011) found that nearly 1 in 5 women and 1 in 17 men reported experiencing rape at some point in their lives (Black et al., 2011). Approximately 1 in 20 women and men (5.6 percent and 5.3 percent, respectively) had experienced sexual violence other than rape.

Several interventions have sought to address sexual assault by providing girls and women tools needed to prevent these acts from occurring. One study focused on the transition of young adult women to the college environment, enlisting their mothers to participate with them the summer prior to their freshmen year (Testa et al., 2010). Mothers in the intervention condition were advised to complete a workbook on alcohol safety with their daughter before the start of school, with participants in the enhanced intervention condition also receiving a workbook chapter on college dating. Both intervention conditions were correlated with decreased incapacitated rape levels during the first year and increased communication among mothers and daughters, which predicted fewer drinking episodes, leading to lower sexual victimization rates involving alcohol.

Another study delivered an intervention for women to promote group responsibility, environmental awareness, and safe personal conduct as groups of college-aged students crossed the border to patronize Tijuana bars. The program led to a significant decrease in reports of sexual victimization (Kelley-Baker et al., 2011). Other strategies have focused on both men and women. A Web-based intervention for college students who were in longer-term relationships advised them on problem solving, communication techniques, and ways to enhance positive relationships, with weekly reminders to employ these skills (Braithwaite and Fincham, 2009). Intervention participants experienced improved mental health and relationship outcomes that continued over time, although anxiety, physical assault, and aggression grew worse before they ultimately improved.

Despite these findings, a meta-analytic Cochrane review of education- and skill-based interventions designed to reduce violence in the context of relationships and dating among youth aged 12-25 found no evidence of a significant effect on relationship violence episodes or on attitudes toward violence (Fellmeth et al., 2013). The 38 interventions included in the review were predominantly educational, and components were delivered in such settings as college classrooms, dorms, and fraternity halls, with sample populations ranging from coed to all-male or all-female. Intervention strategies included group discussions, videos of dramatic vignettes, role playing, problem solving and communication skills, and discussion of rape myths. Despite a trend found in increased knowledge about relationship violence, there was no evidence that these strategies improved participants' attitudes, actions, or proficiency with respect to violence in relationships. The authors highlight that the existing evidence relates primarily to determining changes in attitudes and knowledge, and that interventions both across communities and within families may be needed to reduce relationship violence. Further studies with longer-term follow-up and validated, standardized measures also are required to maximize the comparability of results (Fellmeth et al., 2013).

Mental Health Conditions

Mental health and substance use disorders are public health concerns for numerous reasons. First, they can cause death through the act of suicide. Mental health and substance use disorders also affect families and harm individuals by reducing their ability to achieve social, educational, and vocational goals; increasing the potential for further impairment and compromised functioning throughout life; and imposing costs related to extra care requirements and social disruption (NRC and IOM, 2009; Patel et al., 2007), as well as lost productivity (Birmbaum et al., 2010; Kessler et al., 2006). Of all types of illnesses, moreover, mental health and substance use disorders cause the greatest burden of disability in young adults (IOM and NRC, 2013). Furthermore, given the age of onset of behavioral health conditions, preventing or addressing mental and behavioral health needs in this period of life has the potential to reduce lifelong impact, since many fewer new cases occur after age 24 (Kessler et al., 2005). Timely mental health intervention can reduce morbidity and increase long-term health and well-being.

> "I have severe mental health issues that I haven't addressed yet because I don't want to go to a therapist. I don't feel comfortable. Why am I going to go to this person and tell them my problems? After what I went through, I have a hard time trusting people to talk about my problems."

In addition, although not a psychiatric disorder, the experience of stress is pervasive in young adults (APA, 2013). Compared with older adults, young adults experience greater levels of daily stressors (Stawski et al., 2008) and perceive their lives as more stressful (Scott et al., 2013). One of the benefits of maturity appears to be coping better with stressful situations (Luong and Charles, 2014; Price and Dunlap, 1988; Schilling and Diehl, 2014). Even among young adults, the youngest struggle more with stressful events than their slightly older counterparts (Jackson and Finney, 2002). Psychological stress can contribute to the onset of mental illness (Blazer et al., 1987;

Corcoran et al., 2003; Kendler et al., 1999; Muscatell et al., 2009), and its relationship to physical health is well established (McEwen, 2008; McEwen and Gianaros, 2010).

Although mental health treatment is available and effective (HHS, 1999; NIH, 2009; NIMH, 2000), young people, especially young men and young indigenous and ethnic minorities, are reluctant to obtain professional care for problems relating to mental health (Edlund et al., 2012; Gulliver et al., 2010; Rickwood et al., 2007; Wu et al., 2007). Other studies have found that only about 18-34 percent of young people with depression and anxiety disorders seek professional help (Guilliver et al., 2010). Friends and family members rather than health professionals are preferred sources of help (Rickwood et al., 2007). Likewise, Wu and colleagues (2007) found that approximately 4 percent of full-time college students, 7 percent of part-time college students, and 6 percent of nonstudents aged 18-22 with an alcohol use disorder had sought help within the past year. Gayman and colleagues (2011) found that only about one-third of young adults with a substance use disorder had ever sought help; those in whom the onset of the disorder occurred at 18 or older were less likely to have sought help than those whose onset occurred earlier.

Perceived barriers to young adults' seeking help for behavioral health disorders include stigma and embarrassment, difficulty recognizing symptoms or the need for treatment (i.e., lack of behavioral health literacy), a preference for self-reliance, and lack of confidence that their insurance will pay for treatment (Cellucci et al., 2006; Eisenberg et al., 2007; Gulliver et al., 2010; van der Pol et al., 2013). Perceiving the need for help or being encouraged by family, friends, or others to seek help increases the likelihood of help seeking (Caldeira et al., 2009).

The mental health literacy of young adults is not high (Farrer et al., 2008). Studies in Australia found that fewer than 50 percent of 12- to 25-year-olds could identify depression, and only about 25 percent could identify psychosis (Wright et al., 2005). Rates of recognition are lower in young men than in young women (Cotton et al., 2006). Lack of mental health literacy is regularly given as one of the explanations for missed opportunities to intervene with individuals with serious mental illness (Gulliver et al., 2010; IOM, 2004; Jorm, 2012).

As noted, the stigma attached to having a behavioral health disorder is one important impediment to help seeking by young people, and reducing stigma also is one of the major policy approaches proposed for reducing levels of unmet need for mental health services (HHS, 1999). Public stigma is the reaction of the general population toward a condition; self-stigma is the internalized impact of public stigma, and thus the prejudice people with behavioral health conditions turn against themselves (Corrigan and Watson, 2002); and personal stigma is the reaction of an individual. All three forms of stigma can reduce willingness to seek behavioral health services (Eisenberg et al., 2009; Held and Owens, 2013), with some evidence suggesting that personal stigma may be a stronger disincentive than public stigma for college students (Eisenberg et al., 2009; Lally et al., 2013). Personal stigma also may pose a barrier to help seeking by reducing recognition of the impact of symptoms and thus the need for help (Schomerus et al., 2012). Generally, however, the specific roles of the various forms of stigma in help seeking are not well understood, specifically in young adults with behavioral health conditions. Many of the studies of public and self-stigma and help seeking in young adults examined these issues in general populations, most of whom did not have a behavioral health disorder.

One study illustrates the potential for unexpected and counterproductive consequences of public service announcements designed to reduce stigma; the announcements actually increased self-stigma and reduced help seeking in individuals with depression (Lienemann et al., 2013). In addition, help-seeking intentions have been studied much more thoroughly than actual help seeking. Thus, any public health campaign to reduce the stigma of behavioral health conditions and encourage help seeking for these conditions should be informed by research aimed at understanding the impact of stigma and of various types of public service announcements on help-seeking behavior in a wide range of young adults with behavioral health disorders.

A further impediment to adequate treatment of behavioral health disorders in young adults is that they are more likely than older adults to drop out of treatment once they have started (Edlund et al., 2002; Hadley et al., 2001; Sinha et al., 2003).

The onset of many mental health conditions during the young adult years has prompted a range of strategies aimed at preventing or treating mental health conditions in this population. A review of community-based prevention and early intervention programs found that the majority of interventions for young adults focus on strategies employing cognitive-behavioral therapy (CBT), which has shown the most reliably positive outcomes for treatment of anxiety or depression (Christensen et al., 2010). A later review focused on technology use among 18- to 25-year-old college students found that of diverse strategies employing the Internet, video, and audio, Internet-based strategies using CBT may be particularly useful for targeting anxiety, and to a lesser extent depression (Farrer et al., 2013). The authors conclude that the use of technological interventions targeting certain mental health problems holds promise for students in university settings, although more research is needed to assess the use of technology for other specific mental disorders. A review of 15 interventions targeting prevention of suicide and self-harm among 12- to 25-year-olds found highly limited evidence regarding effective interventions for young adults experiencing suicide attempts, deliberate self-harm, or suicidal ideation (Robinson et al., 2011). While the authors acknowledge that CBT may show some promise, more methodologically rigorous trials of this approach are needed (Robinson et al., 2011).

Motor Vehicle Safety

Motor vehicle safety is a major concern for young adults, particularly since, compared with adolescents and adults aged 26-34, young adults (aged 18-25) are more likely to be injured or die in motor vehicle crashes and have more motor vehicle crash-related hospitalizations and emergency room visits (Neinstein, 2013). Historically, actions to prevent motor vehicle crashes and resulting injuries and deaths have taken an ecological approach, including multiple levels of influence such as policy designed to increase seat belt use. Indeed, the most notable road safety campaigns have promoted and enforced seat belt use (Dinh-Zarr et al., 2001) and have used enforcement campaigns to increase their use (Wakefield et al., 2010). For example, the Click It or Ticket program in North Carolina was associated with an increase in seat belt use from 63 percent to 81 percent and lower rates of highway deaths and injuries (Williams et al., 1996). Increasingly, states also are passing laws banning texting while driving, and in some cases any use of cell phones by drivers under age 18, to address distracted driving, a significant factor in motor vehicle crashes (NHTSA, 2014).

> "The 'Distracted Driving' campaign was interesting and impactful, but I still struggle with being on the phone when driving. Laws about using the phone while driving seem to be making more of an impact than the campaign by itself."

Law enforcement and repeated short-term mass media exposure appear to be important components of effective motor vehicle safety campaigns (Elder et al., 2004; Morrison et al., 2003; Salzberg and Moffat, 2004; Williams and Wells, 2004). The power of mass media also has been harnessed for drinking and driving campaigns. A social norms–based campaign delivered through television, radio, print, and theater advertisements in Montana reduced normative misperceptions about the frequency of drunk driving, increased designated driver use, and decreased drinking and driving rates among 21- to 34-year-olds within the intervention region (Perkins et al., 2010). Another social marketing approach targeting drunk driving in Seattle, Washington, also saw success. A campaign delivered through messaging at taxi stands, at points of alcohol purchase, and in mass media significantly increased the use of designated drivers and taxis among the heaviest drinkers aged 21-34 (Rivara et al., 2011).

Despite the promising results of these campaigns, they may have unintended effects if inappropriate message formats are used. A group of college students that viewed fear-based public service announcements on distracted driving (such as talking on a cell phone, texting, or eating) reported significantly higher intentions to engage in the distracting behaviors after viewing the videos, indicating a boomerang effect (Lennon et al., 2010). The authors caution that fear-based messages may encourage young adults to behave in the opposite way from what is advocated in the message.

Many states are using graduated driver licensing (GDL) systems. Yet the results of a recent study indicate that some of the lives saved by GDL among 15- to 17-year-old novice drivers are offset by associated increases in fatal crashes among 18- to 19-year-old drivers (Fell and Romano, 2013). The reasons for this finding are unclear. It could be due to (1) novice 18- to 19-year-olds beginning to drive without the protective framework of a GDL program as a result of delaying licensure in the "good" GDL states[5]; (2) increased risk taking behaviors by 18- and 19-year-old drivers (e.g., impaired driving, late night driving, driving with teen passengers, lack of seat belt use, distracted driving); and/or (3) lack of exposure to risky situations (e.g., late night driving, driving on high-speed roads) among 18- to 19-year-old drivers in the good GDL states because of the protection from these situations when they were 16 and 17 years old (Fell and Romano, 2013). Further research is required to clarify the finding that those who seek a license in their young adult years actually endanger themselves even more as they lack the checks and family oversight of younger drivers.

Most individual-level driving safety interventions currently focus on educating novice drivers during the high school years as they gain their permit for the first time, often involving parents (Ramirez et al., 2013; Zakrajsek et al., 2013) and working within driver education classes (Zakrajsek et al., 2013). Relatively fewer studies have focused on the driving behaviors of young adults, using various tactics to reduce risky and distracted driving behaviors. An in-car education program involving 23 young men with a history of challenging driving behavior provided coaching sessions and in-car

[5] The Insurance Institute for Highway Safety rated a GDL law "good" if it had five or more of the following components: minimum learner's permit age, mandatory waiting period before applying for an intermediate license, minimum hours of supervised driving, minimum age for an intermediate license, nighttime restriction, passenger limitation, and minimum age for full licensing (Fell and Romano, 2013).

feedback by a monitoring system. The program significantly improved driving skills in the intervention group, leading to positive changes in tailgating and unofficial races with other cars (Tapp et al., 2013). However, other studies with young adults have not shown the same success during actual time on the road. For example, teaching strategies using computer-based training modules to prevent distraction led to a decline in the intervention group's willingness to engage in distracting activities and an increase in perceived risk, but no benefits were seen when the car was in motion (Horrey et al., 2009). Furthermore, a 20-hour prevention program for youth with multiple traffic citations showed no significant change in high-risk traffic behaviors and traffic citations compared with the control group, highlighting the need for further development of behavioral interventions to address high-risk driving behaviors (Nirenberg et al., 2013).

In summary, successful campaigns promoting motor vehicle safety have combined mass media messaging with legal enforcement, often engaging social networks to amplify the message and change norms. Single-component approaches and short-term campaigns have limited impact on intended outcomes.

Multiple Risk Behaviors

In addition to interventions addressing one or a set of related risk behaviors, there may be merit in multicomponent interventions that target various risk behaviors (Jackson et al., 2012). Such interventions may reflect the environmental approach needed to address the multiple transitions young adults experience, and may help focus on building resilience to adversity during these transitions by addressing multiple domains of risk and protective factors (Jackson et al., 2012). For example, a brief intervention among college students consisted of a one-on-one consultation featuring gain- and loss-framed messages tailored to students' specific behaviors, followed by a goal-setting session. This intervention led to significant increases in health-related quality of life, fewer days of poor spiritual health, moderate exercise, and fewer days of driving after drinking compared with controls (Werch et al., 2010). Brody and colleagues (2010) focused on the period leading into the young adult years among African American students in rural counties who were in the past year and a half of secondary school, using a family-based intervention to increase the ability to cope with life stressors associated with the transition to adulthood. The intervention was found to buffer stress and increase resilience, leading to significant decreases in risk behaviors such as marijuana use, alcohol use, and risky sex among the intervention group compared with controls.

Lessons Learned

Although strategies and findings vary by priority area, some overall conclusions can be drawn from this brief review. First, the available evidence provides grounds for systematically investigating the potential utility of multifaceted health and safety campaigns targeting young adults. Single-component interventions focusing on one level, in general, have limited, short-term effects. Evidence of effectiveness as measured by health or safety outcomes at the population level (rather than solely by modification of individual-level beliefs, attitudes, or intentions) is weak for stand-alone interventions in many of the domains with particular application to young adults. By contrast, in the few health areas in which multilevel interventions have been used, the positive effects tend to be larger and long-lasting. Most community-based campaigns have used media but also sought to mobilize different sectors to create environmental and policy supports to facilitate healthy behaviors. Such intersectoral mobilization is exemplified by campaigns on tobacco use, HIV, and youth abuse of alcohol (Ramanadhan et al., 2012; Valente et al., 1993), among other areas. Law enforcement and repeated short-term mass media exposure also appear to be important components of motor vehicle safety campaigns.

Second, the most successful interventions have been those that involve comprehensive, multilevel community initiatives using ecological approaches to influence changes at the individual, organizational, and societal levels, sustained over time through a variety of channels and venues. Community and stakeholder engagement is critical to the sustained effectiveness of interventions. Many successful public health campaigns include such approaches as community-engaged social change and community-based participatory research (Koh et al., 2011; Minkler and Wallerstein, 2008).

Third, and related to the first two points, the most robust effects have been seen in those areas in which policy makers and researchers have collaborated to address the problem and evaluate interventions and, as a result, in which the most experience and evidence have been accumulated.

Fourth, a major limitation of current studies of young adults is that they have largely involved samples of university students. The focus on this population does not fully represent how young adults who do not attend college experience the transition after high school. Given the inequalities between youth and young adults from different socioeconomic and racial and ethnic groups, more information on how to develop and deploy robust interventions among noncollege youth are sorely needed. In particular, rigorous trials using standardized measures are needed so behavioral outcomes can be compared across groups.

This point is related to a broader concern—that public health campaigns that are media based or include a media component are less likely to benefit people from disadvantaged socioeconomic and racial and ethnic groups, a phenomenon characterized as communication inequalities (IOM, 2006; Link and Phelan, 1995; Viswanath, 2006; Viswanath et al., 2013). The reasons for these health campaign inequalities are many, including a lack of access to media; a lack of attention; the complexity of the messages and practices recommended; and the economic, environmental, and social barriers to acting on messages. These inequalities in campaign effects offer a partial but robust explanation for the challenges encountered in attempting to eliminate or ameliorate health inequalities so well documented in the literature (Kawachi and Berkman, 2001; Link and Phelan, 1995; Marmot, 2013; WHO, 2001). It is worth noting, however, that these gaps are less likely to be seen when public health interventions and media campaigns focus explicitly on using strategies to reach different social groups, including minorities and those of lower socioeconomic position.

SOCIAL MEDIA AND THE HEALTH OF YOUNG ADULTS

Social media play an increasing role in curating information and driving audiences. Among those aged 18-29, for example, 97 percent use the Internet, 98 percent have a cell phone, and 83 percent have a smartphone, although income, urbanicity, and education are strongly associated with this phenomenon (Fox and Lee, 2014). More than 70 percent of Internet users use social media, with this number rising to 84 percent among those aged 18-29 (Duggan and Smith, 2013).

At the same time, a steady erosion in audiences for traditional media has occurred. In a Pew survey of online news consumption, for example, 39 percent of respondents reported getting news online—19 percent from social media, 16 percent from email, and 8 percent from podcasts (Pew Research Center, 2013). More germane, 60 percent of those in younger age groups rely on digital sources for their news. And more than one-third of youth aged 18-24 get their news from social media. Ownership of mobile devices, such as mobile phones and tablets, has actually increased news consumption, with people accessing information from multiple platforms (Pew Research Center, 2014). In line with this phenomenon, social media have emerged as key platforms for participation and engagement, particularly among youth.

In light of this dramatic transformation in information and communication technologies and their adoption among youth, it is important to explore the implications of these developments for public health. Social technologies afford new opportunities to reach out to and stay connected with young adults. Social and mobile media, in particular, provide a variety of contexts through which young adults can learn about, contribute to, and engage with developing narratives about public health. These media amplify points of connection with young adults, and they enable broad, rapid, and convenient access to information and a variety of relational interfaces.

The empirical evidence for successful deployment of social media to promote health is nascent, and much of the literature is replete with commentaries and speculation. As these media become more ubiquitous, however, they increasingly are being incorporated into interventions. As the leading social networking site in the United States (Duggan and Smith, 2013), Facebook has been used to promote a number of healthy behaviors among young adults (Carrol and Kirkpatrick, 2011), but with mixed results. Exposure to a Facebook page delivering STI prevention messages to young adults in the community, for example, resulted in increased condom use at 2 months postintervention, although these results were not sustained at 6-month follow-up (Bull et al., 2012). In another study involving college students, using the private message function of Facebook to deliver social norms feedback successfully corrected misperceptions about drinking, reducing the amount and frequency of alcohol consumed postintervention and at 3-month follow-up (Ridout and Campbell, 2014). Enrollment in a Facebook group had no significant effect on increasing physical activity among a group of female undergraduate students (Cavallo et al., 2012). However, Napolitano and colleagues (2013) found significantly greater weight loss among college students exposed to a Facebook Plus intervention group (access to a weight loss–focused Facebook page plus goal setting, self-monitoring, and social support) compared with Facebook-only and control groups. This finding suggests that weight loss material delivered through a social networking platform alone may not be sufficient to effect changes in behavior.

> "In college, lack of sleep is bragged about; if you get less sleep, you're working harder. Until the culture changes, a health campaign isn't going to make a difference."

A systematic review of the use of online social networks for interventions focused on weight loss and physical activity among participants of all ages found that 9 of the 10 articles included in the review reported significant improvements in these behaviors, albeit with small effect sizes (Maher et al., 2014). However, a meta-analysis by Williams and colleagues (2014) found no effects of the use of social media on weight or physical activity levels, citing problems with recruitment, retention, and poorly reported methods among reviewed studies. A systematic review of sexual health interventions among young adults also revealed a lack of evidence for the impact of social media on behavior. While interventions using social media or text messages were found to significantly increase knowledge of STIs among samples of young adults, the evidence for impact on reducing sexual risk behaviors and increasing STI testing was mixed (Jones et al., 2014). Studies emphasize that this field of research is in its infancy, and future studies need to use high-quality research methods and large samples and determine how behavior change can be sustained over time to fully understand the promise of this widely used resource for health behavior change.

Based on experiences from other fields and data from current use, it is possible to formulate some hypotheses about the use of social media for public health interventions. We emphasize that these are hypotheses only that warrant more systematic testing in further research.

"A lot of young adults and teens don't want to trust adults; they want to experiment and experience things themselves. Think about a way to give them the experience without actually giving them the experience."

First, unlike traditional mass media, social technologies afford two- and multiway communication among audiences, especially when the members know each other or share some common interests. The open-ended opportunity for engagement may facilitate personal contributions or the tailoring of campaign content, which is known to result in a stronger impact on outcomes.

Second, social media may allow public health campaign planners to take advantage of the memetic potential for virality embedded within socially oriented technology. Several contemporary health campaigns are premised on the engagement principle, with the Avatars Anonymous project being an example of how health avatars can be personalized to convey health messages more effectively (Wood, 2014). Unlike traditional media, which access people as passive interlocutors, social and mobile media provide opportunities to turn passive audiences into active content producers. By "flipping" traditional roles, social and mobile media suggest new ways of engaging the target audience with public health campaigns. Because of its potential for engagement, the flipping model has become popular in redesigning educational experiences. In the health care and public health sector, the Flip the Clinic model,[6] supported by the Robert Wood Johnson Foundation, is an example of interactive learning and active engagement with routine health care processes. Whether "flipping," in either classroom

[6] See http://fliptheclinic.org/about (accessed October 22, 2014) for details on the Flip the Clinic project.

or clinical settings, is more effective than traditional approaches has yet to be empirically documented.

Third, the storytelling tradition is embedded in a range of cultures, and commercial advertisers often have resorted to this strategy to sell products and services. In social change programs, including those focused on health, narratives and exemplars are frequently used to promote change. Narratives offer both negative and positive examples of influence on health behaviors. Several studies have documented, for example, that exposure to depictions of tobacco use in movies is strongly related to both initiation and sometimes continued smoking among youth in the United States (Dalton et al., 2009; NCI, 2008) and young adults and adults in India (Viswanath et al., 2010a). On the other hand, narratives have also been used to help smokers quit smoking (Strecher et al., 2008). Using social and mobile media to support storytelling invites others to connect with the stories emotionally through the process of adding to, remixing, and reproducing them. This sustained loop of engagement could potentially create a sense of community supportive of health and well-being, a key element in new public health strategic directions.

> "Messages aren't successful when young adults are told what to do. We want to be autonomous, and we want to be treated in a respectful way. Presenting messages in a way that gives young adults the power to choose will be successful."

Fourth, social and mobile media augment points of connection among people, networks, and information. They connect disparate and overlapping networks in ways that sustain existing and enable new connections. In this way, they offer networked "neighborhoods" more accessible to a variety of people than physical places where people traditionally have convened.

Overall, use of social and mobile media appears to hold promise for reaching young adults with public health campaigns. However, the effectiveness of these new technologies in fulfilling this promise has yet to be established. Studies indicate that going beyond the provision of information to include skill-based components may yield the greatest success (Jackson et al., 2012).

PROTECTIVE PUBLIC POLICIES FOR YOUNG ADULTS

Legislatures and public health agencies often adopt protective policies focused on young adults. They may do so for a variety of developmental and behavioral reasons. For example, some risky behaviors that are permitted for adults pose a heightened risk to young people because of the shortsightedness, impulsivity, or other deficits in mature judgment and decision making that often characterize this age group. Legal restrictions are designed either to delay these behaviors until young people mature or to allow a transition period for training and experience. Legal permission to use alcohol and tobacco, to drive a motor vehicle, and to use firearms offers the most pertinent examples.

A key policy issue in all these contexts is where the line should be drawn in formulating these "wait" rules. As discussed in Chapter 2, some of the key policy-relevant features of adolescence, including sensation seeking, impulsivity, and shortsightedness, persist into the early 20s, and there are of course substantial individual variations above and below 18. Although 18 may be a sensible point at which to demarcate the generic "age of majority" for most legal purposes, drawing this line in each setting ultimately requires contextualized value judgments. In the present context, protecting young people from taking unreasonable risks must be balanced with respecting their right to direct their own lives. Cognitive and emotional factors that may affect the maturity of judgment exercised by adolescents and young adults will vary in different social contexts, as will the health and safety consequences of setting the "legal age" at one point or another. It may be sensible to draw the line lower in some health and safety contexts (e.g., obtaining a license to operate a motor vehicle) and higher in others (e.g., lawful access to alcohol) (Bonnie and Scott, 2013; NRC and IOM, 2004).

In recent years, the trend in the United States has been to take a more protective stance toward older adolescents and young adults, a trend that is reinforced by the prolonged transition to economic and social independence described in Chapter 2. In the public health context, this trend is most clearly evident in legislation setting the minimum age for purchasing alcohol, marijuana, and tobacco, and heightened by increasing concern about commercial targeting of young people by manufacturers of these products.

Age of Purchase for Alcohol, Marijuana, and Tobacco

After the repeal of Prohibition in 1933, the vast majority of states set the minimum drinking age at 21. However, when the national voting age was set at 18 by the 26th Amendment in 1971, 29 states changed the drinking age to 18, 19, or 20, which led to a dramatic increase in motor vehicle fatalities related to alcohol among 18- to 20-year-olds (Wagenaar and Toomey, 2002). Many states then raised the minimum age to 21, and a robust literature showed that alcohol-related fatalities declined. In 1984, Congress induced all states to restore the minimum age to 21 by threatening to withhold a percentage of highway funds from noncompliant states (NRC and IOM, 2004). Subsequent studies showed significant decreases among young people in fatal and nonfatal motor vehicle crashes and alcohol-related crashes and arrests (NRC and IOM, 2004). In a comprehensive report published in 2004, the National Research Council (NRC) and the Institute of Medicine (IOM) proposed a strategy for reducing underage drinking and driving based on the idea that, in a world where alcohol is so widespread and aggressively promoted, reducing drinking by adolescents and young adults is a "collective responsibility." Parents and other adults must take the law seriously instead of accepting the idea that teen drinking is a rite of passage to adulthood (NRC and IOM, 2004). Moreover, given the widespread availability of alcohol and easy access by underage drinkers, minimum drinking age laws must be enforced more effectively, along with social sanctions. The effectiveness of underage drinking laws could be enhanced through such approaches as compliance checks, server training, zero tolerance laws, and GDL laws (NRC and IOM, 2004).

Notwithstanding the NRC and IOM report's reaffirmation of the wisdom of setting the minimum drinking age at 21, political efforts are occasionally launched to reduce the minimum drinking age to 18 or 19. Yet a recent literature review reinforces the point that establishing 21 as the minimum drinking age has decreased "alcohol-related traffic crashes and alcohol consumption among youth, while also protecting drinkers from long-term negative outcomes they might experience in adulthood, including alcohol and other drug dependence, adverse birth outcomes, and suicide and homicide" (Dejong and Blanchette, 2014, p. 113). The U.S. Task Force on Community Preventive Services recommends implementing and maintaining a minimum drinking age of 21 based on strong evidence for the effectiveness of doing so, which includes a median 16 percent decrease in underage motor vehicle crashes in states that increased the legal drinking age to 21 (Shults et al., 2001).

The alcohol experience appears to have guided policy makers in states that have chosen to legalize marijuana, where the age of purchase has uniformly been set at 21. Although marijuana policy has been highly controversial since the 1960s (Bonnie and Whitebread, 1974), recent developments have fundamentally changed the regulatory landscape and are likely to have profound effects on the epidemiology of marijuana use (IOM, 1999). The voters of California legalized medical use of marijuana in 1996, and analogous laws have been enacted by more than 20 other states (NCSL, 2014).

Colorado and Washington voters approved initiatives legalizing recreational marijuana use for people over 21 in 2012 and directing state legislatures to license the cultivation and distribution of marijuana and impose taxes on marijuana transactions (American Psychiatric Association, 2014). Although the cultivation, distribution, and possession of marijuana for either medical or recreational purposes remain illegal under federal law, the U.S. Department of Justice has promulgated enforcement guidance to the U.S. Attorneys. That guidance allows for declining to enforce the Controlled Substances Act against persons who comply with the requirements of state law as long as the conduct allowed by the states does not endanger overriding federal interests, such as preventing "distribution of marijuana to minors" and "drugged driving and the exacerbation of other adverse public health consequences associated with marijuana use" (Cole, 2013).

Many questions remain unanswered about the effects of marijuana, especially when used in high-potency preparations. Public health concerns focus on the onset of dependence during adolescence and young adulthood, possible damaging neurodevelopmental effects, and increased risk of psychosis in psychologically vulnerable youth (Volkow et al., 2014). A key question raised by the legalization debate is how different approaches to legalization are likely to affect the prevalence and patterns of marijuana consumption and the extent to which marijuana will be used as a substitute for alcohol. However marijuana policy unfolds, the committee assumes that policy makers will take meaningful steps to discourage its use among youth below the age of purchase, which is nearly certain to be at least 21, and that state and federal public health agencies will establish the surveillance systems necessary to monitor patterns of consumption and the effects of policy changes on the public's health.

The age of purchase for tobacco products also has come under scrutiny. Until the 1990s, the minimum purchase age (typically 16) varied substantially from state to state and was rarely enforced anywhere. In 1992, Congress enacted legislation (known as the Synar Amendment) tying state eligibility for substance abuse prevention and treatment block grant funds to enforcement of youth tobacco access laws, and reports published by the surgeon general (CDC, 1994) and by the IOM (1994) 2 years later highlighted the importance of reducing youth initiation of smoking as a priority component of state tobacco control. In 1996, the U.S. Food and Drug Administration (FDA) promulgated its Tobacco Rule, establishing a federal minimum purchase age of 18 and restricting tobacco advertising and promotion targeting adolescents (Redhead and Burrows, 2009). Although the Supreme Court invalidated the Tobacco Rule in 2000,[7] Congress revived it in the Family Smoking Prevention and Tobacco Control Act of 2009,[8] and the FDA reissued the rule in 2010. While codifying 18 as the federal minimum age of purchase, Congress authorized the states to adopt a higher minimum purchase age and directed the FDA to assemble an expert panel to assess the public health implications of increasing the minimum purchase

[7] *Food and Drug Administration, et al. v. Brown & Williamson Tobacco Corp., et al.* 529 U.S. 120, 2000.

[8] Public Law 111-31, 111th Cong. (June 22, 2009).

age for tobacco products. At the FDA's request, the IOM has convened a panel to assess the effects of raising the minimum age to 19, 21, or 25, and the panel's report is expected in 2015.

Advertising and Promotion of Alcohol, Marijuana, and Tobacco

Recent consideration of marijuana legalization has drawn attention to the challenge of designing a regulatory structure that will adequately protect the public health (American Psychiatric Association, 2014). The shortcomings of current regulatory approaches to alcohol and tobacco are mentioned prominently in the policy debate (Bonnie, 2014), and attention has focused particularly on the effects of advertising and promotional activities targeting young adults. While a review of the effects of advertising and promotion on young adults is beyond the scope of this study, a substantial body of research has accumulated on the exposure of young adults to alcohol advertising, the increasing number of tobacco promotions targeting young adults, the intertwining of alcohol and tobacco advertising, and the rapid acceleration of marijuana advertising in Colorado (Pacula et al., 2014; Richardson et al., 2014; Sepe and Glantz, 2002; Smith and Foxcroft, 2009).

IMPROVING AND COORDINATING PUBLIC HEALTH PROGRAMS

This section examines state and federal public health programs to ascertain whether and to what extent they focus on key issues, such as those presented earlier in Box 6-2, that are relevant for young adults. Although relatively good epidemiological surveillance data are available for many of these issues, information is rarely adequate for evaluating the effectiveness of programs and policies specifically for young adults. This is the case because, while a variety of public health programs and policies have been implemented to improve overall population health, specific data have not been available on whether they have adequately reached young adults and with what effects, or subanalyses of this particular age group have not been conducted. As discussed in Chapter 2, young adults have developmentally distinct characteristics that may require strategies different from those used for children, adolescents, or older adults. Additionally, programs and policies often have been shaped by the needs of distinct groups, as well as resource limitations, resulting in the development of specific eligibility requirements—for example, those at greatest risk of HIV/AIDs. The consequence has been a siloed approach to population health that fails to reflect the fact that the same young adult may be engaged in multiple risk behaviors, such as substance abuse and unprotected sexual activity.

Coordination of State and Local Public Health Programs

The IOM's influential report on the future of public health (IOM, 1988) identifies three core functions performed by state and local public health departments: (1) assess the health of the community (assessment), (2) lead and promote evidence-based policies that are in the public's interest (policy development), and (3) ensure the availability of community and personal health services that are viewed by constituents as appropriate and necessary (assurance). Building on that foundation, recent IOM reports (e.g., IOM, 2011) have endorsed a list of the 10 essential public health services displayed earlier in Box 6-1, which provide the foundation for state and local public health systems that play a lead role in ensuring the delivery of public health services (IOM, 1988, 2003).

The U.S. public health system is made up of 51 state,[9] 2,794 local, and 565 American Indian and Alaska Native tribal public health agencies (Hyde and Shortell, 2012; NACCHO, 2009). The scope of these agencies' duties and authorities and the agencies' organizational structure vary among states (IOM, 2003). Virtually all state public health agencies provide immunizations, conduct infectious disease control and reporting, provide health education, and maintain health statistics (IOM, 2003). At the local level, local health departments are involved in various activities related to public health, such as population-based primary prevention services, immunization, and maternal and child health services. Research describing how these services are delivered is limited (Hyde and Shortell, 2012).

Funding for public health services at the state and local levels comes from a mix of federal, state, local, and private monies. In 2008, about 50 percent of state agency funding came from federal grants, contracts, and cooperative agreements; 24 percent from state general funds; and 26 percent from other sources (ASTHO, 2009). At the local level, in 2007, 25 percent of funds came from local contributions, 20 percent from state contributions, 17 percent from federal pass-through funding, 15 percent from Medicaid and Medicare reimbursements, and 11 percent from fees (NACCHO, 2009). Sources of funding vary widely at both the state and local levels, and agency activities are typically fragmented and siloed, depending on the funding stream. For example, many grantees of the federal Title X Family Planning Program administered by the Office of Family Planning face numerous challenges impacting their ability to provide family planning services because of management and administrative burdens, including funding limitations and increasing supply costs, as well as difficulty coordinating and managing multiple funding sources at the federal, state, and local levels (IOM, 2009). In addition, funding for public health infra-

[9] Including the District of Columbia.

structure is chronically inadequate and tends to decrease during recessions, eroding the capacity of local health departments to provide essential community services (NACCHO, 2014a). Since 2008, local health departments have lost 48,300 jobs as a result of layoffs and attrition, and 36 percent of the population currently lives in a jurisdiction affected by budget cuts (NACCHO, 2014a).

Nonetheless, all state and local public health programs deal at some level with many of the public health priorities for young adults described in this chapter, including tobacco control, obesity prevention, injury prevention, and prevention of unprotected sexual activity. However, fragmentation of organizational structures contributes to inefficiencies and gaps in the performance of the core public health functions, weakening responses to the needs of young adults (among other groups). For instance, the administration of different funding streams, each with its own priorities, eligibility requirements, and scope of work, carried out with little coordination or integration, results in programs reaching some groups of young adults but not providing a comprehensive approach when they are reached, while other young adults may not receive any of the services they need. Thus, for example, young adults may have access to reproductive health services offered through health departments, but may not receive screening for obesity and diabetes. These lost opportunities to take a more comprehensive approach contribute to unevenness in service provision. Furthermore, given the resources available, many young people may not have had the opportunity to access health services—either because their local jurisdiction does not make services available; because eligibility requirements preclude their access to care; or because they lack information about available resources, such as screening for STIs through public health clinics.

States have recognized the importance of integration of services for adolescents, and many state public health agencies have created adolescent topic areas or designated state adolescent health coordinators to help coordinate health programs and policies bearing on the health, safety, and well-being of adolescents (SAHRC, 2012). For example, a number of states have developed comprehensive adolescent health plans to help bring together different funding streams. Most public health departments have had an adolescent health coordinator position over the past 20-30 years, and these coordinators were initially supported directly as part of the Title V Maternal and Child Health (MCH) Block Grants to States Program. Many coordinators continue to work within Title V programs; as state funding and public health structures have changed, however, many are now funded through other divisions within public health agencies, such as family planning and chronic disease divisions.[10] As of June 1, 2014,

[10] See http://nnsahc.org/images/uploads/1-_AHC_Overview.pdf (accessed October 22, 2014).

all states except Alaska, Montana, North Dakota, Tennessee, Utah, and Virginia and the District of Columbia had an adolescent health coordinator in place (SAHRC, 2014). The coordinators' position and role vary greatly by state with respect to their responsibilities and areas of focus, but all are committed to improving the health, safety, and well-being of adolescents (NNSAHC, 2012). In 2012, 54 percent of state adolescent health coordinators had worked in adolescent health and 66 percent in public health for more than 11 years, and 20 percent for more than 20 years. Most take a broad approach to their work, with 64 percent focusing mainly on youth development, 52 percent on general adolescent health, and 38 percent on building health systems for adolescents; more than one-third have engaged adolescents in some way in their work (NNSAHC, 2012).

Very few states have implemented a similar approach for young adults, although some have extended the adolescent health coordinator's role to include young adults. One example is Maine, whose program encompasses ages 10-24 and focuses on the issues of health service access and education and youth development, with the vision that all the state's youth will be healthy, safe, and respected (King, 2014). In Texas, beginning in fiscal year 2015, contractors will be able to serve young adults up to age 24 in their programs. Contractors must select at least one of eight risk areas (motor vehicle safety, juvenile delinquency, substance abuse, dating violence, obesity, mental health issues, HIV/STIs, and access to care) on which to focus their activities. They are also required to facilitate a Youth-Adult Council (ages 12-24) to help guide their program development and incorporate a positive youth development framework.[11]

Two statewide innovations merit careful review and consideration by other states. In Colorado, the public health department convened Colorado 9to25, a partnership of more than 200 organizations, to promote the health, safety, and well-being of youth aged 9-25 (see Box 6-4). And in Maryland, the governor convened an interagency activity—the Transition Age Youth Initiative—to focus on the transition needs of young adults with intellectual disabilities or behavioral health problems (see Box 6-5).

Federal Public Health Programs

Compared with state and local government agencies, the federal government has a limited role in delivering public health services. "Nevertheless, it plays a crucial role in protecting and improving the health of the population by providing leadership in setting health goals, policies, and standards, especially through its regulatory powers" (IOM, 2003, p. 111),

[11] Personal communication, Carol Harvey, Office of Title V & Family Health, Texas Department of State Health Services, July 17, 2014.

BOX 6-4
Convening by the Public Health Department: Colorado 9to25

Colorado 9to25 (CO9to25) is an innovative partnership of youth and adults in Colorado aimed at ensuring that youth aged 9-25 (1) are safe; (2) are physically and mentally healthy; (3) receive a quality education; (4) are connected to caring adults, schools, and their communities; and (5) are contributing to their community (e.g., volunteering, working). CO9to25 is convened by the state's public health department but brings together more than 200 state, local, private, nonprofit, and for-profit organizations to work to improve programs, practices, and policies that impact the health, safety, and well-being of youth. The program recognizes that youth experience difficulties during various transition periods in their lives that can lead to dangerous and unhealthy risks and habits, so the goal of the program is to provide resources and connect youth to statewide initiatives that impact their health and well-being. CO9to25 identifies state problems and then convenes youth, adults, and participating organizations to address them.

Although CO9to25 targets a broad age range, one program focus is on addressing the health needs of young adults as they transition between adolescent and young adult health systems. This work is conducted through social media, webinars, events, and training and by connecting individuals who work with young adults with special health care needs, those with behavioral health needs, those aging out of foster care and at risk of being homeless, and those graduating from high school or completing a General Educational Development credential who need extra learning supports. The program also is working on changing its partner organizations' policies to enable the hiring of young adults as expert advisors instead of their serving in a more limited capacity as interns.

SOURCES: www.co9to25.org; Wood, 2014.

as well as in supporting research. It also contributes operational and financial resources necessary to increase the effectiveness of the public health infrastructure at the federal, state, and local levels (IOM, 2003).

Although few federal programs specifically target young adults, many programs can be utilized to improve the health, safety, and well-being of this population. Table 6-1 illustrates the broad range of current federal public health programs that affect young adults, although, as discussed below, specific data on how many young adults are being served by these programs are not readily available. This table is not exhaustive, but is intended to provide examples within various categories of public health (e.g., substance abuse, reproductive health).

Many programs specifically target adolescents (e.g., the U.S. Department of Health and Human Services' [HHS's] Adolescent Pregnancy and Prevention Grant Programs) or mothers and children (e.g., HHS's Services

BOX 6-5
Convening by the Governor's Office: Maryland Interagency Transition Council for Youth with Disabilities

Maryland's efforts toward providing mental health services to youth and young adults (aged 16-25) initially started under the leadership of the Governor's Office of Disabilities with the goal of establishing a statewide transition plan, the result largely of advocates representing the disability community. While the initial effort was built primarily around the disability community, mental health was added later on. This effort led to a governor's executive order that established an Interagency Transition Council for Youth with Disabilities, with the Mental Health Hygiene Administration and mental health advocates as mandatory partners on the committee. This enabled services for individuals with developmental and intellectual disabilities to be extended to individuals with mental health issues, particularly youth and young adults with emotional and behavioral disabilities.

In 2007, the council was tasked with recommending policies and identifying funding requirements to meet the transition needs of all youth with disabilities within Maryland. Maryland's Transition Age Youth (TAY) initiative was an effort to create a service delivery system for youth and young adults. It started with 12 TAY-specific programs provided through local mental health agencies in 2000; currently there are 24 programs, all tailored to the developmental needs of this population. Funding has come from the state, as well as federal and other resources. While most states situate these programs in the child and youth services division, Maryland's programs are situated in the Office of Adult Services within the Mental Hygiene Administration. This was done intentionally to focus on adult indicators, such as having a job, affordable housing, and relationships with others, that typically are not measured in child and adolescent systems. The programs were designed to provide youth and young adults with skills and supports during the transition phase to minimize further involvement in the adult service system.

Programs leveraged existing services and resources and varied in scope, focus, age range (14-25), type of intervention, and service modality. As knowledge and experience working with this population developed, interventions were refined. Currently, Maryland is in the process of aligning all the services within the

Grant Program for Residential Treatment for Pregnant and Postpartum Women). While young adults meet some of these programs' age eligibility requirements, evidence of whether tailoring has been used in the delivery of care or services has not been formally documented. One notable exception is incorporated as part of the National State-Based Tobacco Control Program, which aims to prevent adolescents and young adults from initiating tobacco use. It is also likely that some other programs, such as the family various programs with the intent of developing expertise in empirically supported approaches that can be brought to scale and replicated statewide.

Key policy changes that have emerged from this initiative include the following:

- Eligibility for TAY was expanded to provide continuous, uninterrupted access to developmentally appropriate services across systems serving youth with disabilities and those with mental health issues so they do not drop off the eligibility cliff upon aging out of child and adolescent services.
- Since employment among this population is a predictor of postschool success, TAY programs were granted access to evidence-based practices supporting employment programs at age 16, prior to graduation from high school.

Many lessons have been learned from the TAY programs that could be useful for other state and local agencies and organizations. These include the following:

- The average length of TAY services is 2 years.
- Among 16- to 25-year-olds in TAY programs, 70 percent are employed, versus 46 percent of those involved in other services in the mental health system.
- The increased number of people eligible for Medicaid under the Patient Protection and Affordable Care Act and children in foster care being able to maintain Medicaid up to age 26 will likely create an increased demand for TAY services.
- Initiatives need to include employment and education as a point of entry to other mental health services.
- Coordination requires pooling of funding and resources among multiple systems of care across government agencies.
- Core competency training is needed for all staff involved in the provision of services.

SOURCE: Reeder, 2014.

planning services provided under Title X funding, which target primarily younger adults (51 percent of Title X clients are in their 20s), may use approaches best suited to young adults (Fowler et al., 2012).

Recently, the National Prevention Council released its Annual Status Report, which describes how federal government departments are collaborating in cross-sector efforts addressing prevention and health.[12] Many of these strategies may impact the young adult population, but the report

[12] See http://www.surgeongeneral.gov/initiatives/prevention/2014-npc-status-report.pdf (accessed October 22, 2014).

TABLE 6-1 Selected Federal Public Health Programs Relevant to Young Adults

Policy/Program	Department/Agency	Population Served	Funding (from the Catalog of Federal Domestic Assistance)[a] (in millions)
FAMILY PLANNING, MATERNITY, PARENTING			
Maternal and Child Health Services Block Grants to States	HHS/HRSA	Mothers and children and their families, especially low-income	FY12 $541 FY13 est. $512 FY14 est. $550
Maternal and Child Health Federal Consolidated Programs	HHS/HRSA	Mothers and children	FY12 $128 FY13 est. $126 FY14 est. $128
Affordable Care Act Maternal, Infant, and Early Childhood Home Visiting Program	HHS/HRSA	Mothers and children; eligibility categories include pregnant women under 21	FY12 $309 FY13 est. $345 FY14 est. $345
Adolescent Pregnancy Prevention Grant Programs	HHS/ACF	Varies by program but primarily 10- to 19-year-old youth and young adults at risk and vulnerable to pregnancy; some programs also include young parents up to 21	FY12 na FY13 na FY14 na
Pregnancy Assistance Fund Program	HHS/Office of the Secretary	Pregnant and parenting teens and women; also supports fathers and families	FY12 $24 FY13 est. $22 FY14 na
Services Grant Program for Residential Treatment for Pregnant and Postpartum Women (PPW)	HHS/SAMHSA	Low-income women aged 18 and over who are pregnant or postpartum and their minor children aged 17 and under	Total funding available: $8,384,000
Family Planning Services (provided under Title X)	HHS/Office of Population Affairs	Universal; priority to people with low income of reproductive age	FY12 $274 FY13 est. $245 FY14 na

TABLE 6-1 Continued

Policy/Program	Department/Agency	Population Served	Funding (from the Catalog of Federal Domestic Assistance)[a] (in millions)
SEXUALLY TRANSMITTED INFECTIONS (STIs)/HIV			
Ryan White HIV/ AIDS Program	HHS/HRSA	Universal, all ages	FY12 $2,392,178,000 FY13 $2,248,638,000[b] FY14 na
HIV Prevention Programs for Women	HHS/Office of the Secretary	Women	FY12 $5 FY13 est. $4 FY14 na
DoD HIV/AIDS Prevention Program	DoD	Universal (includes international)	FY12 $28 FY13 est. $30 FY14 na
SUBSTANCE USE/ABUSE			
Drug-Free Communities	HHS/SAMHSA	Universal	FY12 $84 FY13 est. $59 FY14 est. $39
National State-Based Tobacco Control Programs	HHS/CDC	Universal; focus on youth and young adults	FY12 $0 FY13 est. $0 FY14 est. $58
Tobacco Regulation Awareness, Communication, and Education Program	HHS/FDA	Universal; focus on youth	FY12 $0 FY13 est. $0 FY14 est. $0
Drug Court Training and Technical Assistance	Executive Office of the President	Universal	FY12 $1 FY13 est. $1 FY14 na
Model State Drug Laws Initiative	Executive Office of the President	Universal	FY12 $1 FY13 est. $1 FY14 na
Veterans Rehabilitation Alcohol and Drug Dependence	VA Health Administration Center/ Department of Veterans Affairs	Veterans	FY12 na FY13 na FY14 na

continued

TABLE 6-1 Continued

Policy/Program	Department/Agency	Population Served	Funding (from the Catalog of Federal Domestic Assistance)[a] (in millions)
CHRONIC DISEASE PREVENTION AND HEALTH PROMOTION			
Centers for Research and Demonstration for Health Promotion and Disease Prevention	HHS/CDC	Universal	FY12 $30 FY13 est. $21 FY14 est. $20
INJURY PREVENTION AND CONTROL			
Injury Prevention and Control—Research and State and Community Based Programs	HHS/CDC	Universal	Cooperative agreements: FY12 $70 FY13 est. $68 FY14 est. $71 Project grants: FY12 $12 FY13 est. $11 FY14 est. $11
MOTOR VEHICLE SAFETY			
State and Community Highway Safety	DOT/NHTSA	Universal	FY12 $235 FY13 est. $235 FY14 est. $235
Alcohol Impaired Driving Countermeasures Incentive Grants I	DOT/NHTSA	Universal	FY12 $139 FY13 est. $0 FY14 est. $0

describes only one effort specifically targeting young adults—the launch of HHS's partnership with the American College Health Association and the University of Michigan, which supports the Tobacco-Free College Campus initiative. This initiative resulted in increasing the number of designated smoke-free campuses from 774 to 1,342. The rest of the programs included in the report do not specifically mention young adults, although several federal public health programs (e.g., the Maternal and Child Health Services Block Grant Program, the Ryan White HIV/AIDS Program, Federally Qualified Health Centers) deal with many of the key issues impacting young adults listed earlier in Box 6-2 (see Box 6-6). A similar pattern can be seen at the state and local levels, where, as discussed earlier, numerous public health programs are relevant to young adults.

TABLE 6-1 Continued

Policy/Program	Department/Agency	Population Served	Funding (from the Catalog of Federal Domestic Assistance)[a] (in millions)
Occupant Protection Incentive Grants	DOT/NHTSA	Universal	FY12 $25 FY13 est. $0 FY14 est. $0
Alcohol Open Container Requirements	DOT/NHTSA	Universal	FY12 $115 FY13 est. $0 FY14 est. $0
Incentive Grant Program to Increase Motorcycle Safety	DOT/NHTSA	Universal	FY12 $7 FY13 est. $4 FY14 est. $0
NHTSA Discretionary Safety Grants	DOT/NHTSA	Universal	FY12 $7 FY13 est. $0 FY14 est. $0
National Priority Safety Programs	DOT/NHTSA	Universal	FY13 est. $265 FY14 est. $272

NOTES: ACF = Administration for Children and Families; CDC = Centers for Disease Control and Prevention; DoD = U.S. Department of Defense; DOT = U.S. Department of Transportation; FDA = U.S. Food and Drug Administration; HHS = U.S. Department of Health and Human Services; HRSA = Health Resources and Services Administration; na = not available; NHTSA = National Highway Traffic Safety Administration; SAMHSA = Substance Abuse and Mental Health Services Administration.

[a] For most programs, three fiscal years of funding is available in the Catalog of Federal Domestic Assistance.

[b] See http://hab.hrsa.gov/data/reports/funding.html (accessed October 22, 2014).

The committee found that in most cases, the number of young adults being served by each federal program is not reported as a separate category, reflecting the fact that young adults are not consistently identified as a group with their own set of health conditions, risk factors, and needs. Nor is evidence available on whether programs tailor their efforts to different developmental ages and whether these modifications result in improved outcomes. Moreover, age data are reported differently for each program. As noted throughout this report, young adults should not automatically be combined with adolescents and older adults in public health programs. Breaking down data collection and analyses by adolescents, young adults, and older adults, as well as by gender and race/ethnicity, wherever possible, would help in assessing whether strategies and interventions are

BOX 6-6
Young Adults in Federal Programs: Examples from the Health Resources and Services Administration

The examples below provide a summary of how young adults are currently included in several key public health programs within the Health Resources and Services Administration (HRSA).

Title V Maternal and Child Health Services Block Grant Program (HRSA Title V)

HRSA provides services to mothers, pregnant women, infants, children and youth (including children and youth with special health care needs), and their families by funding states through its Title V program (HRSA, 2014d). Programs range from those that have produced clinical guidelines for child health supervision from infancy through adolescence, standards for prenatal care, and health safety standards for out-of-home child care facilities, to those that are focused on nutrition care during pregnancy and lactation and the incorporation of childhood injury prevention strategies (HRSA, 2000).

Young adults can receive services and support through HRSA's Title V program under the "child" or "mother" category. Title V defines individuals as children until they turn 22. Within that parameter, however, each state can specify how "children" are defined for the purposes of its own block grant program. In Maine, for example, children are defined as ages 1 to 19, but in Louisiana, they are defined as ages 1 to 14. Only Connecticut defines children as up to 22 years of age (HRSA, 2014e). These varying definitions represent states' decisions regarding the population for which they are willing to provide benefits, with states and jurisdictions being required to match every $4 of federal Title V money received with at least $3 of state and/or local money. This matching results in more than $6 billion available annually for maternal and child health programs at the state and local levels (HRSA, 2014d). This state-level variability contrasts with the provision of the Patient Protection and Affordable Care Act that enables children to remain on their parents' health insurance plan until age 26 (KFF, 2011).

Ryan White HIV/AIDS Program

The Ryan White HIV/AIDS Program works with cities, states, and local community-based organizations to provide HIV-related services to more than half

being modified for different developmental age groups, whether diverse eligible populations are actually being served, and what outcomes are being achieved by age group.

Finally, the federal Maternal and Child Health Bureau has established an Adolescent and Young Adult Health Program. This program is designed "to promote comprehensive healthy development, health, safety, and well-being of adolescents and young adults . . . by strengthening the abilities of a million people each year. The program serves those who lack sufficient health care coverage or financial resources for coping with HIV disease (HRSA, 2013), thus filling gaps in care not covered by other sources. The program reaches an estimated 529,000 people, 7 percent of whom are aged 13-24 and 41 percent of whom are aged 25-44, and program components are designed to serve youth (HRSA, 2012, 2013).

In addition to the Ryan White Program, HRSA's HIV/AIDS Bureau supports a range of activities addressing the needs of HIV-positive youth. These include research initiatives and evaluations of innovative models of care focused on HIV-impacted youth, including women of color and young men who have sex with men (HRSA, 2012). In addition, HRSA is working to reduce barriers to early HIV identification and ensure access to health care, as well as engaging in other efforts, including community collaborations with national organizations, such as the National Minority AIDS Council and HealthHIV, that are addressing HIV among youth (HRSA, 2012).

Federally Qualified Health Centers

Federally Qualified Health Centers (FQHCs) are community-based organizations that serve medically underserved areas and/or vulnerable populations to improve public health. In 2012, these HRSA-supported health centers served more than 1 million homeless individuals, more than 900,000 agricultural workers and their families, more than 200,000 individuals in public housing, and almost 7,000 Native Hawaiians (HHS, 2014a).

In 2012, FQHCs served more than 3,700,000 patients aged 18-29, representing 18 percent of their patient population. In addition, approximately 166,000 patients aged 18-29 were served by federal Look-Alikes, representing 17 percent of their patient population (HRSA, 2014b,c).

The U.S. Department of Health and Human Services recently announced the availability of an additional $100 million (under the auspices of the Affordable Care Act) that will support an estimated 150 new FQHC sites in 2015, an expansion intended to increase access to health care in communities with the greatest need for services (HHS, 2014b). The expansion does not specifically target young adults, but if the patterns described above persist, nearly one in five new patients served will be in this age group.

[Title V programs] as well as of public health and clinical health professionals, to better serve these population groups, which range in age from 10 to 25 years" (HRSA, 2014a). The program is an example of a formal effort to recognize young adults as a separate population with their own needs. However, it represents only a small component of public health systems' response to the needs of this population. Where necessary, new data collection efforts, disaggregated by these age groupings and other identifiers, are warranted to support improvements in public health programs and campaigns aimed at improving the health, safety, and well-being of young adults.

Preventive Care Opportunities Under the Affordable Care Act

The Patient Protection and Affordable Care Act (ACA) includes numerous provisions intended to increase access to preventive health care, focused at both the individual and population levels. The architects of the ACA recognized the need for population-level investments that can help modify the environments that are the contexts for public health, as well as reinforce the act's individual preventive focus. The ACA increases incentives for adminstering preventive care and financially supports primary prevention initiatives of communities and public health agencies. The Prevention and Public Health Fund (PPHF), for example, while not specifically focused on young adults, is used to support community and clinical prevention programs, strengthen the public health infrastructure and workforce, and expand public health research and tracking efforts (APHA, 2013). Yet while the ACA includes commitments to prevention, through both an emphasis on the provision of clinical preventive services (see Chapter 7) and the PPHF, the federal government's public health investment would need to be doubled to address current public health needs (IOM, 2012b).

In fiscal year 2012, under the auspices of the PPHF, $401.1 million was set aside to fund community prevention activities proven to reduce health care costs and improve health behaviors. These funds support such initiatives as the Community Transformation Grant (CTG) program, administered by the CDC (APHA, 2012). The CTG program is "designed to address the behavioral, physical, social, and environmental risk factors associated with chronic diseases, such as tobacco use and exposure to secondhand smoke, poor screening systems for disease risks, and lack of access to healthy food and safe environments for physical activity" (Hennrikus, 2013, p. 16).

Ultimately, the CTG program is anticipated to impact 40 percent of the U.S. population (Hennrikus, 2013). CTG grants fund evidence-based programs that address major causes of chronic disease, such as heart disease, diabetes, and cancer, in communities, and promote tobacco-free living, physical activity, healthy eating, services to prevent and control high blood pressure and high cholesterol, social and emotional wellness, and healthy and safe environments (Hennrikus, 2013). State and local government agencies, tribes and territories, and nonprofit organizations are eligible for CTG funds. Thus far, the CTG-funded programs have been implemented in an array of sectors, such as health care, education, and transportation. In 2011, $103 million was distributed among 36 states to 61 state and local government agencies, tribes and territories, and nonprofit organizations for the implementation of evidence-based programs (CDC, 2013a; Hennrikus, 2013). Although many of these programs are likely to improve the contexts in which young people live, their impact on contributing to improved population-level outcomes among young adults cannot be known absent the improvements in data collection and analysis discussed above.

CONCLUSIONS AND RECOMMENDATIONS

Policy makers and practitioners have recognized that the health, safety, and well-being of adolescents can be enhanced, during adolescence and thereafter, by basing policy and practice on an integrated understanding of this distinct period of development. A key conclusion of this report is that the health, safety, and well-being of young adults can similarly benefit from bringing a developmental perspective to bear on public health policies and programs and on the delivery of health care (discussed in Chapter 7). The literature reviewed in this chapter also makes the following points clear:

- The effects of interventions—especially those that include only one component, focus on only one level, and are brief in duration—generally are small and not sustainable. On the other hand, multipronged and reinforcing approaches that target and are tailored to individual behaviors and their social, environmental, and legal contexts and are implemented over a period of at least several years generally are more successful and their effects more sustained.
- Approaches that promote collaboration and participation among multiple stakeholders create the right environment for individual change and foster health-related social change.
- The use of mobile digital media and social networking to implement interventions shows considerable promise, although evidence for the effectiveness of this approach remains to be developed.
- The notable success of some multilevel public health campaigns targeting older adolescents and young adults provides a solid foundation for developing and fielding innovative community initiatives that combine health messages with environmental interventions addressing cross-cutting health and safety challenges for young adults.
- Public health campaigns that are media based or include a media component are less likely to benefit people who are educationally or economically disadvantaged or are from racial and ethnic minorities, as well as young adults who are not in college.
- Formulating an integrated approach to public health policy and practice focused on young adults will require improvements in

the data assembled for surveillance and research, as well as better coordination of federal and state public health programs.
- A major aim of policies focused on improving population health should be to incorporate screening and prevention into primary health care and other health settings for young adults, as well as social settings where at-risk groups congregate (e.g., STI screening in bars or nightclubs).
- The importance of identifying and rectifying health disparities among young adults has received little attention in the design and administration of public health programs, as well as in intervention research.
- Few state or local programs have attempted to coordinate or integrate programs for young adults, although innovations to this end have been undertaken in a handful of states.
- Several recent federal initiatives reflect a nascent effort to promote and support policies and practices reflecting an integrated understanding of young adulthood.

State and Local Coordination Efforts

No states have addressed the needs of young adults aged 18-26 in a large-scale way. Under the new Adolescent and Young Adult Health Program funded by the Health Resources and Services Administration and administered by the MCH Bureau, states and localities will be encouraged to expand care beyond adolescents. To advance this transformation, the committee makes the following recommendation:

Recommendation 6-1: State and local public health departments should establish an office to coordinate programs and services bearing on the health, safety, and well-being of young adults. If a separate office is not established for young adults, these responsibilities should be assigned to the adolescent health coordinator.

The committee is mindful that many state and local public health agencies are underfunded and have limited capacity to take on new responsibilities. Elevating the visibility and importance of young adults may also require additional training and skill development for staff. The committee regards this recommendation as requiring a change in orientation to shape an array of activities that will respond to the documented pressing needs of this population. Aside from bringing together the necessary expertise on the development and needs of young adults, improved coordination of young adult programs and services can also be expected to identify gaps in existing services and opportunities for new services and allow more efficient allocation of resources.

Once an office for coordinating programs and services for young adults is created or linked to an existing office, an evaluation program will be important. Evaluation will provide processes and tools that can be applied to obtain accurate, reliable, and credible data to address program performance questions. Data collection needs to be feasible for health departments and other organizations, which are unlikely to have the resources for elaborate measurements of populations, polices, and environments. Better data will lead to better comparisons across time and may lead to better benchmarks. There are a variety of ways to accomplish this (see the American Evaluation Association's Guiding Principles for Evaluators[13] for examples).

Colorado 9to25, described earlier in this chapter, highlights the potential synergies of a multisectoral model of community mobilization focused on young adults (or adolescents and young adults). The U.S. Department of Education's Promise Neighborhoods and the U.S. Department of Housing and Urban Development's Choice Neighborhoods are analogous initiatives. Building on these models, state public health agencies (or local agencies with adequate staff and authority) should convene multistakeholder initiatives potentially called "Healthy Transitions to Adulthood," as stand-alone activities or a component of already-existing community initiatives. The coalition should reach out to all local organizations with a stake in the healthy, successful development of young adults, including large employers, residential and nonresidential colleges and universities, community colleges, other providers of vocational training, faith-based organizations, and health care systems. A broad scope of activities might be undertaken by such coalitions, encompassing the entire range of transitional tasks in young adulthood and the range of outcomes associated with health and well-being. Young adults should play a pivotal role in these efforts from the outset.

> **Recommendation 6-2: Each community should establish a multistakeholder private-public coalition on "Healthy Transitions to Adulthood," with the goal of promoting the education, health, safety, and well-being of all young adults. State or local public health agencies should take the lead in convening these coalitions. The coalitions should include young adults; colleges and universities; providers of career and technical education; employers; youth organizations; nonprofit organizations; medical specialties providing primary care to young adults; and other community organizations serving, supporting, or investing in young adults. These initiatives should mobilize public and private engagement and support; set priorities; formulate strategies for reaching all groups**

---

[13] See http://www.eval.org/p/cm/ld/fid=51 (accessed October 22, 2014).

of young adults who need services and support; and design, implement, and evaluate prevention activities and programs. Initiatives should also incorporate the valuable input of young adults in shaping their scope and activities to ensure that there is traction among those initiatives aimed at improving their health, safety, and well-being.

The committee is aware of the difficulty of initiating multisector community mobilization efforts and understands that many such efforts do not succeed. However, the creative energy that can be brought to bear on such an initiative provides a solid basis for optimism. Some states may choose to build on the efforts they have devoted to adolescents, extending the purview of those efforts to recognize the importance of the transition into adulthood. The intent is not to dilute existing efforts to improve adolescent health, but to recognize the importance of the young adult years within the life course and the necessity of investing in this particular age group as well.

Finally, once a Healthy Transitions to Adulthood coalition has been formed, stakeholders should be identified and an evaluation process designed with their input so that the evaluations will meet the goals of all stakeholders.

Community Transformation Grants

The CTG program's 5-year measurable performance goals are to decrease all of the following by 5 percent: death and disability due to tobacco use, the rate of obesity through nutrition and physical activity interventions, and death/disability due to heart disease and stroke (CDC, 2013a). While the first two of these areas clearly are congruent with the needs for prevention among young adults, it is not feasible to ascertain how many young adults have benefited directly from these investments to date. As illustrated by Box 6-2, moreover, many priority issues for young adults are not addressed by the CTG program. Since these national investments are currently being made, however, the CTG program presents an opportunity to deal with at least some of the issues that are important for young adults.

Reducing tobacco use is a key issue because smokers who quit before the age of 30 will reverse much of the damage to their health due to tobacco use (HHS, 2012b). Therefore, although much of the focus is appropriately on reducing the initiation rate for tobacco use among people under age 18, the young adult years also are critical for reducing lifelong rates of tobacco use. Similarly, weight gain during young adulthood may be one of the most important determinants of cardiovascular and cancer risk factors, so this time period is critical for reducing rates of obesity through both improved nutrition and physical activity.

Recommendation 6-3: Recipients of Community Transformation Grants—including state and local government agencies, tribes and territories, and nonprofit organizations—should incorporate specific targets for young adults in their plans to reach the 5-year measurable performance goals in the areas of reducing death and disability due to tobacco use and reducing the rate of obesity through nutrition and physical activity interventions.

As communities consider the types of public health interventions they could implement to support young adults, they might make use of two resources—CDC's *The Guide to Community Preventive Services*[14] and the New York Academy of Medicine's *Compendium of Proven Community-Based Prevention Programs*.[15] These resources identify particular programs that have succeeded in reducing obesity and related diseases, including heart disease, hypertension, diabetes, and some forms of cancer—all issues that pose a risk for young adults. Communities also might consider other examples of approaches for impacting young adults. In the area of obesity prevention, for example, HHS, the U.S. Department of Agriculture, the U.S. Department of Defense, and the U.S. Department of Veterans Affairs are engaged in ensuring that federal programs and facilities meet the *Dietary Guidelines for Americans*.[16]

Key Areas for Research

Given existing gaps in the current public health infrastructure for young adults, research is needed in several key areas to inform public health policies and programs:

- **The effectiveness of multilevel interventions in achieving health outcomes, including how to connect with difficult-to-reach young adults.** More research is needed to understand the impact of multilevel interventions, including public health campaigns and initiatives, on prevention and the amelioration of risk factors among young adults. Multidisciplinary researchers can review lessons learned as well as evidence in other relevant areas, such as the use of social marketing for other populations. Most of the young adult population is involved in some type of system (e.g., college, community college, military services), but active outreach to those not connected to these communities, or marginalized in other ways, is

[14] See http://www.thecommunityguide.org/index.html (accessed October 22, 2014).
[15] See http://healthyamericans.org/report/110 (accessed October 22, 2014).
[16] See http://fasinfat.org/national-prevention-strategy (accessed October 22, 2014).

needed. There is limited evidence on these difficult-to-reach populations and on what strategies may be most effective in engaging them so they are better able to recognize and care about the potential risks they create or encounter.

- **The influence of social media on health outcomes.** The dramatic shift to reliance on information and communication technologies and the significant uptake of social media by young adults point to the promise of harnessing this form of communication to better connect this population with health-related content. The nature of social media may allow for a rich, interactive learning environment that can both engage youth and tailor content directly to their perceptions, barriers, and needs. The capability for two-way communication may further engage young adults and may turn passive audiences into active participants. But despite the promise of media for connecting young adults with both health information and resources in their communities, more research is needed to determine how best to integrate this platform into health interventions. Those conducting such research will need to use high-quality research methods and large samples, understand what other resources may be needed to supplement social media content, and determine how behavior change may be sustained over time.
- **Better understanding of how social determinants, mechanisms, and trajectories contribute to health disparities among young adults, including within different groups.** The preponderance of research involving young adults often focuses on college campuses, particularly for priority areas such as alcohol and tobacco consumption. However, the focus on this population fails to fully represent how young adults who do not attend college experience the transition after high school, and thus may obscure how those from different socioeconomic and racial and ethnic groups may be impacted by this transition. More research on how to develop and deploy robust interventions among noncollege youth in diverse community- and work-based settings is sorely needed, including rigorous trials using standardized measures so that behavioral outcomes can be compared across groups. Furthermore, studies with diverse groups may benefit greatly from partnerships with community organizations to increase reach, promote sustainability, account for cultural factors, and tailor the content of interventions more effectively to the needs of the target group.
- **Better understanding of the impact of the advertising and promotion of alcohol, tobacco, and marijuana on the health, safety, and well-being of young adults.** Research is needed to assess the impact, singly and in combination, of the promotion and advertising of al-

cohol, tobacco, and marijuana on the health, safety, and well-being of young adults. The importance of this research is highlighted by the proliferation of new tobacco products, including e-cigarettes, and the combined use of tobacco products and marijuana in jurisdictions that have legalized marijuana's medical or recreational use.

REFERENCES

American Psychiatric Association. 2014. *Resource document on the need to monitor and assess the public health and safety consequences of legalizing marijuana.* http://www.psychiatry.org/learn/library--archives/resource-documents (accessed August 29, 2014).

APA (American Psychological Association). 2013. *Stress in America: Missing the health care connection.* https://www.apa.org/news/press/releases/stress/2012/full-report.pdf (accessed July 15, 2014).

APHA (American Public Health Association). 2012. *The prevention and public health fund: A critical investment in our nation's physical and fiscal health.* Center for Public Health Policy Issue Brief. Washington, DC: APHA.

APHA. 2013. *Get the facts: Prevention and public health fund: Dedicated to improving our nation's public health.* Washington, DC: APHA.

Aronson, R. E., K. L. Rulison, L. F. Graham, R. M. Pulliam, W. L. McGee, J. D. Labban, D. Dingman, and S. D. Rhodes. 2013. Brothers leading healthy lives: Outcomes from the pilot testing of a culturally and contextually congruent HIV prevention intervention for black male college students. *AIDS Education and Prevention* 25(5):376-393.

ASTHO (Association of State and Territorial Health Officials). 2009. *Profile of state public health: Volume one.* Arlington, VA: ASTHO.

ASTHO. 2014. *Profile of state public health: Volume three.* Arlington, VA: ASTHO.

Atkin, C. K., and R. E. Rice. 2012. Theory and principles of public communication campaigns. In *Public communication campaigns*, 4th ed., edited by R. E. Rice and C. K. Atkin. Thousands Oak, CA: Sage Publications. Pp. 3-19.

Birnbaum, H. G., R. C. Kessler, D. Kelley, R. Ben-Hamadi, V. N. Joish, and P. E. Greenberg. 2010. Employer burden of mild, moderate, and severe major depressive disorder: Mental health services utilization and costs, and work performance. *Depression and Anxiety* 27(1):78-89.

Black, M. C., K. C. Basile, M. J. Breiding, S. G. Smith, M. L. Walters, M. T. Merrick, J. Chen, and M. R. Stevens. 2011. *The National Intimate Partner and Sexual Violence Survey (NISVS): 2010 summary report.* Atlanta, GA: National Center for Injury Prevention and Control, CDC.

Blazer, D., D. Hughes, and L. K. George. 1987. Stressful life events and the onset of a generalized anxiety syndrome. *American Journal of Psychiatry* 144(9):1178-1183.

Bonnie, R. J. 2014. The impending collision between first amendment protection for commercial speech and the public health: The case of tobacco control. *Virginia Public Law and Legal Theory Research Paper* No. 2014-34.

Bonnie, R. J., and E. S. Scott. 2013. The teenage brain: Adolescent brain research and the law. *Current Directions in Psychological Science* 22(2):158-161.

Bonnie, R. J., and C. H. Whitebread. 1974. *The marijuana conviction: A history of marijuana prohibition in the United States.* Charlottesville: University Press of Virginia.

Braithwaite, S. R., and F. D. Fincham. 2009. A randomized clinical trial of a computer based preventive intervention: Replication and extension of ePREP. *Journal of Family Psychology* 23(1):32-38.

Brinn, M. P., K. V. Carson, A. J. Esterman, A. B. Chang, and B. J. Smith. 2012. Mass media interventions for preventing smoking in young people. *Evidence-Based Child Health: A Cochrane Review Journal* 7(1):86-144.

Brody, G. H., Y. F. Chen and S. M. Kogan. 2010. A cascade model connecting life stress to risk behavior among rural African American emerging adults. *Development and Psychopathoogy* 22(3):667-678.

Broman, C. L. 2012. Race differences in the receipt of mental health services among young adults. *Psychological Services* 9(1):38-48.

Bronfenbrenner, U. 1979. Contexts of child rearing: Problems and prospects. *American Psychologist* 34(10):844-850.

Brown, J. 2013. A review of the evidence on technology-based interventions for the treatment of tobacco dependence in college health. *Worldviews on Evidence Based Nursing* 10(3):150-162.

Bull, S. S., D. K. Levine, S. R. Black, S. J. Schmiege, and J. Santelli. 2012. Social media-delivered sexual health intervention: A cluster randomized controlled trial. *American Journal of Preventive Medicine* 43(5):467-474.

Caldeira, K. M., S. J. Kasperski, E. Sharma, K. B. Vincent, K. E. O'Grady, E. D. Wish, and A. M. Arria. 2009. College students rarely seek help despite serious substance use problems. *Journal of Substance Abuse Treatment* 37(4):368-378.

Carrol, J. A., and R. L. Kirkpatrick. 2011. *Impact of social media on adolescent behavioral health*. Oakland: California Adolescent Health Collaborative.

Carson, K. V., M. P. Brinn, N. A. Labiszewski, A. J. Esterman, A. B. Chang, and B. J. Smith. 2011. Community interventions for preventing smoking in young people. *Cochrane Database of Systematic Reviews* (7):Cd001291.

Catalano, S. 2013. *Intimate partner violence: Attributes of victimization, 1993-2010*. Washington, DC: U.S. Department of Justice, Office of Justice Programs, Bureau of Justice Statistics.

Cavallo, D. N., D. F. Tate, A. V. Ries, J. D. Brown, R. F. DeVellis, and A. S. Ammerman. 2012. A social media-based physical activity intervention: A randomized controlled trial. *American Journal of Preventive Medicine* 43(5):527-532.

CDC (Centers for Disease Control and Prevention). 1994. *Preventing tobacco use among young people: A report of the Surgeon General*. Atlanta, GA: HHS, Public Health Service, CDC, National Center for Chronic Disease Prevention and Health Promotion, Office on Smoking and Health.

CDC. 2010. *Alcohol and public health*. http://www.cdc.gov/alcohol/ardi.htm (accessed July 14, 2014).

CDC. 2012. Estimated HIV incidence among adults and adolescents in the United States, 2007-2010. *HIV Surveillance Supplemental Report* 17(4)1-26.

CDC. 2013a. *Community transformation grants (CTG)*. http://www.cdc.gov/nccdphp/dch/programs/communitytransformation/ (accessed March 24, 2014).

CDC. 2013b. Homicide rates among persons aged 10-24 years—United States, 1981-2010. *Morbidity and Mortality Weekly Report* 62(27):545-548.

CDC. 2013c. *Incidence, prevalence, and cost of sexually transmitted infections in the United States*. http://www.cdc.gov/std/stats/sti-estimates-fact-sheet-feb-2013.pdf (accessed August 11, 2014).

CDC. 2013d. *Youth violence: National statistics*. http://www.cdc.gov/violenceprevention/youthviolence/stats_at-a_glance/nfa_age-sex.html (accessed July 7, 2014).

CDC. 2013e. *2011 HIV surveillance report*. Vol. 23. http://www.cdc.gov/hiv/topics/surveillance/resources/reports (accessed July 15, 2014).

CDC. 2014a. *Compressed mortality, 1999-2011 data provided by CDC wonder online database*. http://wonder.cdc.gov/cmf-icd10.html (accessed September 4, 2014).

CDC. 2014b. *Fact sheets: Alcohol use and health.* http://www.cdc.gov/alcohol/fact-sheets/alcohol-use.htm (accessed July 9, 2014).

CDC, 2014c. *Fact sheets: Genital HPV infection.* http://www.cdc.gov/std/hpv/stdfact-hpv.htm (accessed August 11, 2014).

CDC. 2014d. *Leading causes of death reports, national and regional, 1999-2011.* http://webappa.cdc.gov/sasweb/ncipc/leadcaus10_us.html (accessed July 10, 2014).

Cellucci, T., J. Krogh, and P. Vik. 2006. Help seeking for alcohol problems in a college population. *Journal of General Psychology* 133(4):421-433.

Chapman, J., C. J. Armitage, and P. Norman. 2009. Comparing implementation intention interventions in relation to young adults' intake of fruit and vegetables. *Psychology and Health* 24(3):317-332.

Chen, P., and K. C. Jacobson. 2012. Developmental trajectories of substance use from early adolescence to young adulthood: Gender and racial/ethnic differences. *Journal of Adolescent Health* 50(2):154-163.

Christensen, H., E. Pallister, S. Smale, I. B. Hickie, and A. L. Calear. 2010. Community-based prevention programs for anxiety and depression in youth: A systematic review. *Journal of Primary Prevention* 31(3):139-170.

Cole, J. M. 2013. *Memorandum for all United States attorneys.* Washington, DC: U.S. Department of Justice.

Corcoran, C., E. Walker, R. Huot, V. Mittal, K. Tessner, L. Kestler, and D. Malaspina. 2003. The stress cascade and schizophrenia: Etiology and onset. *Schizophrenia Bulletin* 29(4):671-692.

Corrigan, P. W., and A. C. Watson. 2002. Understanding the impact of stigma on people with mental illness. *World Psychiatry* 1(1):16-20.

Cotton, S. M., A. Wright, M. G. Harris, A. F. Jorm, and P. D. McGorry. 2006. Influence of gender on mental health literacy in young Australians. *Australian and New Zealand Journal of Psychiatry* 40(9):790-796.

Curtin, S. C., J. C. Abma, S. J. Ventura, and S. Henshaw. 2013. Pregnancy rates for U.S. women continue to drop. *National Center for Health Statistics, Data Brief* (123):1-7.

Dalton, M. A., M. L. Beach, A. M. Adachi-Mejia, M. R. Longacre, A. L. Matzkin, J. D. Sargent, T. F. Heatherton, and L. Titus-Ernstoff. 2009. Early exposure to movie smoking predicts established smoking by older teens and young adults. *Pediatrics* 123(4):e551-e558.

Dejong, W., and J. Blanchette. 2014. Case closed: Research evidence on the positive public health impact of the age 21 minimum legal drinking age in the United States. *Journal of Studies on Alcohol and Drugs* (17):108-115.

DiClemente, R. J., and G. M. Wingood. 1995. A randomized controlled trial of an HIV sexual risk-reduction intervention for young African-American women. *Journal of the American Medical Association* 274(16):1271-1276.

Dinh-Zarr, T. B., D. A. Sleet, R. A. Shults, S. Zaza, R. W. Elder, J. L. Nichols, R. S. Thompson, and D. M. Sosin. 2001. Reviews of evidence regarding interventions to increase the use of safety belts. *American Journal of Preventive Medicine* 21(4):48-65.

DoD (U.S. Department of Defense). 2014. *Department of Defense annual report on sexual assault in the military: Fiscal year 2013.* Washington, DC: DoD.

Duggan, M., and A. Smith. 2013. *Social media update 2013.* http://www.pewinternet.org/2013/12/30/social-media-update-2013 (accessed July 11, 2014).

Edlund, M. J., P. S. Wang, P. A. Berglund, S. J. Katz, E. Lin, and R. C. Kessler. 2002. Dropping out of mental health treatment: Patterns and predictors among epidemiological survey respondents in the United States and Ontario. *American Journal of Psychiatry* 159(5):845-851.

Edlund, M. J., B. M. Booth, and X. Han. 2012. Who seeks care where?: Utilization of mental health and substance use disorder treatment in two national samples of individuals with alcohol use disorders. *Journal of Studies on Alcohol and Drugs* 73(4):635-646.

Eisenberg, D., E. Golberstein, and S. E. Gollust. 2007. Help-seeking and access to mental health care in a university student population. *Medical Care* 45(7):594-601.

Eisenberg, D., M. F. Downs, E. Golberstein, and K. Zivin. 2009. Stigma and help seeking for mental health among college students. *Medical Care Research and Review* 66(5):522-541.

Elder, R. W., R. A. Shults, D. A. Sleet, J. L. Nichols, R. S. Thompson, and W. Rajab. 2004. Effectiveness of mass media campaigns for reducing drinking and driving and alcohol-involved crashes: A systematic review. *American Journal of Preventive Medicine* 27(1):57-65.

Farrer, L., L. Leach, K. M. Griffiths, H. Christensen, and A. F. Jorm. 2008. Age differences in mental health literacy. *BMC Public Health* 8:125.

Farrer, L., A. Gulliver, J. K. Chan, P. J. Batterham, J. Reynolds, A. Calear, R. Tait, K. Bennett and K. M. Griffiths. 2013. Technology-based interventions for mental health in tertiary students: Systematic review. *Journal of Medical Internet Research* 15(5):e101.

Fell, J. C., and E. Romano. 2013. Are strong graduated driver licensing laws having unintended consequences? *Annals of Advances in Automotive Medicine* 57:351-352.

Fellmeth, G. L., C. Heffernan, J. Nurse, S. Habibula, and D. Sethi. 2013. Educational and skills-based interventions for preventing relationship and dating violence in adolescents and young adults. *Cochrane Database of Systematic Reviews* 6.

Fergusson, D. M., L. J. Horwood, E. M. Ridder, and A. L. Beautrais. 2005. Sexual orientation and mental health in a birth cohort of young adults. *Psychological Medicine* 35(7):971-981.

Fowler, C. I., S. Lloyd, J. Gale, J. Wang, and E. McClure. 2012. *Family Planning Annual Report: 2011 National Summary*. Research Triangle Park, NC: RTI International.

Fox, S., and R. Lee. 2014. *The web at 25 in the U.S.* http://www.pewinternet.org/2014/02/27/the-web-at-25-in-the-u-s (accessed May 3, 2014).

Garcia, C. 2010. Conceptualization and measurement of coping during adolescence: A review of the literature. *Journal of Nursing Scholarship* 42(2):166-185.

Gavin, L., A. P. MacKay, K. Brown, S. Harrier, S. J. Ventura, L. Kann, M. Rangel, S. Berman, P. Dittus, N. Liddon, L. Markowitz, M. Sternberg, H. Weinstock, C. David-Ferdon, and G. Ryan. 2009. Sexual and reproductive health of persons aged 10-24 years—United States, 2002-2007. *Morbidity and Mortality Weekly Report Surveillance Summaries* 58(6):1-58.

Gayman, M. D., G. S. Cuddeback, and J. P. Morrissey. 2011. Help-seeking behaviors in a community sample of young adults with substance use disorders. *The Journal of Behavioral Health Services & Research* 38(4):464-477.

Gerend, M. A., M. A. Shepherd, and M. L. Lustria. 2013. Increasing human papillomavirus vaccine acceptability by tailoring messages to young adult women's perceived barriers. *Sexually Transmitted Diseases* 40(5):401-405.

Gow, R. W., S. E. Trace, and S. E. Mazzeo. 2010. Preventing weight gain in first year college students: An online intervention to prevent the "freshman fifteen." *Eating Behaviors* 11(1):33-39.

Greene, G. W., A. A. White, S. L. Hoerr, B. Lohse, S. M. Schembre, D. Riebe, J. Patterson, K. K. Kattelmann, S. Shoff, T. Horacek, B. Blissmer, and B. W. Phillips. 2012. Impact of an online healthful eating and physical activity program for college students. *American Journal of Health Promotion* 27(2):e47-e58.

Gulliver, A., K. M. Griffiths, and H. Christensen. 2010. Perceived barriers and facilitators to mental health help-seeking in young people: A systematic review. *BMC Psychiatry* 10:113.

Ha, E. J., and N. Caine-Bish. 2009. Effect of nutrition intervention using a general nutrition course for promoting fruit and vegetable consumption among college students. *Journal of Nutrition Education and Behavior* 41(2):103-109.

Hadley, D. C., J. R. Reddon, and R. D. Reddick. 2001. Age, gender, and treatment attendance among forensic psychiatric outpatients. *Journal of Offender Rehabilitation* 32(4):55-66.

Han, B., R. McKeon, and J. Gfroerer. 2014. Suicidal ideation among community-dwelling adults in the United States. *American Journal of Public Health* 104(3):488-497.

Harrell, E. 2014. *Crime against persons with disabilities, 2009-2012 statistical tables.* Washington, DC: Bureau of Justice Statistics.

Harris, K. M., P. Gordon-Larsen, K. Chantala, and J. R. Udry. 2006. Longitudinal trends in race/ethnic disparities in leading health indicators from adolescence to young adulthood. *Archives of Pediatrics & Adolescent Medicine* 160(1):74-81.

Hebden, L., A. Cook, H. P. van der Ploeg, L. King, A. Bauman, and M. Allman-Farinelli. 2014. A mobile health intervention for weight management among young adults: A pilot randomised controlled trial. *Journal of Human Nutrition and Dietetics* 27(4):322-332.

Held, P., and G. P. Owens. 2013. Stigmas and attitudes toward seeking mental health treatment in a sample of veterans and active duty service members. *Traumatology* 19(2):136-143.

Hennrikus, D. 2013. *The ACA invests in community health: The community transformation grant program.* http://www.epi.umn.edu/mch/wp-content/uploads/2012/05/HG_Fall20132.pdf (accessed March 24, 2014).

HHS (U.S. Department of Health and Human Services). 1999. *Mental health: A report of the Surgeon General.* Rockville, MD: HHS.

HHS. 2012a. *Healthy people 2020: Core indicators for adolescent and young adults health.* http://www.healthypeople.gov/2020/learn/Draft_Core_Indicators_Web.pdf (accessed July 14, 2014).

HHS. 2012b. *Preventing tobacco use among youth and young adults.* Washington, DC: HHS, CDC, National Center for Chronic Disease Prevention and Health Promotion, Office on Smoking and Health.

HHS. 2012c. *2012 National Strategy for Suicide Prevention: Goals and objectives for action.* Washington, DC: HHS.

HHS. 2014a. *FY 2015 congressional justification for the Health Resources and Services Administration (HRSA).* http://www.hrsa.gov/about/budget/budgetjustification2015.pdf (accessed September 4, 2014).

HHS. 2014b. *HHS announces the availability of $100 million in Affordable Care Act funding to expand access to primary care through new community health centers.* http://www.hhs.gov/news/press/2014pres/07/20140708a.html (accessed July 14, 2014).

HHS. 2014c. Reports of the Surgeon General. In *The health consequences of smoking-50 years of progress: A report of the Surgeon General.* Atlanta, GA: HHS, CDC, National Center for Chronic Disease Prevention and Health Promotion, Office on Smoking and Health.

Hingson, R. W. 2010. Magnitude and prevention of college drinking and related problems. *Alcohol Research & Health* 33(1-2):45.

Hoek, J., A. Hoek-Sims, and P. Gendall. 2013. A qualitative exploration of young adult smokers' responses to novel tobacco warnings. *BMC Public Health* 13(1):1-10.

Holder, H. D., and A. J. Treno. 1997. Media advocacy in community prevention: News as a means to advance policy change. *Addiction* 92(Suppl. 2):S189-S199.

Hopfer, S. 2012. Effects of a narrative HPV vaccination intervention aimed at reaching college women: A randomized controlled trial. *Prevention Science* 13(2):173-182.

Hornik, R. 2002. *Public health communication: Evidence for behavior change.* New York: Lawrence Erlbaum Associates.

Hornik, R., and I. Yanovitzky. 2003. Using theory to design evaluations of communication campaigns: The case of the national youth anti-drug media campaign. *Communication Theory* 13(2):204-224.

Horrey, W. J., M. F. Lesch, and A. Garabet. 2009. Dissociation between driving performance and drivers' subjective estimates of performance and workload in dual-task conditions. *Journal of Safety Research* 40(1):7-12.

HRSA (Health Resources and Services Administration). 2000. *Understanding Title V of the Social Security Act*. Rockville, MD: HRSA.

HRSA. 2012. *The Ryan White HIV/AIDS Program: Population fact sheet*. http://hab.hrsa.gov/abouthab/populations/youthfacts2012.pdf (accessed July 14, 2014).

HRSA. 2013. *The Ryan White HIV/AIDS Program overview*. http://hab.hrsa.gov/abouthab/files/programoverviewfacts2012.pdf (accessed September 4, 2014).

HRSA. 2014a. *Adolescent and Young Adult Health National Resource Center Program*. http://www.acf.hhs.gov/hhsgrantsforecast/index.cfm?switch=grant.view&gff_grants_forecastInfoID=66854 (accessed October 3, 2014).

HRSA. 2014b. *Table 3a—Patients by age and gender*. http://bphc.hrsa.gov/uds/datacenter.aspx?q=t3a&year=2012&state= (accessed July 14, 2014).

HRSA. 2014c. *Table 3a—Patients by age and gender*. http://bphc.hrsa.gov/uds/lookalikes.aspx?q=t3a&year=2012&state=national (accessed September 18, 2014).

HRSA. 2014d. *Title V Maternal and Child Health Services Block Grant Program*. http://mchb.hrsa.gov/programs/titlevgrants/ (accessed September 16, 2014).

HRSA. 2014e. *Title V information system*. https://mchdata.hrsa.gov/tvisreports/MeasurementData/HSCI/HSCI06Search.aspx?measurenum=06B&from=pd (accessed July 14, 2014).

Hyde, J. K., and S. M. Shortell. 2012. The structure and organization of local and state public health agencies in the U.S.: A systematic review. *American Journal of Preventive Medicine* 42(5, Suppl. 1):S29-S41.

IOM (Institute of Medicine). 1988. *The future of public health*. Washington, DC: National Academy Press.

IOM. 1994. *Growing up tobacco free: Preventing nicotine addiction in children and youths*. Washington, DC: National Academy Press.

IOM. 1999. *Marijuana and medicine: Assessing the science base*. Washington, DC: National Academy Press.

IOM. 2002. *Guidance for the national healthcare disparities report*. Washington, DC: The National Academies Press.

IOM. 2003. *The future of the public's health in the 21st century*. Washington, DC: The National Academies Press.

IOM. 2004. *Health literacy: A prescription to end confusion*. Washington, DC: The National Academies Press.

IOM. 2006. *Examining the health disparities research plan of the National Institutes of Health: Unfinished business*. Washington, DC: The National Academies Press.

IOM. 2007. *Ending the tobacco problem: A blueprint for the nation*. Washington, DC: The National Academies Press.

IOM. 2009. *A review of the HHS Family Planning Program: Mission, management, and measurement of results*. Washington, DC: The National Academies Press.

IOM. 2011. *For the public's health: The role of measurement in action and accountability*. Washington, DC: The National Academies Press.

IOM. 2012a. *Accelerating progress in obesity prevention: Solving the weight of the nation*. Washington, DC: The National Academy Press.

IOM. 2012b. *For the public's health: Investing in a healthier future*. Washington, DC: The National Academies Press.

IOM. 2012c. *How far have we come in reducing health disparities?: Progress since 2000: Workshop summary*. Washington, DC: The National Academies Press.

IOM and NRC (National Research Council). 2013. *Improving the health, safety, and well-being of young adults: Workshop summary*. Washington, DC: The National Academies Press.

Israel, B. A., A. J. Schulz, E. A. Parker, A. B. Becker, A. J. Allen III, and J. R. Guzman. 2008. Critical issues in developing and following CBPR principles. In *Community-based participatory research for health: From process to outcomes*, edited by M. Minkler and N. Wallerstein. San Francisco, CA: Jossey-Bass. Pp. 56-73.

Jackson, C. A., M. Henderson, J. W. Frank, and S. J. Haw. 2012. An overview of prevention of multiple risk behaviour in adolescence and young adulthood. *Journal of Public Health* 34(Suppl. 1):i31-i40.

Jackson, P. B., and M. Finney. 2002. Negative life events and psychological distress among young adults. *Social Psychology Quarterly* 65(2):186-201.

Johnston, J. D., A. P. Massey, and R. L. Marker-Hoffman. 2012. Using an alternate reality game to increase physical activity and decrease obesity risk of college students. *Journal of Diabetes Science and Technology* 6(4):828-838.

Jones, K., P. Eathington, K. Baldwin, and H. Sipsma. 2014. The impact of health education transmitted via social media or text messaging on adolescent and young adult risky sexual behavior: A systematic review of the literature. *Sexually Transmitted Diseases* 41(7):413-419.

Jones, R., D. R. Hoover, and L. J. Lacroix. 2013. A randomized controlled trial of soap opera videos streamed to smartphones to reduce risk of sexually transmitted human immunodeficiency virus (HIV) in young urban African American women. *Nursing Outlook* 61(4):205-215.e203.

Jorm, A. F. 2012. Mental health literacy: Empowering the community to take action for better mental health. *American Psychologist* 67(3):231-243.

Kawachi, I., and L. F. Berkman. 2001. Social ties and mental health. *Journal of Urban Health* 78(3):458-467.

Kelley-Baker, T., M. B. Johnson, E. Romano, E. A. Mumford, and B. A. Miller. 2011. Preventing victimization among young women: The SafeNights intervention. *American Journal of Health Studies* 26(4):185-195.

Kendler, K. S., L. M. Karkowski, and C. A. Prescott. 1999. Causal relationship between stressful life events and the onset of major depression. *American Journal of Psychiatry* 156(6):837-841.

Kennedy, S. B., S. Nolen, Z. Pan, B. Smith, J. Applewhite, and K. J. Vanderhoff. 2013. Effectiveness of a brief condom promotion program in reducing risky sexual behaviours among African American men. *Journal of Evaluation in Clinical Practice* 19(2):408-413.

Kessler, R. C., P. Berglund, O. Demler, R. Jin, K. R. Merikangas, and E. E. Walters. 2005. Lifetime prevalence and age-of-onset distributions of DSM-IV disorders in the National Comorbidity Survey Replication. *Archives of General Psychiatry* 62(6):593-602.

Kessler, R. C., H. S. Akiskal, M. Ames, H. Birnbaum, P. Greenberg, R. M. Hirschfeld, R. Jin, K. R. Merikangas, G. E. Simon, and P. S. Wang. 2006. Prevalence and effects of mood disorders on work performance in a nationally representative sample of U.S. workers. *American Journal of Psychiatry* 163(9):1561-1568.

Kester, L. M., R. B. Shedd-Steele, C. A. Dotson-Roberts, J. Smith, and G. D. Zimet. 2014. The effects of a brief educational intervention on human papillomavirus knowledge and intention to initiate HPV vaccination in 18-26 year old young adults. *Gynecologic Oncology* 132(Suppl. 1):S9-S12.

KFF (The Henry J. Kaiser Family Foundation). 2011. *The uninsured: A primer—key facts about Americans without health insurance.* http://obamacarefacts.com/obamacare-docs/kisair-people-without-health-insurance.pdf (accessed September 16, 2014).

King, B. A., S. Alam, G. Promoff, R. Arrazola, and S. R. Dube. 2013. Awareness and ever use of electronic cigarettes among U.S. adults, 2010-2011. *Nicotine & Tobacco Research.*

King, M., J. Semlyen, S. S. Tai, H. Killaspy, D. Osborn, D. Popelyuk, and I. Nazareth. 2008. A systematic review of mental disorder, suicide, and deliberate self harm in lesbian, gay and bisexual people. *BMC Psychiatry* 8:70.

King, S. 2014. *Teen and young adult health program.* http://www.maine.gov/dhhs/mecdc/population-health/tya/index.html (accessed July 14, 2014).

Koh, H. K., J. J. Piotrowski, S. Kumanyika, and J. E. Fielding. 2011. Healthy people: A 2020 vision for the social determinants approach. *Health Education & Behavior* 38(6):551-557.

Krebs, C. P., C. H. Lindquist, T. D. Warner, B. S. Fisher, and S. L. Martin. 2009. College women's experiences with physically forced, alcohol- or other drug-enabled, and drug-facilitated sexual assault before and since entering college. *Journal of American College Health* 57(6):639-647.

Kypri, K., T. Vater, S. J. Bowe, J. B. Saunders, J. A. Cunningham, N. J. Horton, and J. McCambridge. 2014. Web-based alcohol screening and brief intervention for university students: A randomized trial. *Journal of the American Medical Association* 311(12):1218-1224.

Lally, J., A. O'Conghaile, S. Quigley, E. Bainbridge, and C. McDonald. 2013. Stigma of mental illness and help-seeking intention in university students. *The Psychiatrist* 37(8):253-260.

Laska, M. N., J. E. Pelletier, N. I. Larson, and M. Story. 2012. Interventions for weight gain prevention during the transition to young adulthood: A review of the literature. *Journal of Adolescent Health* 50(4):324-333.

Lennon, R., R. Rentfro, and B. O'Leary. 2010. Social marketing and distracted driving behaviors among young adults: The effectiveness of fear appeals. *Academy of Marketing Studies Journal* 14(2):95-104.

Lienemann, B. A., J. T. Siegel, and W. D. Crano. 2013. Persuading people with depression to seek help: Respect the boomerang. *Health Communication* 28(7):718-728.

Link, B. G., and J. Phelan. 1995. Social conditions as fundamental causes of disease. *Journal of Health and Social Behavior* Spec. No. 80-94.

Luong, G., and S. T. Charles. 2014. Age differences in affective and cardiovascular responses to a negative social interaction: The role of goals, appraisals, and emotion regulation. *Developmental Psychology* 50(7):1919-1930.

Mack, K. A. 2013. Drug-induced deaths—United States, 1999-2010. *Morbidity and Mortality Weekly Report Surveillance Summaries* 62(Suppl. 3):161-163.

Maher, C. A., L. K. Lewis, K. Ferrar, S. Marshall, I. De Bourdeaudhuij, and C. Vandelanotte 2014. Are health behavior change interventions that use online social networks effective? A systematic review. *Journal of Medical Internet Research* 16(2):e40.

Marcus, B. H., D. M. Williams, P. M. Dubbert, J. F. Sallis, A. C. King, A. K. Yancey, B. A. Franklin, D. Buchner, S. R. Daniels, and R. P. Claytor. 2006. Physical activity intervention studies: What we know and what we need to know: A scientific statement from the American Heart Association Council on Nutrition, Physical Activity, and Metabolism (Subcommittee on Physical Activity); Council on Cardiovascular Disease in the Young; and the Interdisciplinary Working Group on Quality of Care and Outcomes Research. *Circulation* 114(24):2739-2752.

Marmot, M. 2013. Universal health coverage and social determinants of health. *Lancet* 382(9900):1227-1228.

Martin, J., B. Hamilton, M. Osterman, S. Curin, and T. J. Mathews. 2013. *Births: Final data for 2012.* Washington, DC: HHS.

May, A. L., D. Freedman, B. Sherry, and H. M. Blanck. 2013. Obesity—United States, 1999-2010. *Morbidity and Mortality Weekly Report Surveillance Summaries* 62(Suppl. 3):120-128.

McEwen, B. S. 2008. Central effects of stress hormones in health and disease: Understanding the protective and damaging effects of stress and stress mediators. *European Journal of Pharmacology* 583(2-3):174-185.

McEwen, B. S., and P. J. Gianaros. 2010. Central role of the brain in stress and adaptation: Links to socioeconomic status, health, and disease. *Annals of the New York Academy of Sciences* 1186:190-222.

Mevissen, F. E., R. A. Ruiter, R. M. Meertens, F. Zimbile, and H. P. Schaalma. 2011. Justify your love: Testing an online STI-risk communication intervention designed to promote condom use and STI-testing. *Psychology and Health* 26(2):205-221.

Milstein, B., J. Homer, P. Briss, D. Burton, and T. Pechacek. 2011. Why behavioral and environmental interventions are needed to improve health at lower cost. *Health Affairs* 30(5):823-832.

Minkler, M., and N. Wallerstein. 2008. *Community-based participatory research for health: From process to outcomes*, 2nd ed. San Francisco, CA: Jossey-Bass.

Moore, G. F., A. Williams, L. Moore, and S. Murphy. 2013. An exploratory cluster randomised trial of a university halls of residence based social norms marketing campaign to reduce alcohol consumption among 1st year students. *Substance Abuse Treatment, Prevention, and Policy* 8:15.

Morrison, D. S., M. Petticrew, and H. Thomson. 2003. What are the most effective ways of improving population health through transport interventions? Evidence from systematic reviews. *Journal of Epidemiology and Community Health* 57(5):327-333.

Mosher, W., J. Jones, and J. C. Abma. 2012. *Intended and unintended birth in the United States*. Hyattsville, MD: National Center for Health Statistics.

Mulye, T. P., M. J. Park, C. D. Nelson, S. H. Adams, C. E. Irwin, Jr., and C. D. Brindis. 2009. Trends in adolescent and young adult health in the United States. *Journal of Adolescent Health* 45(1):8-24.

Muscatell, K. A., G. M. Slavich, S. M. Monroe, and I. H. Gotlib. 2009. Stressful life events, chronic difficulties, and the symptoms of clinical depression. *The Journal of Nervous and Mental Disease* 197(3):154-160.

NACCHO (National Association of County and City Health Officials). 2009. *National profile of local health departments*. Washington, DC: NACCHO.

NACCHO. 2014a. *Local health department budget cuts and job losses: Findings from the 2014 forces of change survey*. http://www.naccho.org/topics/research/forcesofchange/upload/Budget-Cuts.pdf (accessed July 14, 2014).

NACCHO. 2014b. *National profile of local health departments*. http://nacchoprofilestudy.org/chapter-2 (accessed July 14, 2014).

Napolitano, M. A., S. Hayes, G. G. Bennett, A. K. Ives, and G. D. Foster. 2013. Using Facebook and text messaging to deliver a weight loss program to college students. *Obesity* 21(1):25-31.

Natelson, R. 2009. A case for federal oversight of military sexual harassment. *Clearinghouse Review: Journal of Poverty Law and Policy* 43:277-573.

NCAVP (National Coalition of Anti-Violence Programs). 2013. *Lesbian, gay, bisexual, transgender, queer and HIV-affected hate violence in 2012*. New York: New York City Gay and Lesbian Anti-Violence Project, Inc.

NCI (National Cancer Institute). 2008. *The role of the media in promoting and reducing tobacco use*. Tobacco Control Monograph No. 19. Bethesda, MD: NCI.

NCSL (National Conference of State Legislatures). 2014. *State medical marijuana laws.* http://www.ncsl.org/research/health/state-medical-marijuana-laws.aspx (accessed August 29, 2014).

Neinstein, L. S. 2013. *The new adolescents: An analysis of health conditions, behaviors, risks, and access to services among emerging young adults.* Executive Summary. http://www.usc.edu/student-affairs/Health_Center/thenewadolescents/doc/TheNewAdolescents_Final_Locked.pdf (accessed September 5, 2014).

NHTSA (National Highway Traffic Safety Administration). 2013. *Alcohol-impaired driving.* Washington, DC: NHTSA's National Center for Statistics and Analysis.

NHTSA. 2014. *Distracted driving 2012.* Washington, DC: NHTSA's National Center for Statistics and Analysis.

NIH (National Institutes of Health). 2009. *DrugFacts: Treatment approaches for drug addiction.* http://www.drugabuse.gov/publications/drugfacts/treatment-approaches-drug-addiction (accessed July 15, 2014).

NIH. 2014. *Abuse of prescription (Rx) drugs affects young adults most.* http://www.drugabuse.gov/related-topics/trends-statistics/infographics/abuse-prescription-rx-drugs-affects-young-adults-most (accessed July 10, 2014).

NIHCM (National Institute for Health Care Management). 2007. *Reducing health disparities among children: Strategies and program for health plans.* Washington, DC: NIHCM.

NIMH (National Institute of Mental Health). 2000. *Treatment of children with mental disorders.* Bethesda, MD: NIMH.

Nirenberg, T., J. Baird, R. Longabaugh, and M. J. Mello. 2013. Motivational counseling reduces future police charges in court referred youth. *Accident Analysis & Prevention* 53:89-99.

NNSAHC (National Network of State Adolescent Health Coordinators). 2012. *State adolescent health coordinator survey.* http://nnsahc.org/images/uploads/2012NNSAHC_SurveySummary.pdf (accessed July 14, 2014).

Norton, W. E., J. D. Fisher, K. R. Amico, J. F. Dovidio, and B. T. Johnson. 2012. Relative efficacy of a pregnancy, sexually transmitted infection, or human immunodeficiency virus prevention-focused intervention on changing sexual risk behavior among young adults. *Journal of American College Health* 60(8):574-582.

NRC and IOM. 2004. *Reducing underage drinking: A collective responsibility.* Washington, DC: The National Academies Press.

NRC and IOM. 2009. *Preventing mental, emotional, and behavioral disorders among young people: Progress and possibilities.* Washington, DC: The National Academies Press.

Pacula, R. L., B. Kilmer, A. C. Wagenaar, F. J. Chaloupka, and J. P. Caulkins. 2014. Developing public health regulations for marijuana: Lessons from alcohol and tobacco. *American Journal of Public Health* 104(6):1021-1028.

Park, M. J., T. Paul Mulye, S. H. Adams, C. D. Brindis, and C. E. Irwin, Jr. 2006. The health status of young adults in the United States. *Journal of Adolescent Health* 39(3):305-317.

Park, M. J., J. T. Scott, S. H. Adams, C. D. Brindis, and C. E. Irwin. 2014. Adolescent and young adult health in the United States in the past decade: Little improvement and young adults remain worse off than adolescents. *Journal of Adolescent Health* 55(1):3-16.

Paschall, M. J., T. Antin, C. L. Ringwalt, and R. F. Saltz. 2011a. Effects of AlcoholEdu for college on alcohol-related problems among freshmen: A randomized multicampus trial. *Journal of Studies on Alcohol and Drugs* 72(4):642-650.

Paschall, M. J., T. Antin, C. L. Ringwalt, and R. F. Saltz. 2011b. Evaluation of an Internet-based alcohol misuse prevention course for college freshmen: Findings of a randomized multi-campus trial. *American Journal of Preventive Medicine* 41(3):300-308.

Patel, V., A. J. Flisher, S. Hetrick, and P. McGorry. 2007. Mental health of young people: A global public-health challenge. *Lancet* 369:1302-1313.

Paus, T., M. Keshavan, and J. N. Giedd. 2008. Why do many psychiatric disorders emerge during adolescence? *Nature Reviews Neuroscience* 9(12):947-957.

Perkins, H., J. W. Linkenbach, M. A. Lewis, and C. Neighbors. 2010. Effectiveness of social norms media marketing in reducing drinking and driving: A statewide campaign. *Addictive Behaviors* 35(10):866-874.

Pew Research Center. 2013. *State of the news media 2013*. http://stateofthemedia.org/2013/overview-5/ (accessed September 15, 2014).

Pew Research Center. 2014. *State of the news media 2014*. http://www.journalism.org/packages/state-of-the-news-media-2014 (accessed April 3, 2014).

Planty, M., L. Langton, C. Krebs, M. Berzofksy, and H. Smiley-McDonald. 2013. *Female victims of sexual violence, 1994-2010*. Washington, DC: Bureau of Justice Statistics.

Poobalan, A., L. Aucott, E. Precious, I. Crombie, and W. Smith. 2010. Weight loss interventions in young people (18 to 25 year olds): A systematic review. *Obesity Reviews* 11(8):580-592.

Price, D., and L. Dunlap. 1988. Stress and coping of adults and young adults in economically uncertain rural areas. *Lifestyles* 9(2):123-144.

Ramanadhan, S., C. Salhi, E. Achille, N. Baril, K. D'Entremont, M. Grullon, C. Judge, S. Oppenheimer, C. Reeves, C. Savage, and K. Viswanath. 2012. Addressing cancer disparities via community network mobilization and intersectoral partnerships: A social network analysis. *PLoS ONE* 7(2):e32130.

Ramirez, M., J. Yang, T. Young, L. Roth, A. Garinger, L. Snetselaar, and C. Peek-Asa. 2013. Implementation evaluation of steering teens safe: Engaging parents to deliver a new parent-based teen driving intervention to their teens. *Health Education & Behavior* 40(4):426-434.

Randle, A. A., and C. A. Graham. 2011. A review of the evidence on the effects of intimate partner violence on men. *Psychology of Men & Masculinity* 12(2):97-111.

Randolph, W., and K. Viswanath. 2004. Lessons learned from public health mass media campaigns: Marketing health in a crowded media world. *Annual Review of Public Health* 25:419-437.

Ray, S., V. Bhaskar, S. Bhandari, and C. Kodange. 2012. Impact of a behaviour change intervention model for promotion of condoms amongst young adult males in an occupational setting. *Medical Journal Armed Forces India* 68(4):316-321.

Redhead, C. S., and V. K. Burrows. 2009. *FDA tobacco regulation: The Family Smoking Prevention and Tobacco Control Act of 2009*. Washington, DC: Congressional Research Service.

Reeder, S. 2014. *Innovative state and local approaches: The Maryland transition age youth system change experience*. Presentation at IOM Workshop to Explore the Current and Potential Roles of State Policies and Programs and Media and Information Technology, Washington, DC. http://www.iom.edu/~/media/Files/Activity%20Files/Children/ImprovingYoungAdultsHealth/Reeder%20Presentation.pdf (accessed September 5, 2014).

Richardson, A., V. Williams, J. Rath, A. C. Villanti, and D. Vallone. 2014. The next generation of users: Prevalence and longitudinal patterns of tobacco use among U.S. young adults. *American Journal of Public Health* 104(8):1429-1436.

Rickwood, D. J., F. P. Deane, and C. J. Wilson. 2007. When and how do young people seek professional help for mental health problems? *Medical Journal of Australia* 187(Suppl. 7):S35-S39.

Ridout, B., and A. Campbell. 2014. Using Facebook to deliver a social norm intervention to reduce problem drinking at university. *Drug and Alcohol Review* (2014):1-7.

Rivara, F. P., D. Boisvert, A. Relyea-Chew, and T. Gomez. 2011. Last call: Decreasing drunk driving among 21-34-year-old bar patrons. *International Journal of Injury Control and Safety Promotion* 19(1):53-61.

Robinson, J., S. E. Hetrick, and C. Martin. 2011. Preventing suicide in young people: Systematic review. *Australian and New Zealand Journal of Psychiatry* 45(1):3-26.

SAHRC (State Adolescent Health Resource Center). 2012. *What is a state adolescent health coordinator?* http://nnsahc.org/images/uploads/1-_AHC_Overview.pdf (accessed September 4, 2014).

SAHRC. 2014. *State adolescent health coordinators & contacts.* http://nnsahc.org/images/uploads/StateAHCwebroster.pdf (accessed July 14, 2014).

Sallis, J. F., N. Owen, and E. B. Fisher. 2008. Ecological models of health behavior. In *Health behavior and health education: Theory, research, and practice*, Vol. 4. San Francisco, CA: John Wiley & Sons, Inc. Pp. 465-485.

Salzberg, P. M., and J. M. Moffat. 2004. Ninety five percent: An evaluation of law, policy, and programs to promote seat belt use in Washington state. *Journal of Safety Research* 35(2):215-222.

SAMHSA (Substance Abuse and Mental Health Services Administration). 2012. *2010-2011 National Survey on Drug Use and Health: Model-based prevalence estimates (50 states and the District of Columbia).* http://www.samhsa.gov/data/NSDUH/2k11State/NSDUHsae2011/ExcelTabs/NSDUHsaeTables2011.pdf (accessed September 2, 2014).

SAMHSA. 2013. *Results from the 2012 National Survey on Drug Use and Health: Summary of national findings.* NSDUH series H-46, HHS publication no. (SMA) 13-4795. Rockville, MD: SAMHSA.

SAMHSA. 2014. *The CBHSQ report: Serious mental health challenges among older adolescents and young adults.* Washington, DC: Center for Behavioral Health Statistics and Quality, SAMSHA.

Santelli, J. S., K. Sivaramakrishnan, Z. R. Edelstein, and L. P. Fried. 2013. Adolescent risk-taking, cancer risk, and life course approaches to prevention. *Journal of Adolescent Health* 52(5):S41-S44.

Schilling, O. K., and M. Diehl. 2014. Reactivity to stressor pile-up in adulthood: Effects on daily negative and positive affect. *Psychology and Aging* 29(1):72-83.

Schmidt, S., and H. M. Parsons. 2014. Vaccination interest and trends in human papillomavirus vaccine uptake in young adult women aged 18 to 26 years in the United States: An analysis using the 2008-2012 National Health Interview Survey. *American Journal of Preventive Medicine* 104(5):946-953.

Schomerus, G., C. Auer, D. Rhode, M. Luppa, H. J. Freyberger, and S. Schmidt. 2012. Personal stigma, problem appraisal and perceived need for professional help in currently untreated depressed persons. *Journal of Affective Disorders* 139(1):94-97.

Schulenberg, J. E., and J. L. Maggs. 2002. A developmental perspective on alcohol use and heavy drinking during adolescence and the transition to young adulthood. *Journal of Studies on Alcohol and Drugs* (14):54.

Scott, S. B., M. J. Sliwinski, and F. Blanchard-Fields. 2013. Age differences in emotional responses to daily stress: The role of timing, severity, and global perceived stress. *Psychology and Aging* 28(4):1076-1087.

Sepe, E., and S. A. Glantz. 2002. Bar and club tobacco promotions in the alternative press: Targeting young adults. *American Journal of Public Health* 92(1):75-78.

Shults, R. A., R. W. Elder, D. A. Sleet, J. L. Nichols, M. O. Alao, V. G. Carande-Kulis, S. Zaza, D. M. Sosin, and R. S. Thompson. 2001. Reviews of evidence regarding interventions to reduce alcohol-impaired driving. *American Journal of Preventive Medicine* 21(4):66-88.

Sims, T. H., T. McAfee, D. L. Fraser, T. B. Baker, M. C. Fiore, and S. S. Smith. 2013. Quitline cessation counseling for young adult smokers: A randomized clinical trial. *Nicotine & Tobacco Research* 15(5):932-941.

Sinha, R., C. Easton, and K. Kemp. 2003. Substance abuse treatment characteristics of probation-referred young adults in a community-based outpatient program. *American Journal of Drug and Alcohol Abuse* 29(3):585-597.

Skov-Ettrup, L., L. Ringgaard, P. Dalum, T. Flensborg-Madsen, L. C. Thygesen, and J. S. Tolstrup. 2014. Comparing tailored and untailored text messages for smoking cessation: A randomized controlled trial among adolescent and young adult smokers. *Health Education Research* 29(2):195-205.

Smith, E. L., and A. Cooper. 2013. *Homicide in the U.S. known to law enforcement, 2011.* Washington, DC: Bureau of Justice Statistics.

Smith, L., and D. Foxcroft. 2009. The effect of alcohol advertising, marketing and portrayal on drinking behaviour in young people: Systematic review of prospective cohort studies. *BMC Public Health* 9(1):51.

Snyder, L. B., M. A. Hamilton, E. W. Mitchell, J. Kiwanuka-Tondo, F. Fleming-Milici, and D. Proctor. 2004. A meta-analysis of the effect of mediated health communication campaigns on behavior change in the United States. *Journal of Health Communication: International Perspectives* 9(Suppl. 1):71-96.

Sorensen, G., E. Barbeau, M. K. Hunt, and K. Emmons. 2004. Reducing social disparities in tobacco use: A social-contextual model for reducing tobacco use among blue-collar workers. *American Journal of Public Health* 94(2):230-239.

Spalter-Roth, R., T. A. Lowenthal, and M. Rubio. 2005. *Race, ethnicity, and the health of Americans.* http://www2.asanet.org/centennial/race_ethnicity_health.pdf (accessed August 18, 2014).

Stawski, R. S., M. J. Sliwinski, D. M. Almeida, and J. M. Smyth. 2008. Reported exposure and emotional reactivity to daily stressors: The roles of adult age and global perceived stress. *Psychology and Aging* 23(1):52-61.

Stewart, D. E., and G. E. Robinson. 1998. A review of domestic violence and women's mental health. *Archives of Women's Mental Health* 1(2):83-89.

Strecher, V. J., J. B. McClure, G. L. Alexander, B. Chakraborty, V. N. Nair, J. M. Konkel, S. M. Greene, L. M. Collins, C. C. Carlier, C. J. Wiese, R. J. Little, C. S. Pomerleau, and O. F. Pomerleau. 2008. Web-based smoking-cessation programs: Results of a randomized trial. *American Journal of Preventive Medicine* 34(5):373-381.

Tapp, A., A. Pressley, M. Baugh, and P. White. 2013. Wheels, skills and thrills: A social marketing trial to reduce aggressive driving from young men in deprived areas. *Accident Analysis & Prevention* 58:148-157.

Testa, M., J. H. Hoffman, J. A. Livingston, and R. Turrisi. 2010. Preventing college women's sexual victimization through parent based intervention: A randomized controlled trial. *Prevention Science* 11(3):308-318.

Valente, S. M., J. M. Saunders, and M. Z. Cohen. 1993. Evaluating depression among patients with cancer. *Cancer Practice* 2(1):65-71.

van der Pol, P., N. Liebregts, R. de Graaf, D. J. Korf, W. van den Brink, and M. van Laar. 2013. Facilitators and barriers in treatment seeking for cannabis dependence. *Drug and Alcohol Dependence* 133(2):776-780.

Villanti, A. C., H. S. McKay, D. B. Abrams, D. R. Holtgrave, and J. V. Bowie. 2010. Smoking-cessation interventions for U.S. young adults: A systematic review. *American Journal of Preventive Medicine* 39(6):564-574.

Viswanath, K. 2006. Public communications and its role in reducing and eliminating health disparities. In *Examining the health disparities research plan of the National Institutes of Health: Unfinished business*, edited by G. E. Thomson, F. Mitchell, and M. B. Williams. Washington, DC: The National Academies Press. Pp. 215-253.

Viswanath, K., and J. R. Finnegan. 2002. Reflections on community health campaigns: Secular trends and the capacity to effect change. In *Public health communication: Evidence for behavior change*, edited by R. C. Hornik. Mahwah, NJ: Lawrence Erlbaum Associates. Pp. 289-313.

Viswanath, K., L. K. Ackerson, G. Sorensen, and P. C. Gupta. 2010a. Movies and TV influence tobacco use in India: Findings from a national survey. *PLoS ONE* 5(6):e11365.

Viswanath, K., R. S. Herbst, S. R. Land, S. J. Leischow, and P. G. Shields. 2010b. Tobacco and cancer: An American association for cancer research policy statement. *Cancer Research* 70(9):3419-3430.

Viswanath, K., R. McCloud, S. Minsky, E. Puleo, E. Kontos, C. Bigman-Galimore, R. Rudd and K. M. Emmons. 2013. Internet use, browsing, and the urban poor: Implications for cancer control. *Journal of the National Cancer Institute Monographs* 2013(47):199-205.

Volkow, N. D., R. D. Baler, W. M. Compton, and S. R. Weiss. 2014. Adverse health effects of marijuana use. *New England Journal of Medicine* 370(23):2219-2227.

Wagenaar, A. C., and T. L. Toomey. 2002. Effects of minimum drinking age laws: Review and analyses of the literature from 1960 to 2000. *Journal of Studies on Alcohol* (Suppl. 14):206-225.

Wakefield, M. A., B. Loken, and R. C. Hornik. 2010. Use of mass media campaigns to change health behaviour. *Lancet* 376(9748):1261-1271.

Werch, C. E. C., M. J. Moore, H. Bian, C. C. DiClemente, I. Huang, S. C. Ames, D. Thombs, R. M. Weiler, and S. B. Pokorny. 2010. Are effects from a brief multiple behavior intervention for college students sustained over time? *Preventive Medicine* 50(1):30-34.

WHO (World Health Organization). 2001. *The world health report 2001—Mental health: New understanding, new hope*. Geneva, Switzerland: WHO.

Williams, A. F., and J. K. Wells. 2004. The role of enforcement programs in increasing seat belt use. *Journal of Safety Research* 35(2):175-180.

Williams, A. F., D. Reinfurt, and J. K. Wells. 1996. Increasing seat belt use in North Carolina. *Journal of Safety Research* 27(1):33-41.

Williams, G., M. P. Hamm, J. Shulhan, B. Vandermeer, and L. Hartling. 2014. Social media interventions for diet and exercise behaviours: A systematic review and meta-analysis of randomised controlled trials. *BMJ Open* 4(2)1-16.

Wingood, G. M., R. J. DiClemente, K. Villamizar, D. L. Er, M. DeVarona, J. Taveras, T. M. Painter, D. L. Lang, J. W. Hardin, E. Ullah, J. Stallworth, D. W. Purcell, and R. Jean. 2011a. Efficacy of a health educator-delivered HIV prevention intervention for Latina women: A randomized controlled trial. *American Journal of Public Health* 101(12):2245-2252.

Wingood, G. M., J. J. Card, D. Er, J. Solomon, N. Braxton, D. Lang, P. Seth, J. Cartreine, and R. J. Diclemente. 2011b. Preliminary efficacy of a computer-based HIV intervention for African-American women. *Psychology & Health* 26(2):223-234.

Wolfson, M., H. Champion, T. P. McCoy, S. D. Rhodes, E. H. Ip, J. N. Blocker, B. A. Martin, K. G. Wagoner, M. C. O'Brien, E. L. Sutfin, A. Mitra, and R. H. DuRant. 2012. Impact of a randomized campus/community trial to prevent high-risk drinking among college students. *Alcoholism: Clinical and Experimental Research* 36(10):1767-1778.

Wood, S. 2014. *Colorado9to25*. Presentation at IOM's Improving the Health, Safety, and Well-Being of Young Adults: A Workshop on State Policies and Programs and Social Media and Information Technology, Washington, DC. http://www.iom.edu/~/media/Files/Activity%20Files/Children/ImprovingYoungAdultsHealth/Wood%20Presentation.pdf (accessed September 5, 2014).

Wright, A., M. G. Harris, J. H. Wiggers, A. F. Jorm, S. M. Cotton, S. M. Harrigan, R. E. Hurworth, and P. D. McGorry. 2005. Recognition of depression and psychosis by young Australians and their beliefs about treatment. *Medical Journal of Australia* 183(1):18-23.

Wu, L. T., D. J. Pilowsky, W. E. Schlenger, and D. Hasin. 2007. Alcohol use disorders and the use of treatment services among college-age young adults. *Psychiatric Service* 58(2):192-200.

Zakrajsek, J. S., J. T. Shope, A. I. Greenspan, J. Wang, C. R. Bingham, and B. G. Simons-Morton. 2013. Effectiveness of a brief parent-directed teen driver safety intervention (checkpoints) delivered by driver education instructors. *Journal of Adolescent Health* 53(1):27-33.

7

The Health Care System

Key Findings

- Young adults have significantly lower rates of health care system utilization compared with other groups, but significantly higher emergency room visit rates compared with those immediately younger and older than them. These lower utilization rates do not necessarily indicate better health; for example, the use of specialty psychiatric services by those with mental health conditions falls from approximately 20 percent of adolescents to about 10 percent of young adults.
- The transition from child to adult medical and behavioral health care often is associated with poor outcomes among young adults. Challenges include discontinuities in care, differences between the child/adolescent and adult health systems, a lack of available adult providers, difficulties in breaking the bond with pediatric providers, lack of payment for transition support, a lack of training in childhood-onset conditions among adult providers, the failure of pediatric providers to prepare adolescents for an adult model of care, and a lack of communication between pediatric and adult providers and systems of care.
- Young adulthood provides an important opportunity for prevention. Serious illnesses and disorders can be avoided or man-

aged better if young adults are engaged in wellness practices and screened for early signs of or untreated illness, and the risk taking that is common during these years can impact lifelong functioning. Yet young adults rarely receive preventive counseling on important issues for this age group, such as smoking and mental health, and there is no consolidated package of preventive medical, behavioral, and oral health guidelines specifically focused on the young adult population.

- While there are effective behavioral health treatments and strategies for adults, the efficacy of these treatments specifically for young adults is largely undemonstrated because typical clinical trials and research studies (e.g., studies of adults aged 18-55) are insufficient to establish efficacy in young adults.
- Young adults without health insurance or with gaps in insurance coverage are less likely to access health services than young adults who are continuously insured. Health insurance coverage rates for young adults, however, have historically been the lowest of any age group. Certain groups of young adults—such as young adults exiting the foster care system, young adults involved in the justice system, and unauthorized immigrants—have particular difficulties in obtaining health care coverage. The Patient Protection and Affordable Care Act and state-level efforts are increasing coverage for many young adults, including young adults who age out of the foster care system, but others, such as unauthorized immigrants, remain outside the system.

Young adults often are perceived as healthy and as low users of health care, and recent attention has focused primarily on enrolling young adults in health care insurance to offset the higher costs associated with care for older adults. However, while young adults are clearly an important priority population for health insurance coverage, there also needs to be an expanded focus on improving the health care system's ability and capacity to serve them. Important opportunities exist within the health care system to improve young adults' health, safety, and well-being in both the short and long terms. Yet many young adults face serious challenges in accessing and navigating the health care system, with potentially serious repercussions.

Young adulthood provides an important opportunity for prevention. Serious illnesses or disorders can be avoided or managed better if young adults are engaged in wellness practices and screened for early signs of or untreated illness. Furthermore, as described in earlier chapters, young adulthood is an age not only of opportunities, but also of risks that can impact lifelong functioning. Keeping young adults as healthy as possible during this critical stage of life may support more positive pathways into mature adulthood. Young adulthood also provides an opportunity to help young adults access and learn to navigate the adult health care system and develop the ability to work directly with health care providers to manage their health care more effectively.

Among the many young adults who are parents, moreover, there is an opportunity to minimize the potential impact of their behavioral and physical health problems on their children. For example, alcohol, tobacco, or drug use during pregnancy increases the likelihood of long-term cognitive and emotional development problems, such as attention-deficit hyperactivity disorder (ADHD), conduct problems, and lower school achievement, in the child (Knopik, 2009; Minnes et al., 2011). And children of depressed parents have three times the risk of anxiety disorders, major depression, and substance dependence compared with children of nondepressed parents (Weissman et al., 2006). Use of cognitive-behavioral therapies with parents with mental illness can help reduce mental health disorders in their children (Siegenthaler et al., 2012).

In addition to the challenges that almost all adults face in accessing and navigating a complicated health system, two challenges are particularly relevant for young adults: the transition from child to adult systems and the onset of certain health conditions, such as serious mental illness. Young adults are transitioning from pediatric to adult health care providers and from the child to the adult behavioral health system, and these new systems of care often differ significantly from those they used as children and adolescents. Some struggle as they assume primary responsibility for their health care for the first time. The health system may not be set up in ways that young adults find easy to use, and providers sometimes lack young adult–specific content knowledge and the skills needed to work effectively with this age group. This transition is widely recognized as challenging for those with

> "Even with insurance, it is still hard to access health care. It is so complicated and you don't really learn in school how to navigate it."*

* Quotations are from members of the young adult advisory group during their discussions with the committee.

chronic illness, but it is also essential that all young adults make a successful transition to the adult health care system to ensure they receive preventive services that help them remain in good health, as well as the comprehensive array of physical and behavioral health services many of them need. Box 7-1 summarizes barriers discussed in the remainder of this chapter that impede young adults from accessing and continuing to use health care.

BOX 7-1
Barriers to Optimal Health Care for Young Adults

The following are barriers faced by young adults in accessing care and/or continuing to receive care in the health care system:

- Transitions
  - navigating the differences between pediatric and adult health care providers, including differences in treatment culture, family involvement, and care coordination;
  - discontinuity of care caused by age-based changes in eligibility criteria or target populations for behavioral health services and management of chronic medical conditions; and
  - changes in insurance coverage.
- Content
  - no unified set of young adult preventive care guidelines; and
  - significant gaps in interventions and treatments with strong evidence of efficacy for young adults, particularly in preventive and behavioral health.
- Cost and difficulty of obtaining health care coverage.
- Young adults' lack of health literacy and knowledge of how to access and complete the enrollment process, identify providers in the community, and navigate the health system.
- The stigma of behavioral health and substance abuse problems.
- Systems issues
  - few incentives to provide transition care, preventive care, counseling, and health education, particularly about treatment for or early signs of mental health problems and risk behaviors such as substance use;
  - inconsistency among pediatric systems in offering adolescent patients and their families preparation and planning for the transition to adult systems and for an adult model of care;
  - adult systems' being unfamiliar with how to engage and integrate young adults into their practice;
  - inadequate health care provider training and skills for caring for adult manifestations of childhood diseases; and
  - confidentiality concerns.

Health systems are currently undergoing significant changes that affect both young adults and the general population. A key provision of the Patient Protection and Affordable Care Act (ACA) is the requirement that health insurance plans extend dependent coverage so that young adults can be added to a parent's plan until they turn 26; several states also had initiated expansion of insurance coverage before the ACA was enacted (Blum et al., in press). Driven by advocacy goals and the fiscal need to enroll healthy individuals to offset the cost of older and sicker individuals, the White House, states, health insurance companies, and advocacy organizations across the country have recently developed campaigns to increase young adult enrollment in insurance plans (e.g., Colorado Consumer Health Initiative and ProgressNow Colorado Education, 2014; HealthSource RI, 2014; Ostrom, 2014; Young Invincibles, 2014). Results of a 2013 survey indicate that of 15 million 19- to 25-year-olds who enrolled in a parent's plan, 7.8 million would not have been able to do so prior to the ACA (Collins et al., 2013). In addition, federal surveys suggest that 1-3 million previously uninsured young adults have gained coverage since this provision took effect (Blumenthal and Collins, 2014). This change is likely to have a significant impact on young adults' relationship with the structure and content of the health care system for years to come, and the evolving system offers opportunities for integrating further changes to benefit young adults.

In this chapter, we examine young adults in the health care system and provide recommendations for improving the system's role in enhancing their health, safety, and well-being. As described in Chapter 1, the term health care is used broadly in this report to include both physical and behavioral health, and the term behavioral health encompasses the promotion of emotional health; the prevention of mental and substance use disorders; and treatments and services for substance abuse, addiction, and mental and substance use disorders (SAMHSA, 2011). Since the epidemiology of young adults is covered in greater depth in Chapters 2 and 6, this chapter focuses on health care delivery.

We first briefly describe where young adults currently receive health care services and what services they use. We then explore in turn transitions from pediatric to adult medical health care systems and from child to adult behavioral health care systems, preventive care for young adults, behavioral health interventions for young adults, health care coverage, and systems issues related to young adults. The chapter ends with conclusions and recommendations for improving health care for young adults. Note that the primary recommendations offered in this chapter are applicable to health systems in a variety of forms and are not restricted to specific implementations of the ACA. Some of our suggestions are not exclusive to young adults, but with the current large influx of young adults into the system, there is an opportunity to think about how to get the system right for them and then extend it to others.

CURRENT USE OF HEALTH CARE BY YOUNG ADULTS

Comprehensive care with a medical home does not appear to characterize the health care delivery system for young adults as compared with children and adults (for a discussion of medical homes for 10- to 17-year-olds, see Adams et al., 2013).[1] An analysis of health care utilization conducted before the passage of the ACA found that young adults had significantly lower health care system utilization rates than other groups (see Table 7-1). Specifically, this age group had significantly lower rates of office-based and dental visits. Of interest is that young adults had significantly higher emergency room visit rates compared with those immediately younger and older than them. In addition, the use of specialty psychiatric services by those with mental health conditions falls from approximately 20 percent of adolescents to about 10 percent of young adults (Copeland et al., in press). The use of services in general—including medical care, educational and job services, and services provided through organizations such as Big Brother—by individuals with mental health conditions drops from about half of adolescents to a quarter of young adults.

> "I would like to receive my health information from my doctor. The problem here is that I only go to the doctor when things go wrong, as do many other young adults."

The prevalence and trends of the major health-related problems affecting young adults are discussed extensively in Chapters 2 and 6. Table 7-2 highlights the percentages of young adults utilizing the various types of health care services. This table shows that small percentages of young adults received care for substance use and mental health disorders, even though more than 50 percent reported having a usual source of care and having received a routine general checkup within the past 12 months, and even though early young adulthood is often when the burden of illness emerges for substance abuse and mental health conditions. Emergency rooms represent a major component of care for young adults, utilized by an estimated 15 to 20 percent of this age group (Fortuna et al., 2010; Lau et al., 2014a), although evidence from three states suggests that the ACA

[1] The patient-centered medical home is a model for primary care that promotes effective care coordination, accessibility, quality, and safety (AAFP et al., 2007; IOM, 2013a).

TABLE 7-1 Past-Year Health Care Utilization Rates by Age Group: 2009 Medical Expenditure Panel Survey (rates adjusted for pregnancy)

	Children (aged 0-11)	Adolescents (aged 12-17)	Young Adults (aged 18-25)	Adult (aged 26-44)	Adult (aged 45-64)	Adult (aged 65+)
Utilization						
% had any health care utilization	88%***	83%***	72%	78%***	89%***	97%***
Office-based visits						
% had visit(s)	77%***	67%***	55%	65%***	79%***	91%***
Hospital outpatient visits						
% had visit(s)	7%	5%*	7%	12%***	20%***	30%***
Emergency room visits						
% had visit(s)	15%	12%**	15%	12%**	12%***	17%
Inpatient hospitalizations						
% had visit(s)	2%***	4%***	5%	6%	7%*	19%***
Prescription medications						
% had prescription(s)	50%	49%	48%	57%***	75%***	92%***
Dental visits						
% had visit(s)	44%***	53%***	34%	37%*	47%***	44%***

NOTES: Hospital outpatient visits are to general clinics that are hospital-based. ***$p<0.001$, **$p<0.01$, *$p<0.05$.
SOURCES: Adapted from Lau et al., 2013a, 2014a.

TABLE 7-2 Health Service Utilization by Type of Service

Variable	Year	%	Source
Preventive Care: Attended a preventive care visit within the past 12 months (ages 18-25)	2011	48	MEPS
Mental Health: Received any mental health treatment/counseling in the past year (does not include substance abuse treatment) (ages 18-25)	2012	12	NSDUH
Substance Abuse: Received treatment at any location for illegal drug or alcohol use in the past year (ages 18-25)	2012	2.4	NSDUH
Reproductive Health: Among all women (ages 20-24), used sexual and reproductive health services	2006-2010	72	NSFG
Reproductive Health: Among sexually experienced women (ages 20-24), used	2006-2010		NSFG
Any sexual and reproductive health services		81	
Contraceptive services		64	
Services for sexually transmitted infections (STIs)		30	
Emergency Care: Proportion of young adults' (ages 20-29) health care visits occurring in the emergency department	2006	22	NAMCS
Dental Care: Had a dental visit in the past 12 months (ages 19-25)	2012	59	NHIS

NOTE: MEPS = Medical Expenditure Panel Survey; NAMCS = National Ambulatory Medical Care Survey; NHIS = National Health Information Survey; NSDUH = National Survey on Drug Use and Health; NSFG = National Survey of Family Growth.
SOURCES: MEPS: Lau et al., 2014b; NAMCS: Fortuna et al., 2010; NHIS: Vujicic et al., 2014; NSDUH: SAMHSA, 2013a,b; NSFG: Hall et al., 2012.

has reduced emergency department use (Hernandez-Boussard et al., 2014). There appear to be no population data documenting the use of services for management of chronic medical or mental health conditions for young adults.

TRANSITIONS

Most young adults face the challenge of accessing a new health care system and new health care team independently of their parents or guardians. In addition to the differences between pediatric and adult health care systems and the possibility that the adult system is less well suited to their developmental stage, they may have changes in insurance coverage and face confidentiality concerns. These challenges are amplified when the young

> "Even if you have private insurance and you are transitioning from pediatric care to adult care, you are just kind of on your own in terms of finding doctors, in terms of figuring out how the system works. I didn't particularly have anybody to help me go through that process. I had to figure it out on my own. I am still figuring it out."

adult has a chronic physical or mental health condition that requires ongoing coordinated care. Pediatric providers may not prepare adolescents for an adult model of care, and there is a lack of adult providers who are familiar with managing the adult progression of childhood chronic diseases (AAP et al., 2011). In this section, we first examine the transition from pediatric to adult medical health care for young adults with chronic health conditions, and we then we explore transitions in behavioral health care and substance abuse treatment. While much of the published literature focuses on the transition challenges for those with chronic illness, requiring close medical care, there appears to be no systematic coordination of the transition to adult care for those without chronic medical conditions. It is important to improve the transition process for all youth moving to the adult health care system, not just those who have identified chronic medical conditions.

Transitions for Young Adults with Chronic Health Conditions

As noted, most transition research has focused on young adults with chronic health conditions, including cystic fibrosis, rheumatological diseases, diabetes mellitus, sickle cell anemia, acute lymphocytic leukemia (ALL), organ transplant, inflammatory bowel disease, and congenital heart disease (CHD). In this context, transition has been defined as "the purposeful, planned movement of adolescents and young adults with chronic physical and medical conditions from child-centered to adult-oriented health care systems" (Blum et al., 1993, p. 570). Although it is recommended that transition planning begin during early adolescence, expert consensus suggests that the actual transfer should generally occur during the early young adult years, between ages 18 and 21 (AAP et al., 2011). Before young adults reach the age at which they can legally make their own decisions regarding their care, which could include discontinuing or not accepting available treatment, it is important that they understand their own health conditions and have the tools needed to make such decisions.

The transition from pediatric to adult care is a time of vulnerability that can result in poor outcomes among individuals with chronic health conditions. Poor health outcomes can result from discontinuities of care during the transition process itself, including difficulties identifying a new care team. In a survey of more than 900 adults with CHD, 42 percent reported a lapse of care of more than 3 years, and 8 percent reported a lapse of greater than 10 years; the most frequent age at which lapses occurred was 20 (Gurvitz et al., 2013). Further, a study of 360 young adults (aged 19-21) in Canada with CHD showed that more than one-quarter had not seen a cardiologist since the age of 18 (Reid et al., 2004). These health care lapses among young adults with CHD result in poor health outcomes (Kovacs and McCrindle, 2014).

Concerns also arise regarding young adults' health outcomes after they have transitioned into adult care. For example, a study of 185 participants found that young adults with diabetes had poor glycemic control after they transitioned from pediatric to adult care compared with those young adults who did not make this transition (Lotstein et al., 2013). A large retrospective study of sickle cell disease–related emergency department visits and hospitalizations found that young adults aged 18-30 had higher rates of acute care encounters and rehospitalizations compared with those immediately younger and older (Brousseau et al., 2010). A longitudinal study of individuals with sickle cell disease also found that deaths most frequently occurred after age 18 and after the transfer to adult care (Quinn et al., 2010), although stronger data are needed to fully support the conclusion that the transfer caused the poorer outcomes (DeBaun and Telfair, 2012). In addition, a recent study found increased intubation risk and longer lengths of stay for those young adults (aged 16-25) with sickle cell disease and acute chest syndrome who were cared for in adult hospitals versus those who were cared for in pediatric hospitals (Jan et al., 2013).

Barriers to implementing an effective system to improve transitions have been well documented (e.g., McManus et al., 2008). Some of the critical barriers include those mentioned above: a lack of trained adult providers able to accept young adults with adult manifestations of childhood chronic illnesses, apprehension among patients and families and pediatric providers that care will be compromised during transition, lack of reimbursement for recommended transition practices, a lack of tools with which to assess readiness for transition, and a lack of time for the provider (McManus et al., 2008). The uptake of better practices also has been hampered by the lack of widespread dissemination of research findings.

Despite these challenges, it is possible to plan for a smooth transition with good outcomes. In the case of cystic fibrosis, a chronic illness for which more programs have been implemented for transition care relative to most childhood conditions, a recent study contradicts many previous studies, finding that those who transitioned to adult care had a less rapid decline in respiratory status than patients with similar characteristics who stayed in pediatric care (Tuchman and Schwartz, 2013). These inconsistent research results necessitate greater focus on what constitutes the content of the most effective health care for these and other populations of young adults.

Along with increases in life expectancy in recent decades, many more children with serious childhood-onset diseases are now living into the young adult years. For example, 25 years ago, approximately 30 percent of people with cystic fibrosis were age 18 or older, whereas today approximately half of people with cystic fibrosis are adults, and the median predicted survival age is over 40 (CFF, 2012). This change underscores the need for a successful transition to adult health care. Next we further explore reasons behind the poor outcomes associated with that transition.

Limitations of Adult Health Care Providers' Familiarity with the Disease Process and Developmental Needs of Young Adults

Because many individuals with serious congenital and childhood-onset diseases are now living into the young adult years, many are now receiving care from adult-focused health professionals who previously did not see patients with these diseases and may not have received training in these areas (e.g., Tuchman et al., 2010). From a neurosurgery perspective, for example, caring for an individual with childhood-onset hydrocephalus is very different from caring for an adult in whom this condition emerged as a result of hemorrhage, infection, or tumor (Simon et al., 2009). In a survey, only 15 percent of general internists felt comfortable providing primary care to adults with cystic fibrosis, and 32 percent felt comfortable providing primary care to adults with sickle cell disease (Okumura et al., 2008). In another survey, a lack of training was cited by 24 percent of general internists as a significant or severe limitation on their ability to treat young adults with childhood-onset chronic diseases, although these reports were not statistically associated with physicians' perceived quality of care (Okumura et al., 2010).

In addition, disease manifestation in young adults may differ from that in older adults. Health care providers who provide care for conditions that most commonly affect older adults, such as cancer, may be less familiar with the disease process in young adults. Studies on adolescent and young adult oncology training for health professionals have emphasized the importance of understanding tumor biology, pointing out that the epidemiology and biology are different for many cancers in adolescents and young adults compared with children and older adults (Bleyer and Barr, 2009; Bleyer et al., 2008; Hayes-Lattin et al., 2010).[2] Similarly, young adults may have different concerns and psychosocial needs than older adults. For example, fertility preservation is a great concern for young adults with cancer (Gupta et al., 2013). Young adults with cancer also have a high desire for information and services in the areas of cancer diagnosis, nutrition, physical activity, complementary and alternative services, and health insurance assistance (Gupta et al., 2013; Zebrack, 2008). However, research also indicates that these needs frequently go unmet; in a survey of 217 young adults with cancer, 40-50 percent of respondents indicated that these needs were unmet (Zebrack, 2008). These young adults also expressed needs for or interests in services and supports such as "camp programs and retreats, counseling or guidance related to sexuality, counseling for family members, infertility treatment and adoption services, transportation assistance, child care, and alcohol or drug abuse counseling" (Zebrack, 2008, p. 1). Again, more than 50 percent reported that these needs were unmet. A comparison by age showed that young adults aged 18-29 had greater unmet needs than those aged 30-40.

Differences Between the Child and Adult Medical Care Systems

In pediatric longitudinal studies over the last few decades, the 5-year survival rate for pediatric ALL has increased to 90 percent (Robison, 2011). Unfortunately, there has been no similar increase for adolescent and young adult ALL; currently, the overall survival rate for adults is 30-40 percent (Narayanan and Shami, 2012). Yet there is evidence that treatment in a pediatric cancer center increases survival for adolescents and young adults (De Bont et al., 2004; Peppercorn et al., 2004; Ramanujachar et al., 2006). Box 7-2 examines potential reasons for this difference. In the case of cancer treatment, it may be that the transition to adult care should be based not on age but on disease outcome, meaning that some people may need to have pediatric subspecialty care even though they have transitioned to adult primary care and taken on adult roles in other areas of life.

Like some adult providers, adult health systems are new to providing care to large numbers of young adults with serious childhood-onset diseases. Until the 1980s, for example, only childhood cystic fibrosis centers existed (Tuchman et al., 2010). Now that many more individuals with the disease are living well into adulthood, adult programs have been developing, but in many cases they are provided in the same location as pediatric programs, and adult patients often are hospitalized in pediatric settings

[2] In this field, "adolescents and young adults with cancer" are typically defined as those aged 15-39 (NCI, 2014).

BOX 7-2
Caring for Young Adults with Chronic Diseases in Pediatric Versus Adult Settings

Adolescents and young adults with chronic diseases such as cancer and sickle cell disease generally have better outcomes if treated in pediatric rather than adult centers (De Bont et al., 2004; Jan et al., 2013; Peppercorn et al., 2004; Ramanujachar et al., 2006). This difference persists even when young adults are treated in the adult system using pediatric protocols. The factors that account for this difference are not yet clear, but the following may be factors: wraparound care, a developmental approach, and familiarity with the disease in pediatric care systems. The latter is especially the case with diseases such as acute lymphocytic leukemia (ALL) that can be considered pediatric diseases that either persist into adulthood or have their onset in late adolescence or young adulthood (Narayanan and Shami, 2012).

An important question is whether young adults should be kept longer in pediatric settings or changes can be made to the adult health care system. An argument for the former approach is that adult care systems are burdened with a growing elderly population and lack the resources to care for young adults. On the other hand, one could argue that keeping young adults in pediatric centers does not facilitate their being treated as adults with appropriate preventive care and confidentiality, and that adult systems are not being encouraged to develop appropriate systems of care based on a life span approach. Additional research on this question is needed.

Despite this open question, institutions are already reacting to the evidence of past poorer outcomes in adult systems by building systems within children's hospitals to care for adolescents and young adults. Examples include the Adolescent and Young Adult Cancer Program at Seattle Children's Hospital (Seattle Children's Hospital, 2014) and the Adolescent and Young Adult Program at MD Anderson Children's Cancer Hospital in Texas (MD Anderson Cancer Center, 2014).[a] In addition, some adult systems are creating follow-up clinics especially for those with pediatric-onset diseases. An example is the Thriving After Cancer clinic at the George Washington Cancer Institute/George Washington University Medical Faculty Associates, which provides care that addresses young adults' needs in an appropriate adult setting (GW Cancer Institute, 2014; personal communication, September 17, 2014, April Barbour, M.D., The George Washington Medical Faculty Associates).

[a] For additional examples of care programs for adolescents and young adults with cancer, see IOM (2013b).

(Tuchman et al., 2010). Thus the age-appropriateness of care offered for adult patients in a pediatric setting is a concern (AAP et al., 2011). In the survey by Okumura and colleagues, physicians responded that a lack of subspecialty access and having an office structure that did not facilitate coordination of care for young adults with special health care needs had the greatest negative impact on their perceived quality of care (Okumura et al., 2010). In another study, internists saw a need to obtain the consent of young adults for family involvement in their care (Peter et al., 2009).

Studies on the perspectives of patients, providers, and families underscore the general discomfort with and lack of a structured process for the transition to adult health care (Peter et al., 2009; Reiss et al., 2005). Some pediatric providers who have developed successful relationships with patients and their families delay transitioning young adults to adult care because of "difficulty letting go," previous experiences with difficult patient transitions, and the perception that the transfer will result in negative health outcomes (Reiss et al., 2005). An American Academy of Pediatrics (AAP) survey of pediatric providers' activities related to transition found that few offered youth and their families preparation for transitioning to an adult model of care at age 18, communicated directly with the adult provider, offered medical summaries for the youth/family and the adult provider, and/or created a medical transition plan (McManus et al., 2008). Also of note is the internist perspective that there is a need for better training in congenital and childhood-onset conditions and an urgent need for more training for adult subspecialists (Peter et al., 2009). The perspectives of patients and physicians, coupled with concern for financial support to care for these complex patients, are important factors in successful planning for transition by all concerned (Peter et al., 2009).

Efforts to Improve the Transition Process

The transition from pediatric to adult care has been identified as a problem for decades. Yet there has been minimal systematic implementation and evaluation of institutional change to address concerns about the increasing numbers of pediatric patients with chronic conditions who are now living into adulthood.

> "At my age—19—my friends and I don't even know the first thing about looking into health care services. I think that it would be very beneficial to start educating us about these things now rather than later."

Multiple consensus studies have been published on the transition from pediatric to adult care, starting with a Surgeon's General Conference in 1989 (AAP, 1996; AAP et al., 2002, 2011; Blum et al., 1993; Magrab and Millar, 1989). The 2011 recommendations of the AAP, American Academy of Family Physicians (AAFP), and American College of Physicians (ACP) identify best practices in transitions (see Box 7-3)

BOX 7-3
Recommendations for Successful Transitions from the American Academy of Pediatrics (AAP), American Academy of Family Physicians (AAFP), and American College of Physicians (ACP)

AAP, AAFP, and ACP have together developed a health care transitions planning algorithm for all youth and young adults in medical home settings. The plan components are (a) assess for transition readiness, (b) plan a dynamic and longitudinal process for accomplishing realistic goals, (c) implement the plan through education of all involved parties and empowerment of the youth in areas of self-care, and (d) document progress to enable ongoing reassessment and movement of medical information to the receiving (adult care) provider. These apply to all youth and young adults, and the guidelines provide additional information for youth and young adults with special health care needs.

The document also identifies the following educational and policy recommendations for the transition from pediatric to adult health care systems:

- enhanced payment for transition services;
- case finding of those in need of transition services who are not receiving them;
- insurance coverage for patients in need of transition planning;
- standards of care and credentialing of providers;
- training for primary care physicians and medical subspecialists to promote transitions within the medical home; and
- promotion of training and clinical learning experience on transition and transfer of youth and young adults (both with and without special needs) for trainees in all medical fields.

SOURCE: AAP et al., 2011.

and state that additional elements of health care delivery and reimbursement systems are needed to achieve a successful transition (AAP et al., 2011). Recently, the Agency for Healthcare Research and Quality (AHRQ) published a technical brief on transition for children with special health care needs that reiterates many of the same findings published in 1989 (McPheeters et al., 2014). Efforts also have been made to apply the Institute for Healthcare Improvement's Triple Aim[3] framework to this transition (Benson et al., 2014; Berwick et al., 2008).

[3] The Institute for Healthcare Improvement's Triple Aim framework is aimed at achieving three goals: "Improving the patient experience of care (including quality and satisfaction); improving the health of populations; and reducing the per capita cost of health care" (IHI, 2014).

Various federal agencies support transition-related activities. For example, the Got Transition initiative/Center for Health Care Transition Improvement, a cooperative agreement between the Health Resources and Services Administration's (HRSA's) Maternal and Child Health Bureau and the National Alliance to Advance Adolescent Health, aims to improve health care transitions by developing and expanding the use of transition materials, training the workforce, enhancing youth and parent leadership, promoting health system changes, and serving as a resource clearinghouse (The National Alliance to Advance Adolescent Health, 2014a). This initiative has developed updated recommended core elements (Six Core Elements of Transition) for pediatric, internal medicine, family medicine, and med-peds[4] practices (The National Alliance to Advance Adolescent Health, 2014b):

- establishing a transition policy,
- tracking and monitoring transition progress,
- conducting transition readiness assessments,
- planning for adult care,
- transferring into adult care (if applicable), and
- integrating the young adult into an adult practice.

Materials are organized and customized for three different situations, with corresponding types of health care providers:

- transitioning youth to adult health care providers (pediatric, family medicine, and med-peds providers);
- transitioning to an adult approach to health care without changing providers (family medicine and med-peds providers); and
- integrating young adults into adult health care (internal medicine, family medicine, and med-peds providers) (The National Alliance to Advance Adolescent Health, 2014b).

These recommended core elements and available customizable tools are based on the AAP/ACP/AAFP Clinical Report (2011) and were created using the quality improvement approach outlined by the Institute for Healthcare Improvement's change framework. This approach may set the stage for less fragmentation of care in transition, with clear guidance for coordination and communication between pediatric and adult providers, improved preparation for the transfer to adult health care, improved integration of young adults as a special population into the adult health care setting, and ways to evaluate the transition process.

[4] Combined internal medicine and pediatric practice.

Similarly, the Substance Abuse and Mental Health Services Administration (SAMHSA) sponsors the Emerging Adulthood Initiative. This initiative is focused on improving outcomes among adolescents and young adults with serious mental health conditions as they transition to adulthood, including transitions in health care (Georgetown University Center for Child and Human Development, 2014).

Beyond the transition issues for children with chronic medical conditions, health systems need to accommodate the needs of young adults who do not have a chronic condition but still have increased health care needs due to their stage of development and heath behaviors and the emergence of new mental and physical health conditions. The increased emergency room utilization noted above may speak to the difficulty experienced by young adults in transitioning to the adult health care system and their unmet health needs.

Behavioral Health Care Transitions

Behavioral health care systems typically are separate from medical health care systems, and include both mental health and substance abuse systems. The 1999 Surgeon General's report on mental health describes the "de facto" mental health system as comprising four sectors (a description that applies equally well to substance abuse services): "the specialty mental health sector, the general medical/primary care sector, the human services sector, and the voluntary support network sector" (HHS, 1999, p. 73).

Funding of this de facto system generally is split between public/government sources (e.g., Medicaid, Medicare, state funding) and private sources (including services provided through private funding and services provided directly by private agencies, such as employer-provided insurance) (HHS, 1999). Behavioral health services may be office based (typically 1-6 hours/week), home based (usually more intensive than office-based treatment), intensive outpatient (in which clients sleep at home but receive treatment for several hours per day), residential/inpatient, and intensive inpatient (which includes more extensive medical care, typically for a relatively brief period of time). Until recently, private insurance often limited payment for treatment to a restrictive amount that was easily exceeded by more serious treatment needs. Individuals then either paid out of pocket or applied to the public sector for services (HHS, 1999).

The Mental Health Parity and Addiction Equity Act, enacted in 2008, targets reducing the large disparity in insurance coverage for behavioral and physical health treatment. The legislation requires insurance groups to provide the same level of benefits they provide for general medical treatment for mental health or substance use disorders. Under final rules for this act, effective July 1, 2014, deductibles for behavioral health must be on par with those for similar services for other medical conditions, and treatment limits or co-pays more restrictive than those for medical/surgical services are prohibited. Standards for reimbursement for psychosocial treatments also are being discussed, and the Institute of Medicine (IOM) has been asked to conduct a study to develop a framework for establishing efficacy standards for psychosocial interventions used to treat mental disorders; the results of these discussions will have important implications for young adults (Insel, 2014; IOM, 2014). In addition, the ACA now prohibits lifetime or annual dollar limits for essential health benefits, which include mental health and substance abuse care (CMS, 2014a). Future research examining the impact of these new rules and requirements will help determine the extent to which needed behavioral health care is more affordable and accessible to young adults.

Aging Out of Child-Serving Systems

For young adults with mental health or substance use treatment needs, an additional factor that complicates service delivery is the many funding streams, state-funded services, and ways of organizing treatment that are age defined (Davis et al., 2009). Age-defined services and systems include special education (ending at age 21), foster care (typically ending at age 18 or 21), juvenile justice (typically ending at age 17 or 18), and adult criminal justice (starting at ages 16, 17, or 18). Public mental health systems also are typically divided organizationally and fiscally between child and adult services (Davis, 2003; Davis et al., 2006). Each of these systems may provide or coordinate behavioral health services. Thus, young adulthood marks an age when particularly vulnerable individuals' behavioral health services are disrupted by "aging out" of children's service systems. Continuity of care as individuals age out is dependent on access and strong connections to behavioral health services from adult systems. In addition, within public mental health services, policies that define eligibility criteria or target populations for services are distinctly different for child and adult mental health (Davis and Koroloff, 2006), with adult criteria typically being more narrow. This produces a barrier to access based on changing age, not changing need.

> "It took me about 6 months to get an intake appointment. My psychologist left after 2 months."

Another factor that contributes to discontinuities in care for any young adult with health care needs is the age-based eligibility criteria for Medicaid and Supplemental Security Income (SSI).[5] Medicaid has different eligibility criteria for children (dependent members of a household) and adults. Those who age out can fail to meet the adult criteria (Pullman et al., 2010). Qualifying for Medicaid by meeting the Social Security Administration's (SSA's) definition of disability also is impacted by age-based definitions of "disability" (e.g., ADHD is a qualifying mental disorder for children but not for adults). According to SSA, each year tens of thousands of child SSI recipients reach age 18, and their medical eligibility is redetermined according to adult disability standards (Hemmeter, 2012). Overall, about one-third of these children (37 percent) lose eligibility (Hemmeter, 2012). Among youth with mental health disorders that fall under the "other mental disorders" category (e.g., anxiety, affective, and disruptive behavior disorders)—who make up 28 percent of all children receiving SSI after reaching age 18—more than half (53 percent) lose eligibility upon redetermination (Hemmeter, 2012). Overall, these age-based criteria contribute to higher risk of Medicaid disenrollment during young adulthood, even among highly vulnerable clinical populations (Davis et al., 2014; Pullman et al., 2010), and may contribute to reduced access to needed behavioral health care (Slade et al., 2014). Although discussed here in the context of behavioral health transitions, many of these same discontinuities apply more generally to health care coverage issues for young adults.

Differences Between Child and Adult Mental Health Systems

Several typical treatment culture differences characterize child and adult mental health systems. The first is the manner in which parental figures are involved. In their seminal work defining system-of-care principles for children with emotional disturbance, Stroul and Friedman (1986) focus on the importance of partnering with parents to provide appropriate treatment and supports for their child. Since that work was published, child mental health systems have largely changed to work more closely with parental figures in developing and implementing treatment and service plans for their children (Stroul, 2002). Approaches such as the wraparound process (VanDenBerg and Grealish, 1996) and multisystemic therapy (Henggeler et al., 1998) are formalized means of partnering with family members to address the child's mental health condition and resulting functional impairments. However, family involvement is less emphasized in adult mental health systems, and once they turn 18, youth can legally restrict providers from sharing any treatment information with family members. Yet client factors that facilitate shared decision making often are still immature in the

[5] In most states, SSI beneficiaries are automatically eligible for Medicaid, while other states require a separate application and determination of eligibility (SSA, 2014).

youngest adults (Delman, 2012; Joseph-William et al., 2014). Given the unique role parents can play in the lives of young adults (as described in Chapter 3) and the help they could provide with decision making, excluding their potential supports may compromise the efficacy of treatment for a young adult needing behavioral health services. Indeed, family cognitive-behavioral treatment appears to be an important component of early intervention in psychosis (Gleeson et al., 2009).

Another substantial difference in practice between child and adult mental health systems is related to care coordination. Children with serious mental health conditions often are involved in multiple systems, including child welfare, juvenile justice, special education, and mental health. Providers in these systems typically are aware of the involvement of other systems, and often communicate and coordinate with them. Adult mental health, by contrast, is often insular, so that services such as vocational rehabilitation or drug treatment are provided within the mental health system rather than in partnership with those systems (Davis et al., 2012b). Disconnects in cross-system connections, especially between child and adult systems, can cause disruptions or redundancies in services, especially for 18- to 21-year-olds who are still involved in child systems.

Finally, adult mental health systems often fail to recognize the unique needs of young adults, and there are few interventions with strong evidence of efficacy for this age group (GAO, 2008). With the exception of interventions to treat early psychosis, few interventions have been devised specifically for this age group, and all are in early stages of development (Davis, 2012a). Evidence of the efficacy of evidence-based adult or child interventions with a young adult population is limited (Davis et al., 2012a). Clinical trials including this age group as part of a larger age group (e.g., studies of adults in general) cannot sufficiently establish efficacy in the young adult population. For an age effect to be detected, a large sample size of the young adult age group is needed, and few age group comparisons have been conducted thus far in published studies. However, some studies have reported significant differences in outcomes or relative effectiveness of psychosocial interventions between older and younger age groups (e.g., Burke-Miller et al., 2012; Haddock et al., 2006; Kaplan et al., 2012; Rice et al., 1993). Applying interventions that have been established in older or younger populations and adapting those interventions for young adults is a reasonable starting point for research and service provision. For example, the individual placement and support model for adults with severe mental illness (Bond, 1998) has been adapted and tested for use with young adults with first or early episodes of psychosis (Killackey et al., 2008; Major et al., 2010; Porteous and Waghorn, 2007), with results providing support for its use in this age group.

Substance Abuse Care Transitions

Many of the issues of transition faced by young adults with mental health conditions are also faced by those with substance use disorders: involvement in multiple child systems that end variably between ages 18 and 21, adolescent and adult treatment providers who are trained to work with one but not the other age group, stricter diagnostic criteria for adult than child Medicaid coverage for substance abuse-based eligibility, and few interventions with efficacy for reducing substance use specifically in young adults. Several of the unique aspects of the substance use system are worth noting, however. Foremost is the heightened stigma of substance abuse problems. Most substance use is illegal, and alcohol use is illegal for young adults under age 21. Recreational use of marijuana also is illegal except in Washington and Colorado for those over the age of 21. Moreover, use of substances often is seen as a moral issue, and problematic substance use is viewed as a volitional problem rather than a chronic illness. The legal issues and moral values have two major consequences—reducing funding for treatment and posing a barrier to treatment seeking (Cutcliffe and Saadeh, 2014; Drucker, 2012). The result is a scarcity of substance abuse services and long wait lists for those services.

Brief substance use treatments for which there is growing evidence of efficacy are increasingly available on college campuses, but for the many young adults with substance use problems that are not in college or the military, or for college students whose substance abuse problems require more than brief treatment, the challenge of finding a provider after the significant step of acknowledging the need for help is a formidable barrier to care. The scarcity of treatment resources, in combination with the need for young adults to advocate on their own behalf despite their inexperience in doing so, can lead to a large unmet need for treatment in this age group (Tighe and Saxe, 2006). Mental health and substance use disorders can further impede young adults' abilities to advocate for themselves. Young adults' inexperience with self-advocacy also means that simply providing them with information about how and where to obtain health insurance or care, while important, is not sufficient. Also necessary are active and effective preparation of adolescents and young adults and outreach by the health care system to help them access and complete needed treatment.

PREVENTIVE CARE FOR YOUNG ADULTS

The majority of health problems during young adulthood are preventable, and behaviors associated with negative health outcomes have high prevalence among young adults, as described in Chapter 6. These behaviors often are also responsible for the onset of many chronic health conditions (e.g., obesity, diabetes, addiction to substances, mental health disorders) that lead not only to functional impairment throughout adulthood but also to a shortened life span. Many of these behaviors represent an opportunity for cessation of harmful behaviors, the development of healthy alternatives, or further entrenchment of the behaviors that threaten adult health.

Use of Preventive Care in Young Adults

Knowledge of the use and delivery of preventive services for young adults is limited by the lack of attention to this age group in clinical delivery systems and health services research noted throughout this report. A few recent studies, either population-based assessments or based within health care delivery systems, have documented the relatively low rates of preventive services in this population (Fortuna et al., 2009; Lau et al., 2013b; see Table 7-3). Considerable variation is related to gender, race/ethnicity, and having a usual source of care. With the exception of influenza vaccination, young females are more likely than males to receive preventive services (Lau et al., 2013b). Young adults who have a source of care they typically use also are more likely to receive preventive services. Black young adults are more likely than their white counterparts to receive the full range of sexually transmitted infection (STI), cholesterol, and diet counseling (Lau et al., 2013b). Compared with whites, Asians are less likely to receive STI

TABLE 7-3 Percentage of Visits During Which Preventive Counseling Was Provided to Young Adults (aged 20-29), 1996-2006

	All Specialties (%)	Primary Care (%)	Ob/Gyn (%)
Any	30.6	32.7	33.6
Injury[a]	2.4	3.1	0.8
Smoking	3.1	4.2	3.1
Exercise	8.2	9.4	8.2
Weight reduction[b]	3.0	3.8	3.4
Mental health	4.1	4.2	1.3
STI/HIV[c]	2.7	2.6	7.1

NOTES: "Mental health" does not include substance abuse or use; STI = sexually transmitted infection.
Primary care includes internal medicine, pediatrics, family practice, general practice, general preventive medicine, or public health or general preventive medicine.
[a] Data were available for 1996-2000 and 2005-2006.
[b] Data were available for 2001-2006.
[c] Data were available for 1996-2000.
SOURCE: Adapted from Fortuna et al., 2009.

TABLE 7-4 Past-Year Receipt of Screening or Preventive Services Among Young Adults Aged 18-25 Who Had a Past-Year Visit, National Health Interview Survey, 2011

	Blood Pressure Check	Fasting Blood Sugar Check	Talked About Diet	Talked About Smoking If a Smoker	Pap Screen for Women	Flu Shot
% Who received screening or preventive service	87.3	22.3	22.8	52.0	66.5	26.2

SOURCE: Analysis done by Sally H. Adams @ University of California, San Francisco, Division of Adolescent & Young Adult Medicine.

and emotional health screening, and Latinos/as are more likely to receive cholesterol and diet counseling (Lau et al., 2013b).

Analysis of National Health Interview Survey (NHIS) data from 2011 reveals that among young adults who had a clinical visit during the past year, access to a range of preventive services ranged in frequency from 87 percent receiving a blood pressure check to 22 percent receiving a fasting blood sugar check (see Table 7-4). It is important to note that such preventive screening can take place during any clinical encounter with a provider or in alternative delivery systems (e.g., pharmacies, work or school sites). Providers need to be encouraged to use any visit as an opportunity to address a component of preventive care.

Guidelines for Preventive Care for Young Adults

This section examines existing guidelines, their implementation, and monitoring of adherence.

Existing Guidelines

There continue to be no specific medical, behavioral, or oral health guidelines focused specifically on the young adult population. The clinical preventive services recommendations[6] of the U.S. Preventive Services Task Force (USPSTF) consist of evidence-based recommendations across several specific health areas. For the past two decades, there has been a strong movement toward developing consensus-based guidelines for care for adolescents, starting with the American Medical Association's Guidelines for

[6] See http://www.uspreventiveservicestaskforce.org/recommendations.htm for details (accessed October 22, 2014).

Adolescent Preventive Services: Recommendations and Rationale (Elster and Kuznets, 1994) and Bright Futures: Guidelines for Health Supervision of Infants, Children, and Adolescents (Green, 1994). The most recent Bright Futures edition includes preventive care recommendations up to age 21 (Hagan et al., 2008). A revision of Bright Futures is expected to be released in 2015.

Several groups have called for the development of care guidelines for young adults (Callahan and Cooper, 2010; Fortuna et al., 2009; Irwin, 2010; Ozer et al., 2012). Recently, Ozer and colleagues (2012) conducted an analysis to identify evidence-based guidelines for young adults by reviewing professional consensus guidelines and the evidence-based guidelines from the USPSTF that include young adults (aged 18-26). They found that four groups—AAP, the American Congress of Gynecologists and Obstetricians (ACOG), AAFP, and ACP—had developed guidelines relevant to young adults.

> "Most young adults don't want to pay for anything if they can, so even though preventive care is for your benefit and you can access it at any time, some people don't realize that that is the case. They think they may not be covered and may have to pay for services."

Increasingly, health care plans have incorporated an annual preventive care visit with limited or no co-pays as part of the core benefits for subscribers. The ACA has expanded the opportunity for young adults to receive an annual preventive visit with no associated co-payments, and a recent study documents an increase in young adults' receipt of a general checkup in the first year of implementation of the ACA—48 percent in 2011 as compared with 44 percent in 2009 (Lau et al., 2014b). Table 7-5, adapted from Ozer et al. (2012), lists the preventive services that most private plans must cover under the ACA, which include the evidence-based screening and counseling services rated highly in either Category A or B by the USPSTF,[7] the Advisory Committee on Immunization Practices' recommended immunizations, the Bright Futures recommendations, and the services specified in the Women's Preventive Services Guidelines (HHS, 2012). The Women's Preventive Services Guidelines (HRSA, 2014; IOM, 2011) specify that in addition to the services provided for all adults, the services

---

[7] The USPSTF defines Category A as follows: "The USPSTF recommends the service. There is high certainty that the net benefit is substantial." Category B is defined as follows: "The USPSTF recommends the service. There is high certainty that the net benefit is moderate or there is moderate certainty that the net benefit is moderate to substantial" (USPSTF, 2012).

TABLE 7-5 Preventive Health Care Services for Young Adults (aged 18-26) Covered Under the Affordable Care Act

Services Covered for All Young Adults (ages 18-26)	Additional Services Covered for Young Adults Ages 18-21	Additional Services Covered for Women (ages 18-26)
Alcohol misuse screening and counseling	Annual wellness visit	Well-woman visits
Tobacco use screening	Screening and counseling for illicit drugs	Contraception
Blood pressure screening	Suicide screening	Folic acid supplements
Diabetes (Type 2) screening for those with high blood pressure*	Safety/violence screening	Domestic and interpersonal violence screening and counseling (women of all ages)
Diet counseling*	Family/partner violence (male and female)	Cervical cancer screening (if sexually active)
Obesity screening and counseling	Fighting	Chlamydia infection screening
Cholesterol screening*	Use of helmets	Gonorrhea screening*
Depression screening	Use of seat belts	Breast cancer genetic test counseling (BRCA)*
HIV screening	Driving under the influence	Breast cancer chemoprevention counseling*
STI prevention counseling*	Use of firearms	Hepatitis B screening for pregnant women
Syphilis screening*	Bullying	Rh incompatibility screening for pregnant women
Immunizations	Polio immunization	Anemia screening for pregnant women
Hepatitis A		Gestational diabetes screening
Hepatitis B		Urinary tract or other infection screening for pregnant women
Human papillomavirus		Comprehensive support and counseling for breastfeeding
Influenza		
Measles, mumps, rubella		
Meningococcal		
Pneumococcal		
Tetanus, diphtheria, pertussis		
Varicella		

* If at higher risk.
NOTE: STI = sexually transmitted infection.
SOURCES: Adapted from Ozer et al., 2012, 2013. Original sources are the evidence-based screening and counseling services rated highly either in Category A or B by the USPSTF, immunizations recommended by the Advisory Committee on Immunization Practices, the Bright Futures recommendations, and the services specified in the Women's Preventive Services Guidelines.

listed in Table 7-5 must be provided to women by private plans without cost sharing (Armstrong, 2012a,b; HHS, 2012; HRSA, 2014). Note that Table 7-5 summarizes what evidence-based services are currently covered, and does not provide a comprehensive list of what this committee deems should be covered.

Comprehensive dental guidelines for young adults could not be identified, although the American Academy of Pediatric Dentistry recommends that a dental home be established when the adolescent patient, family, and dentist agree that it is time to transition to adult dental care (AAPD, 2013).

Implementation of Guidelines

Multiple approaches can be used to incorporate preventive guidelines into clinical practice for young adults. At present, however, there is no consensus among health professional organizations, the USPSTF, health care plans, and state and federal agencies on guidelines that should be used as the starting point for implementation.

Barriers that impede the delivery of preventive services in clinical settings include both clinician factors (e.g., lack of knowledge of guidelines; attitudes toward the efficacy of preventive services; and lack of training, skills, and confidence to deliver the services) and external factors (e.g., time constraints, lack of screening tools, lack of reimbursement) (e.g., Ozer et al., 2005). Efforts comparable to those over the past two decades to increase the delivery of preventive services to adolescents are just beginning for young adults. Multiple models shown to increase preventive screening in adolescents could be adapted for use for young adults (Boekeloo and Griffin, 2007; Boekeloo et al., 2003; Klein et al., 2003; Olson et al., 2009; Ozer, 2007; Ozer et al., 2005; Sanci et al., 2012; Stevens et al., 2008; Tylee et al., 2007).

Monitoring of Adherence to Guidelines for Young Adult Preventive Care

No mechanisms for monitoring adherence to guidelines relevant to young adult preventive care currently exist. With the implementation of preventive care under the ACA, it will be necessary to identify national- and state-level datasets that can be used to monitor the implementation of these guidelines. Monitoring guideline adherence for young adult preventive care is important in both the public health and health care domains. Below are identified existing datasets that could be used for this purpose and describe associated challenges.

Four nationally representative ongoing surveys that include some measures of preventive screening and counseling for adults in general can be accessed to obtain estimates specifically for young adults: the NHIS, a survey of health status and health care access; the Medical Expenditures Panel Survey (MEPS), a household survey of health, health care, and health care expenditures; the National Ambulatory Medical Care Survey, which monitors the services patients receive from clinicians in ambulatory settings; and the Behavioral Risk Factor Surveillance System, a survey of behavioral risk factors associated with major morbidity and mortality (AHRQ, 2014; CDC, 2014a,b,c). In addition, the Centers for Medicare & Medicaid Services (CMS) is developing and implementing a revised set of adult health care quality measures in conjunction with AHRQ (CMS, 2014e; GPO, 2012; Mann, 2012). Many of these measures are applicable to young adults (e.g., influenza vaccinations, body mass index assessment, screening for clinical depression) and will be of use in assessing the implementation of clinical preventive screening in Medicaid-enrolled young adults. The use of these measures is encouraged by CMS but is optional for the states. It is not clear how states will choose the measures on which they will report and what capability they will have to access data specific to young adults.

Despite the availability of these data, researchers, policy makers, funders, and other stakeholders need to have the expertise to break out the specific ages that make up young adulthood, examine state-level data, and differentiate specific subpopulations. Moreover, some of these datasets are more readily accessible than others. In many cases, online analysis can be carried out, but there usually are restrictions on the specificity of age groups and the breadth of subgroup analyses possible. In addition, most national survey data centers allow analysis of state-level data upon request, but the datasets are not always sufficiently large to study the states with smaller populations.

For both national- and state-level data analysis, data elements that help differentiate special populations may be insufficient. Gaps may exist for youth who have been in foster care or were recently homeless or incarcerated. For the CMS data, only young adults enrolled in Medicaid will be able to be assessed with the new adult core measures.

Some of the survey procedures also may introduce bias into the survey responses. For example, the MEPS data collection procedures identify the adult respondent for the entire household, including young adults, as the adult who is most knowledgeable about the health care utilization and expenditures of all household members (AHRQ, 2014). For many young adults, parents may be unaware of health care accessed confidentially; through college health services; or through other systems of care, such as public health clinics and pharmacies (Lau et al., 2014a).

In addition, current adult health care monitoring efforts do not cover many key topics relevant to young adult screening and counseling, such as obesity-related issues, substance use, and reproductive health issues. When these topics are assessed, a lack of specificity often limits the utility of the assessment. For example, the USPSTF recommends that young adults have their blood pressure screened every 2 years when it is is below 120/80 mm Hg (NAHIC, 2014). Yet surveys such as the NHIS asking about the recency of blood pressure monitoring do not always ask respondents to report their blood pressure, so adherence to this guideline cannot be determined.

Preventive Care for Behavioral Health Conditions

There are fewer rigorously tested approaches for preventing behavioral health disorders than exist for many physical disorders (e.g., encouraging diet or exercise in all patients to reduce the likelihood of their developing cardiovascular disease). One example of an accessible behavioral health prevention approach is encouraging aerobic physical activity to prevent the development of depression (Mammen and Faulkner, 2013).

Most prevention approaches for behavioral health target children and adolescents based on the young ages at which many behavioral health conditions develop and the ready access to these populations in schools (IOM, 1994; Stice et al., 2009). Studies of prevention interventions for conditions common to young adults—including Web-based technologies to reduce the risk of developing depression (Van Voorhees et al., 2011) and anxiety (Braithwaite and Fincham, 2007; Christensen et al., 2010; Cukrowicz and Joiner, 2007)—have targeted primarily college students. SAMHSA funds the Campus Suicide Prevention Grants[8] to support efforts at postsecondary institutions to prevent suicide and to improve services for students with problems that put them at risk of suicide, such as depression, substance abuse, and other behavioral health issues; however, there are currently no rigorously tested interventions to implement. A growing body of research documents brief interventions for reducing college binge drinking with some evidence of efficacy (e.g., Kulesza et al., 2013). Preliminary evidence also suggests that parents who talk with their children about binge drinking before they depart for college can decrease excessive drinking and alter drinking perceptions (Turrisi et al., 2001).

Instead of going to college, some young adults enter the military after high school. As discussed in Chapter 5, military personnel who have been deployed are at heightened risk of developing posttraumatic stress disorder and other mood and anxiety disorders and for suicide. While several interventions have been developed for use both before and during deployment to prevent the development of posttraumatic stress disorder or suicide, none have as yet been rigorously tested (Hoge and Castro, 2012; Hourani et al., 2011). Predeployment mental health screening also has been used to either divert some individuals from deployment or provide additional mental health support (mainly medication) during deployment (Warner et al., 2011). There is evidence of reduced mental health needs in brigades with screening compared with those without (Warner et al., 2011).

For civilian young adults not enrolled in college or in colleges that offer some preventive interventions, most interventions are designed for

---

[8] See http://www.samhsa.gov/grants/2013/sm-13-009.aspx for details (accessed October 22, 2014).

individuals at high risk of developing a mental health disorder or with conditions that increase this risk. For example, cognitive-behavioral interventions can reduce the risk of developing posttraumatic stress disorder if administered within days or weeks after a traumatic event (Agorastos et al., 2011). Given the high risk of violent victimization in young adulthood, including sexual violence and witnessing violence, prevention of trauma symptoms and posttraumatic stress disorder is particularly relevant in this age group.

The experience of psychological stress is pervasive in young adults and may contribute to the subsequent development of behavioral or physical health disorders, as described in Chapter 6. A variety of stress reduction techniques are available for which there is evidence of efficacy in adults, such as mindfulness-based approaches or cognitive therapy (Abbott et al., 2014; Querstret and Cropley, 2013), cognitive-behavioral techniques (Cruess et al., 1999), and relaxation techniques (Shah et al., 2014). Some of these techniques can reduce symptoms of behavioral health conditions (Chiesa and Serretti, 2014; Khoury et al., 2013; Shah et al., 2014), although findings on the benefits for physical conditions are more mixed (Abbott et al., 2014; Fordham et al., 2013; Hughes et al., 2013; Lauche et al., 2013; Reiner et al., 2013). As with other behavioral health interventions, direct evidence of the efficacy of these stress reduction approaches specifically in young adults is limited, and studies have focused primarily on college students (Bodenlos et al., 2013; Tanis, 2012).

There are also approaches for reducing the development of depression in high-risk groups, such as adolescent children of parents with depression or adolescents with elevated depression symptoms (Beardslee et al., 2013; Clarke et al., 1995, 2001). One such approach has been adapted for Web-based intervention and has shown moderate effects in young adults (Clarke et al., 2009). In addition, pharmacological treatment combined with psychotherapy reduces the likelihood of suicide in individuals who have unipolar or bipolar affective disorders (Rihmer and Gonda, 2013). And since young adulthood is a common age for becoming a parent, preventing postpartum depression is particularly relevant in this age group. While cognitive-behavioral therapies reduce postpartum depression, evidence is currently insufficient regarding approaches for identifying those at risk and providing preventive interventions (Nardi et al., 2012).

Finally, because young adulthood is the peak age of onset of psychosis (Copeland et al., 2011), prevention of these most serious mental illnesses is a high priority. There is growing evidence that cognitive-behavioral therapies and complex psychotherapies can delay the transition from symptoms indicating high risk of developing psychosis to the development of a psychotic disorder, while pharmacotherapy does not appear to be beneficial for this purpose (Stafford et al., 2013). Both psychotherapies and pharmacotherapies can, however, help reduce the likelihood of a second episode of psychotic illness in those who have recently experienced a first episode (Álvarez-Jiménez et al., 2011).

BEHAVIORAL HEALTH INTERVENTIONS FOR YOUNG ADULTS

Effective behavioral health treatments and strategies exist for adults. The efficacy of these treatments specifically for young adults, however, is largely undemonstrated because they typically group young and other adults together (Davis et al., 2012a).

Pharmacological interventions are expected to be as efficacious in young as in older adults, although noncompliance may be greater in young adults (Baillargeon et al., 2000; Kessing et al., 2007). Psychosocial interventions, however, cannot be assumed to be as efficacious in young as in older adults, as they can be influenced by many of the factors that are changing or less mature in young compared with older adults. Such factors include responsibility taking, response to authoritative figures, changing roles within the family, and responses to behavioral contingencies. Indeed, young and older adults even perceive various qualities of their interaction with physicians differently (Bradley et al., 2001). Consequently, psychosocial interventions need to be explicitly tested in young adults. To this end, the young adult sample size needs to be large enough to detect an age effect compared with older or younger age groups (Davis et al., 2012a). Few published studies have compared age groups, although some have yielded significant findings comparing young and older adults with respect to outcomes or the effiacy of psychosocial interventions (e.g., Burke-Miller et al., 2012; Haddock et al., 2006; Kaplan et al., 2012; Rice et al., 1993; Sinha et al., 2003). With the exception of interventions to treat early psychosis, few interventions have been developed specifically for young adults; all are in early stages of development, and there are few for which efficacy has been demonstrated in this age group.

HEALTH CARE COVERAGE FOR YOUNG ADULTS

Young adults without health insurance or with gaps in insurance coverage are less likely to access health services compared with young adults who are continuously insured (see Figure 7-1). Health insurance coverage rates for young adults, however, have historically been the lowest of any age group. In 2010 and 2011, for example, young adults aged 19-25 had an uninsured rate of 28 percent and were the age group most likely to be uninsured (Todd and Sommers, 2012). The rate of uninsurance among empoyed young adults also is one-third higher than that among older

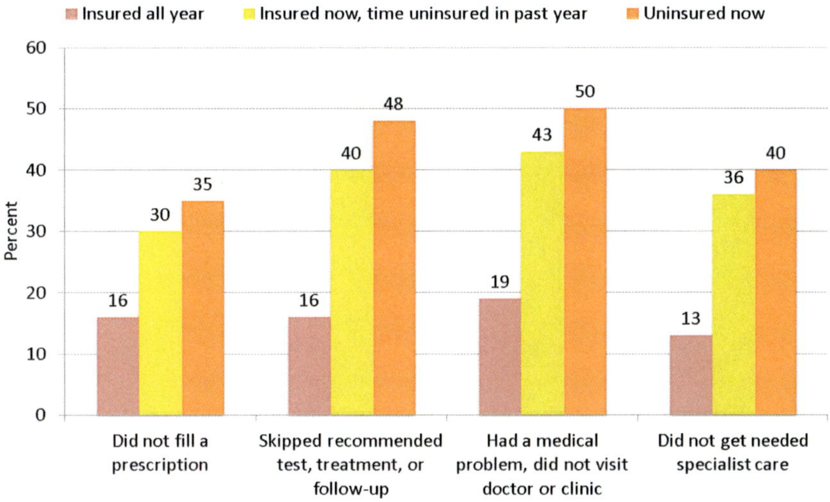

FIGURE 7-1 Percentage of young adults aged 19-29 who experienced different types of health care access problems in the past year because of cost (2010 data).
SOURCE: Collins et al., 2012.

employed adults because the part-time, entry-level, seasonal, and small-business jobs held more commonly by young versus older adults often do not include health benefits (CMS, 2014d).

> "My boss took the time to discuss general health care information with me, which helped me understand my choices better."

In this section, we describe state-level efforts to enhance coverage for young adults and the impact of the ACA on this population. We also discuss several groups of young adults who have particular difficulty accessing care, including unauthorized immigrants, those exiting the foster care system, those involved in the justice system, and those with mental illness. The focus is primarily on financial barriers, but we identify additional barriers as well. It is important to keep in mind that access to adult care that fails to effectively engage and retain young adults or address their particular needs also is insufficient. A recent study showed that even though young adults' coverage increased following enactment of the ACA, the impact on their health status and the care they received was limited (Kotogal et al., 2014), although their use of emergency departments for care does appear to have decreased (Hernandez-Boussard et al., 2014).

State-Level Efforts to Improve Young Adults' Health Care Coverage

Prior to passage of the ACA, laws extending dependent coverage for young adults were passed in 37 states (Collins and Nicholson, 2010). These laws vary considerably in scope. For example, the age of dependency ranges from 23 in Oregon and Wyoming to 31 in New Jersey (Collins and Nicholson, 2010). Dependency criteria also vary by student, financial, and marital status, with some laws covering only young adults who are full-time students, financially dependent, living in the same state as their parents, or unmarried (Collins and Nicholson, 2010). In addition, under an option included in a 1999 federal law, 33 states took action to extend Medicaid coverage from age 18 to age 21 for youth exiting foster care (English et al., 2006; Lehmann et al., 2012).

The Patient Protection and Affordable Care Act

The ACA includes four principal pathways for increasing health insurance coverage for young adults—one specific to this age group (coverage under their parents' employer-sponsored health plans) and the others shared with other age groups (health insurance for college students, Medicaid expansion, and insurance exchanges).

Providing for continued coverage for young adults is the intent of the ACA requirement that employer plans providing coverage for dependent children extend that coverage to young adults up to the age of 26. This employer mandate has had a notable impact on retention of young adults already covered by parental plans as well as new enrollment. The Health Insurance Tracking Survey of Young Adults found in 2013 that 19- to 25-year-olds on parental employer plans increased from 13.7 million to 15 million between November 2011 and March 2013, and that 7.8 million of these young adults who joined a parent's plan would not have been eligible for coverage in the absence of the employer mandate (Collins et al., 2013). The survey also found notable increases (from 17 percent to 26 percent in 2013) among lower-income young adults, although this demographic group also is less likely to have parents with employer-sponsored health insurance (Collins et al., 2013).

The ACA addresses the high degree of variation in coverage and oversight of student health insurance by making these plans subject to the same protections as health insurance exchange plans. The act does not, however, require guaranteed availability and guaranteed renewal because of the unique transient status of students (CMS, 2014b). As many as 3 million students may be covered under student health insurance plans at institutions of higher learning (CMS, 2014f).

Medicaid expansion and health insurance exchanges under the ACA are the major pathways for increasing coverage among lower-income young adults. Adults with incomes up to 133 percent of the federal poverty level (FPL) ($15,521 for an individual, $31,721 for a family of four for 2014) are now eligible for Medicaid or for coverage in new health insurance exchanges, with graded subsidies for incomes between 100 percent of the FPL ($11,670 for an individual, $23,850 for a family of four) and 400 percent of the FPL ($46,680 for an individual, $95,400 for a family of four) (FamiliesUSA, 2014). In 2013, 15.7 million 19- to 29-year-olds were uninsured for at least part of the prior year, and of these individuals, 82 percent had household incomes qualifying either for Medicaid under the ACA expansion or subsidized coverage in insurance exchanges (Collins et al., 2013). By the end of the first full ACA enrollment period in April 2014, there were 2.2 million young adults (aged 18-34) among the 8 million total enrollees in state-based or federally facilitated insurance exchanges (ASPE, 2014). Medicaid expansion in 27 states and the District of Columbia will increase the number of eligible insured young adults (KFF, 2014a).

Despite increases in young adult coverage under the ACA, young adult enrollment has been modest compared with the total estimated number of uninsured young adults. Moreover, it remains uncertain how many of the young adults newly enrolled in the exchanges will actually pay premiums to acquire, use, and sustain their coverage. Lack of awareness and knowledge of eligibility for subsidized insurance and concerns about affordability among young adults have been cited as major reasons for the slow uptake in this age group (Collins et al., 2013).

In addition, as of this writing, 21 states are not moving forward with Medicaid expansion, and 2 are in open debate on the issue (KFF, 2014a). An estimated 4.8 million adults who are uninsured, poor, and nonelderly could fall into the coverage gap in the states not expanding Medicaid, but it is not known how many of these individuals are young adults (KFF, 2014b). This failure to participate in Medicaid expansion will adversely impact the ability of lower-income young adults, particularly those of color, to obtain health insurance. These states provide much less Medicaid coverage than states adopting Medicaid expansion; for example, parents in a family of three have median eligibility limits of 46 percent and 138 percent of the FPL, respectively (KFF, 2014b). Nearly half of all nonelderly adults with family incomes below 138 percent of the FPL live in these states (KFF, 2014b).

Insurance exchanges at the state and federal levels are required to offer a range of health plans that provide specific levels of coverage defined by the proportion of eligible expenses the plan will pay (actuarial value). These proportions range from 60 percent to 90 percent of eligible expenses—bronze, silver, gold, or platinum—with premiums rising accordingly. Premiums also are higher if the individual is a smoker, enrolls a family, or is over age 24 (GPO, 2013). Coverage of prevention services is mandatory (GPO, 2013), as is coverage for mental health, maternity, and newborn care and prescription medications—all especially relevant to young adults. Coverage of dental care is not required for adults, but may be offered as part of a health plan or as an independent policy. It has been estimated that the ACA could reduce dental uninsurance in all adults by approximately 5 percent, compared with about 55 percent in children younger than 19, for whom dental care is an essential health benefit (ADA, 2013).

Concern about affordability as an enrollment barrier for young adults, who generally are more financially constrained, healthier, and less likely to utilize health care services compared with older adults, prompted the addition of a fifth health plan category under the ACA. This "catastrophic coverage" entails low premiums, but very high deductibles that translate to little coverage until considerable out-of-pocket expenses have been incurred (CMS, 2014c). In the state of Connecticut, for example, a single young adult aged 27 earning $32,000 per year could purchase a catastrophic plan at $115.10 per month net of an ACA premium tax credit of $60.20 per month, and receive free preventive services and three free primary care visits. However, this plan requires that $6,350 of out-of-pocket expenses be incurred before any additional coverage is provided.[9] "Catastrophic plans" were not a major contributor to increased young adult enrollment during the first enrollment period, with only 5 percent of 18- to 34-year-old young adult enrollees in federally facilitated exchanges selecting such a plan (ASPE, 2014).

Approximately 67 percent of young adult workers (aged 19-29) are enrolled in health insurance as a result of employer health benefits (Collins et al., 2013). Enrollment rates are higher among those aged 26-29 (79 percent) than those aged 19-25 (52 percent) (Collins et al., 2013). This differential may reflect the finding that up to half of 19- to 25-year-olds not enrolling in their employer plan are receiving coverage under their parental (34 percent) or spousal (19 percent) plan, while others may not be working enough hours to be eligible for employer benefits. Of those not enrolled in employer, parental, or spousal plans, most report unaffordability (22 percent) rather than lack of need (5 percent) as the principal reason for nonenrollment (Collins et al., 2013).

[9] Calculation performed on access health CT, the Connecticut health insurance exchange, using these parameters during the first ACA enrollment cycle for 2014 coverage.

Young Adults Who Have Difficulty Accessing or Maintaining Care

As noted above, certain groups of young adults—including those exiting the foster care system, those involved in the justice system, those with mental illness, and unauthorized immigrants—face particular difficulty accessing care. Chapter 8 provides a broader look at these groups and other marginalized young adults and examines programs and policies that can support their well-being.

Young Adults Exiting Foster Care

Young people in foster care have higher rates of serious health problems compared with the general population of adolescents and young adults (English et al., 2014). They are also disproportionately members of racial and ethnic minority groups (English et al., 2014). Higher rates of both physical and mental health issues are found among children and youth in foster care, including birth defects, developmental delays, emotional adjustment problems, chronic medical problems such as asthma, dental caries, and substance abuse (AAP, 2012; CMHS and CSAT, 2013; Halfon et al., 1995). And it is estimated that more than 30 percent of older adolescents in foster care have a disability or chronic illness (Rosenbach et al., 2001). A portion of their health concerns are directly related to the issues that led to their placement in foster care, such as physical or sexual abuse; other health concerns arise during placement (English et al., 2014).

In 2012, approximately 23,396 individuals left foster care by "emancipation," or "aging out" (Children's Bureau, 2013). Up until 2008, most individuals in foster care exited at 18, although the exit age was older in some states (English et al., 2014). Thus, many youth face an abrupt ending to social, educational, and health services, including Medicaid services, for which virtually all foster care children and adolescents are eligible (English et al., 2014). In 2008, the federal Fostering Connections to Success and Increasing Adoption Act (P.L. 110-351) was signed into law. This act offers federal payments for young adults aged 18 or older who meet certain requirements related to their placement and who are working toward independence through activities such as educational programs, certain programs related to obtaining employment, and employment (Children's Bureau Training and Technical Assistance Network, 2008). Many foster youth transitioning into young adulthood face a variety of problems, including poor or absent family support; problems with employment and low income; problematic living arrangements; medical, dental, and mental health issues; and lack of health care coverage. Therefore, continuation of support has been noted as crucial to successful transitions (AAP, 2012).

The ACA is expected to lead to significant changes in access to health care for these youth. Starting in 2014, the ACA requires states to provide Medicaid coverage up to the age of 26 for most individuals aging out of foster care. Still, health care coverage accessibility challenges will likely remain for the foster care population, given their need for help in the enrollment process and the need to identify appropriate providers in their community (English and Park, 2012). Barriers such as lack of transportation and low health literacy may pose challenges as well.

Young Adults Involved in the Justice System

In the United States, millions of young adults have some form of contact with the justice system, ranging from arrest without prosecution to detention or incarceration in an adult facility (as discussed in greater detail in Chapter 8). A variety of studies have documented increased health concerns, particularly mental health and substance abuse issues, for this population, as well as vast disparities in access to needed health care (English et al., 2014). Many of these young adults have long-standing preexisting physical and mental health problems. For example, approximately 65-70 percent of the adolescent juvenile justice system population has a mental health disorder, and more than 25 percent of these disorders are considered serious enough to require significant and immediate treatment (Shufelt and Cocozza, 2006). These and other health profile data do not apply only to young adults involved in the juvenile justice system; adults in the criminal justice system generally experience many of the same health problems.

Access to health care for young adults is determined by many different factors, both while they are in the justice system and afterward. These factors can include their socioeconomic circumstances, their geographic location, and the particular part of the justice system in which they are involved. Young adults involved in the justice system frequently are living in poverty or come from families with very low incomes. Prior to enactment of the ACA, many young adults were not eligible for Medicaid unless they were pregnant or disabled, and in most states the Medicaid eligibility income threshold for adults was extremely low (Heberlein et al., 2012). Moreover, Medicaid funds may not be used for services to "inmates of public institutions" (Zemel and Kaye, 2009). Health care for this population is provided at the state and local levels, and its quality varies significantly. Even among those who are living in nonsecure residential placements or on probation or parole, health insurance coverage under both Medicaid and private plans is uneven (English et al., 2014).

Future effects of the ACA on low-income young adults in the justice system will depend primarily on their state's decision about whether to expand Medicaid. As discussed above, young adults who do not qualify for Medicaid because of higher incomes may have access to health insurance through a parent's employer-based policy until they turn 26 or through the health insurance exchanges. Agencies and facilities in the justice system can play a critical role in ensuring that young adults enroll in insurance coverage for which they are eligible, particularly as they exit the system (NACo, 2012; National Conference of State Legislatures, 2014). Some states have taken steps to facilitate this coordination. For example, legislation in Nevada allows the director of the Department of Corrections to apply for determination of Medicaid eligibility on a prisoner's behalf.[10] Having health insurance in place before exiting the system is key so that follow-up health care appointments can proceed immediately thereafter. Among other benefits, this can help prevent recidivism, particularly for those with mental health and substance abuse issues (English et al., 2014).

Young Adults with Behavioral Health Disorders

Utilization of behavioral health care is lower among young adults relative to children and older adults (Hower et al., 2013; Pottick et al., 2008, 2014; Ringeisen et al., 2009). Beginning in 2014, the implementation of Medicaid expansion and insurance exchanges under the ACA, in addition to the 2008 legislation mandating parity for behavioral health care discussed above, improvements in Medicaid disenrollment rates and more continuous and integrated behavioral and physical health care can be expected for young adults. Many states are establishing administrative processes intended to simplify health care plan enrollment (KFF, 2013; Koyanagi and Alfano, 2013). Examples of these processes include using a single application for both Medicaid and exchange plans and designing exchange plans specifically for youth under age 21. In addition, states can choose to make adults without children with incomes up to 133 percent of the FPL eligible for Medicaid, with a much higher match from the federal government than for other populations, and to make those who have been uninsured for more than 6 months potentially eligible for federally subsidized, high-risk state insurance plans that provide coverage for individuals with preexisting conditions (Koyanagi and Alfano, 2013).

The potential effectiveness of these reforms for young adults with substantial behavioral health issues is unknown. For example, the application process for health care coverage can be a barrier to treatment for young adults. Studies of Massachusetts' health care reform have found that young adults enrolled in Medicaid and health care exchanges at higher rates

[10] Nevada S.B. 519. An Act relating to Medicaid; authorizing the Director of the Department of Corrections to apply on behalf of a prisoner for a determination of Medicaid eligibility; and providing other matters properly relating thereto.

(Gettens et al., 2011; Long et al., 2010), but those with behavioral health issues had lower enrollment rates (Capoccia et al., 2013).

Young adults also are much more likely than more mature adults to drop out of outpatient psychotherapy (Davis, 2013; Edlund et al., 2002). It is unclear to what extent the reasons for treatment dropout are similar and simply more prevalent in young than in older adults (e.g., insurance loss due to more frequent job change/loss), or the reasons are qualitatively different (e.g., related to peer influence in young adults but to spousal influence in mature adults). It is intriguing, however, that at least one study of a large-scale effort to tailor mental health care to the needs and characteristics of young people found much higher treatment enrollment rates in those settings than in standard adult settings (Gilmer et al., 2012).

Unauthorized Immigrants

An estimated 11-12 million unauthorized immigrants reside in the United States, representing about 17 percent (one in six) of all uninsured Americans (Gusmano, 2012; Passel et al., 2013). The age distribution of this population differs from the legal immigrant or U.S.-born population, with 18- to 39-year-old males making up 35 percent of unauthorized immigrants, compared with 18 percent of legal immigrants and 14 percent of the U.S.-born (Passel and Cohn, 2009). Overall, in 2008 unauthorized immigrants represented 4 percent of the population in the United States and 5.4 percent of the workforce (Passel and Cohn, 2009). The children of unauthorized immigrants may be unauthorized immigrants or U.S. citizens, and together they account for 6.8 percent of elementary and secondary school students (Passel and Cohn, 2009).

On average, this population has used subsidized medical care and other forms of public assistance less than legal immigrants and U.S.-born citizens (Wallace et al., 2013). Unauthorized immigrants represent approximately 13 percent of the uninsured; they remain ineligible for Medicaid and may not participate in the health exchanges or receive tax credits (KFF, 2014c). While there are important questions about whether and how this population and the communities in which they live would benefit from health insurance coverage, research suggests a positive relationship between extending coverage to all uninsured residents (regardless of legal status) and the more general health and well-being of everyone living in those communities (IOM, 2009; Pauly and Pagán, 2007).

The Obama Administration established the Deferred Action for Childhood Arrivals (DACA) program in 2012 (HHS, 2014a). Under this program, children who came to the United States without authorization before age 16 and were under age 31 as of June 15, 2012, may request relief from deportation for a period of 2 years, during which they are eligible for work authorization (HHS, 2014a). Consideration of deferred action is available for individuals who "are currently in school, have graduated or obtained a certificate of completion from high school, have obtained a general education development (GED) certificate, or are an honorably discharged veteran of the Coast Guard or Armed Forces of the United States" and have no significant criminal record (HHS, 2014a). Approximately 1.7 million individuals nationally, primarily Hispanic youth (85 percent), were eligible for the DACA program when it started (Passel and Lopez, 2012). However, DACA recipients are specifically excluded from the ACA's Medicaid expansion and health insurance exchanges (Brindis et al., 2014).

SYSTEMS ISSUES RELATED TO YOUNG ADULTS

While young adults have lower health care utilization than other age groups, this is not necessarily because they have less need for health care. In this section, we examine how several issues raised earlier can be adddressed to improve the health care system for young adults and help ensure that they enter and remain in the system to receive the care they need. Specifically, we consider the health care workforce providing care to young adults, confidentiality concerns, the need for better integration of behavioral and medical health care, and innovative approaches to care delivery that may better address young adults' needs and preferences. The section ends with proposed frameworks for young adult health care.

The Health Care Workforce

As noted earlier in the discussion of transitions, health care providers require both biomedical and psychosocial knowledge and training to provide high-quality care to young adults. Some adolescent-focused medical boards, professional associations, and researchers have started to include young adults within their population of interest, although their primary focus remains on adolescence. Yet little attention has been given to the skills and training needed by both pediatric health care professionals and systems that provide adult health care to provide high-quality care to young adults; most youth with special health care needs are still with their pediatrician at age 18 (the lower end of the age definition for young adults for this report). The limited research in this area is focused primarily on care for young adults with special health care needs.

Over the past 50 years, the need to train a health care workforce to work with adolescents has increasingly been recognized, although important gaps and inadequacies remain (see, for example, Emans et al., 2010; Fox et al., 2010; Hergenroeder et al., 2010; NRC and IOM, 2009). Postgraduate fellowship training in adolescent medicine is available for those

TABLE 7-6 Inclusion of Young Adults in Training Programs and Materials

Training Program/Materials	Incorporation of Young Adults
Child- and Adolescent-Focused Training	
Accreditation Council for Graduate Medical Education (ACGME) program requirements for graduate medical education in pediatrics	Young adults are mentioned in the program description: "Pediatrics encompasses the study and practice of physical and mental health promotion, disease prevention, diagnosis, care, and treatment of infants, children, adolescents and young adults during health and all stages of illness" (ACGME, 2012, p. 2). However, there is no educational unit on young adults as there is for adolescents.
	Within the content outline for the adolescent medicine examination, young adults are mentioned only in a highly specific context: candidates should be able to "develop a plan of transition from child-centered to adult-centered health care for young adults with cystic fibrosis" (ABP, 2010, p. 4).
ACGME program requirements for child and adolescent psychiatry	Young adults are not mentioned (ACGME, 2007).
Board certification in clinical child and adolescent psychology	Young adults are not mentioned in the examination manual (American Board of Clinical Child and Adolescent Psychology, 2013).
National Association of Social Workers, Standards for the practice of social work with adolescents	Young adults are not mentioned (NASW, 1993).

who have completed accredited residency training in pediatrics, family medicine, or internal medicine. After the fellowship, candidates take an exam to be certified with a subspecialty in adolescent medicine. Among formal training programs and materials in medicine, public health, social work, and behavioral health, there is no comparable recognition of the uniqueness of young adulthood. Similarly, for example, the National Association of Social Workers has published standards for the practice of social work with adolescents (NASW, 1993).

Some adolescent-focused professional associations and training programs have begun to incorporate a greater focus on young adults. For example, the Society for Adolescent Health and Medicine includes both

TABLE 7-6 Continued

Training Program/Materials	Incorporation of Young Adults
Adult-Focused or All-Ages Training	
ACGME program requirements for graduate medical education in family medicine, internal medicine, and obstetrics and gynecology	Young adults are not mentioned in the ACGME program requirements for these relevant adult specialties. In contrast, family medicine residents must experience caring for adolescents (ACGME, 2013). The internal medicine program uses an encompassing definition "from adolescence to old age" (ACGME, 2009, p. 1), while the obstetrics and gynecology program mentions no specific age groups (ACGME, 2008b). As noted above, for those in family and internal medicine who seek board certification in adolescent medicine, preparing adolescents with cystic fibrosis for the transition to adult care is mentioned in the examination content guide (ABP, 2010).
ACGME program requirements for graduate medical education in hospice and palliative medicine	Young adults are mentioned among the types of patients with whom residents should work (ACGME, 2008a).
Maternal and child health leadership competencies	Adolescents are highlighted as a specific group of focus, but young adults are not (MCH Leadership Competencies Workgroup, 2009).
Association of Social Work Boards licensing examination	"Young adult behavior and development" is a topic on the bachelor's examination (ASWB, 2014).
National Certification Examination for Addiction Counselors	Unlike adolescents and geriatric adults, young adults are not included as a special population in the examination manual (NCCAP, 2011).

adolescents and young adults within its vision statement (SAHM, 2014). And its *Journal of Adolescent Health* also has recently recognized the importance of young adults by changing its tagline to "Improving the Lives of Adolescents and Young Adults." As noted throughout this report, however, it is important to keep in mind that young adults have needs distinct from those of both adolescents and older adults and often are cared for by different health care providers from those who care for adolescents; therefore, the workforce training needs also are distinct. Table 7-6 provides

BOX 7-4
Kaiser Permanente Northern California's Young Adult Specialist Model

The Kaiser Permanente Group in Northern California has developed a targeted effort for young adults that includes four critical steps: (1) develop a personalized transition from pediatric to adult medicine, (2) enhance the health insurance plan's relationship with young adults, (3) develop a cadre of primary care providers trained through the plans with targeted skills and knowledge who are enthusiastic about young adult members, and (4) enable access to care and information around the clock through both virtual and physical paths (personal communication, Calvin Gordon, M.D., Kaiser Permanente Northern California). This Young Adult Specialist Model represents a unique approach to increasing both the skills of practitioners and the navigation skill of young adults.

examples of training programs and materials in medicine, public health, social work, and addiction counseling, along with information about how young adults are explicitly mentioned, if at all. It is important to note that training specific to young adults also is lacking in other areas relevant to young adults' health. For example, few adult correctional settings provide staff members with training in the mental health needs of this age group (Fagan and Zimring, 2000). Of interest as well is the Young Adult Specialist Model developed by the Kaiser Permanente Group in Northern California, described in Box 7-4.

Resources and training materials for young adult health care are limited. Various curriculums and training materials are available that address adolescents and young adults together (EuTEACH, 2014; Neinstein, 2014; Partnership for Male Youth, 2014). However, reflecting the availability of material, the majority of videos, case studies, and cited references focus more on adolescents than on young adults. The National Adolescent and Young Adult Health Information Center has collected clinical preventive screening guidelines for young adults aged 18-26, extracting recommendations from the USPSTF, Bright Futures, and ACOG (NAHIC, 2014).

Confidentiality Concerns

While much has been written about the need for confidential care among adolescents, less attention has been paid to that need among young adults, even though they similarly seek and use sensitive services, such as those related to sexual health, substance use, and mental health. Research has documented that adolescents will forego medical care if confidentiality is not ensured (NRC and IOM, 2009); serious consequences, such as unprotected sex, unintended pregnancy, untreated STIs, and mental health issues, can result (Ford et al., 2004; Lehrer et al., 2007; Slive and Cramer, 2012). This is particularly true for those adolescents most at risk. As more young adults are insured through the ACA, many more are expected to seek and receive services that entail senstive issues (Tebb et al., 2014), such as discussion of sexual behavior and provision of contraception; screening and treatment for STIs; and screening, counseling, and treatment related to mental health or substance use disorders.

At the same time, a number of important changes are occurring in how patient health care data are collected, stored, accessed, and shared. While these changes hold promise for improving care and keeping consumers better informed, they may result in breaches of confidentiality for both adolescents and young adults covered through their parents' plans (Tebb et al., 2014). The general rule of the Health Insurance Portability and Accountability Act (HIPAA) is that individually identifiable health information cannot be released by a health care provider or insurer without written authorization if the patient is 18 or older. Yet a number of exceptions allow or require a provider or insurer to release individually identifiable health information without written authorization, giving insurance companies the discretion to share otherwise protected information with an insurance holder if the disclosure is for billing and payment purposes. Thus even though a parent/insurance holder does not have a right to demand full access to protected information, the insurer can provide that individual with information related to billing and payment (termed Explanation of Benefits [EOB]). The objective is to reduce insurance fraud and abuse by informing policy holders of insurance claims made and actions taken on their account by anyone covered under their policy (including dependents) (Tebb et al., 2014). There is no legal mandate to send this information; however, claims reflecting services received in a doctor's office that are denied because they may not be part of the insurance benefits package need to be reported to the policy holder (Tebb et al., 2014). Thus, there is inherent tension between the importance of confidentiality and the need for policy holders to be informed about the costs of health care services and benefits under their health plan. This issue is less of a problem for individuals enrolled in Medicaid, because most state Medicaid programs do not send EOB information at all or withhold it for sensitive services (although policy holders must be notified when claims are denied) (Tebb et al., 2014).

The HIPAA regulations do give individuals the right to request that their insurers send such communications by alternative means or to an alternative location rather than by mail to the home address. However, insurers need accept such a request only if it "clearly states" that disclosing the information involved might "endanger the individual." Confidential conversations with several insurance companies suggest they receive very few such requests each year (Gudeman, 2013).

Creative solutions to this issue are emerging. In Massachusetts, New York, and Wisconsin, for example, plans are not required to send an EOB when no additional payment is required for services (Tebb et al., 2014). This might happen if an adolescent or young adult receiving services paid the co-pay or if a service were one of the preventive services for which co-pays cannot be imposed under the ACA. Some health care systems also are designing systems to protect confidentiality in multiple areas, such as the making of appointments, lab and pharmacy procedures, and electronic medical records and billing. The state of California passed the Confidential Health Information Act (SB138), scheduled to take effect in January 2015, which will enable patients to request that EOB information be sent to the beneficiary (in this case, the young adult) rather than the policy holder (Gudeman, 2013; Tebb et al., 2014).

Confidentiality issues will be different for young adults with intellectual disabilities, for whom guardianship and decision-making support may be appropriate. The Got Transition initiative has developed an overview of options for guardianship and alternative options for decision-making support (Center for Health Care Transition Improvement, 2012). In addition, special concerns have been raised regarding situations in which parents or other family members are serving caregiving roles for young adults with mental illness, leading to efforts to allow providers to make disclosures when necessary to prevent clinical deterioration or harm to the patient or others.[11]

Better Integration of Behavioral and Medical Health Care

Emphasis is increasing on integrating the medical and behavioral health care systems. The ACA endorses collocated, collaborative care.

There is no one model of integrated care. Rather, there are three basic dimensions that vary in different models: collocation, integration, and collaboration (Blount, 2003; Perrin and Sheldrick, 2012). Collocation refers to physicians and mental health clinicians sharing space and having at least somewhat overlapping hours. Integrated practice includes sharing medical records; going to the same meetings; sharing office staff for scheduling and billing; sharing medical charts, referrals, and scheduling; and the like. Collaborative practices incorporate more purposeful strategies for ensuring coordinated care, including shared decision making across practices, shared

---

[11] For example, Rhode Island Code § 40.1-5-27.1.

care of the same patients, and a single plan of treatment that incorporates both physical and behavioral health. Collocation is not required for integration and collaboration to occur. Integrated care can emphasize physical health care while linking patients to behavioral health care, or emphasize behavioral health care while linking patients to physical health care.

Given the health profile of young adults as described in Chapter 2, integrated behavioral and physical health care would be particularly beneficial to this age group. Having easy access to behavioral health services through primary care settings could increase early use of such services (i.e., before symptoms worsen) among a population in which, as discussed above, utilization of these services is low relative to other age groups. Moreover, one study found that about half of individuals with common behavioral health conditions were seen exclusively in primary care settings (Regier et al., 1993). Thus, better integration of services also could improve general medical practitioners' treatment of common behavioral health conditions. And because going to a primary care setting is less stigmatizing than going to a behavioral health clinic (Bower, 2002; Bower et al., 2001; Kramer and Garralda, 2000), a primary care clinic with integrated behavioral health services could decrease dropping out of behavioral health treatment among young adults. Thus, access to primary care that offers prevention or early intervention for behavioral health problems could help reduce early mortality in young adults and prevent future conditions.

However, no studies have examined access to care or care outcomes for integrated care in young adults. In general, evidence indicates that collaborative care models based in primary care targeting depressive and anxiety disorders are more effective than usual care in reducing symptoms in adults (Archer et al., 2012). These models have demonstrated improved employment rates, functioning, and quality of life, as well as cost-effectiveness (Schoenbaum et al., 2001, 2002, 2004; Simon et al., 2001, 2002). Far less research has been conducted on other mental health disorders. Evidence on the benefit of connecting individuals receiving behavioral health care to physical health care interventions also is less clearly established, although randomized controlled trials have found some benefit (van Hasselt et al., 2013). Thus, while integrated care holds promise for better behavioral health care delivery and early intervention with physical health conditions that contribute to early mortality, research is needed to test this promise.

Innovative Approaches to Care Delivery

There is burgeoning interest in how to get young adults to come "in the door" and then stay engaged in the system. Unfortunately, little research has examined how young adults prefer to access and interact with the health system, limiting health care systems' ability to improve the system design for young adults. As noted above, for example, young adults receive care in emergency departments at higher rates than those immediately younger and older than them. However, it is unclear whether this is related to payment issues, a lack of knowledge about how to access care in other settings, or certain features of the emergency department that make it a more attractive place for young adults to seek care. Further research could investigate which features of emergency departments and/or urgent care are appealing to young adults so that these features could be incorporated into other care settings.

> "Having a representative for health care organizations who is also a young adult would be a good way to engage other young adults. This person could go where other young adults are, promote health care, and get them to take an interest in their own health."

One potential idea is to provide care to young parents and their children together. This could be accomplished through programs that focus explicitly on two generations together (see Glied and Oellerich, 2014). Or, for example, when young adult parents take their children in for preventive/well-child visits, there could be an opportunity to provide them with information on adult preventive/wellness services that may apply to them. In the U.S. health care system, however, structural barriers impede the development of such two-generation approaches to health. Glied and Oellerich (2014) identify as the primary barrier that most physicians specialize in treating children or adults and are not used to providing care to a whole family. Other barriers include financing constraints related to health insurance, access to care, and benefits.

Below we briefly describe research on technology-based and peer-led approaches to health care for young adults.

Harnessing Technology for Young Adult Health Care

The emerging field of "mHealth" focuses on innovative approaches to using social media and mobile technology for public health and health care delivery (see, for example, the annual mHealth Summit [2014], the mHealth Alliance [2014], the U.S. Department of Health and Human Services' [HHS's] mHealth initiatives [HHS, 2014b], and Jones et al. [2014]). While there is little evidence on the question of whether these approaches are effective generally, let alone for young adults, they appear to hold promise for this population, who, as discussed earlier in this report, are heavy users of these media. Therefore, further research in this area is warranted.

The limited research on harnessing technology to enhance the care provided to young adults suggests that caution and careful design are needed. Although young adults are heavy users of social and mobile media and the Internet, including to search for and receive health-related information, research suggests that they generally prefer face-to-face interaction with health care providers over interaction via telephone, webcam, email, or text message (Garrett et al., 2011; Labacher and Mitchell, 2013; Lindstrom Johnson et al., 2012). To explain this preference, young adults cite confidentiality concerns, and in one study, many participants said they thought they would receive more individualized and credible information during face-to-face interaction (Lindstrom Johnson et al., 2012). Young adults' preferences are not homogenous: Cunningham and colleagues (2014) examined young adults' preferences for how to receive information about anxiety and depression and found that they fell into three groups, one of which preferred working independently on the Internet to obtain this information.

> "Having social media apps for health would be appealing to young people, yet there is definitely a concern about privacy. If I lose my phone and someone sees that I ate five ice cream sandwiches today, I don't really care. But if I lose my phone and someone can see that I am taking an antibiotic for an STI or something, that is really embarrassing."

It is important to recognize that the research described in the preceding paragraph has limitations with respect to determining the preferences of young adults in the United States. First, most of this research focuses on young adults with chronic health conditions, and their preferences and needs may not be applicable to all young adults. Second, there is little research to enable the exploration of commonalities and differences across subgroups of young adults. Third, some of the research in this area comes from Canada, European countries, and Australia, and cross-cultural differences may be relevant. In addition, the care delivery system in these countries is very different from that in the United States.

Research is needed in this area to address several key questions. First, would enhancing confidentiality/security policies and assurances increase young adults' preferences for using technology for health care purposes? Second, would technology be particularly helpful for young adults who would otherwise lack access to services, such as those who are geographically remote from providers or otherwise unable to access care? Third, would offering technology approaches as an option work well for certain subgroups of young adults? Fourth, how can technology be integrated to supplement face-to-face interactions?

The Quantified Self

A growing body of research on preventive health care, self-diagnosis, self-monitoring of health-related behaviors, and health awareness examines how technology can be used to track, store, and analyze data on an individual's daily behaviors (Fox and Duggan, 2013). This research and the technologies that support it can be loosely summarized by the term "the quantified self." This form of self-tracking is enhanced by wearable devices and by networked platforms that facilitate the collection and sharing of data, and is also referred to as "lifestreaming," "lifelogging," "lifehacking," "self-quantifying," or "personal informatics" (Marwick, 2013). The idea is to monitor one's behaviors so as to improve both behavioral and physical health.

The sociotechnical environments and devices that support the quantified self may be described as "human augmentics." The term describes technologies that are designed to assist sensory, cognitive, and physical systems in evolving beyond their limits (Kenyon and Leigh, 2011). Human augmentics include devices that connect and sustain the human augmentics ecosystem, such as displays, robots, sensors (wearable and not), and a variety of cognitive amplifiers (Kenyon and Leigh, 2011). They also include compensatory devices for both healthy and disabled populations, such as a variety of prostheses and brain-machine interfaces. At this time, however, there are no studies indicating whether young adults as a group are relying on such technology and how and under what circumstances they are using such devices and with what outcomes.

Peer-Led Approaches

Given the vital role of peer influence in the lives of young adults, peer-led approaches to health care are intuitively appealing. Although such approaches are offered with increasing frequency, however, research is limited on their efficacy among adults in general, and even more so among young adults. In a systematic review, Lloyd-Evans and colleagues (2014) found that the existing body of research on peer-led approaches among adults with severe mental health conditions is weak, with inconsistencies in both methods and reporting. Peer-led approaches appear to be as effective as, but no better than, usual behavioral health services provided to adults (Lloyd-Evans et al., 2014).

Another evidence-based health care approach that utilizes peer support is the chronic disease self-management model for adults (Lorig et al., 2009).

This model has been extended to address the health status of adults with serious mental illness, with promising results (Druss et al., 2010).

In the past, a lack of funding has served as a barrier to offering peer-led health services. However, many states now reimburse peer specialists under Medicaid (Kaufman et al., 2012). Because of the importance of peer influence among young adults, developing and rigorously testing well-specified peer-led interventions is an important area for future research.

Characteristics of High-Quality Health Care for Young Adults

In Box 7-5, we draw on two frameworks developed by the World Health Organization (WHO, 2001, 2009) and the IOM (2001) to identify the characteristics of high-quality care for young adults. The WHO framework, originally developed for adolescent-friendly services, is adapted here to the needs of young adults. Of course, the health care system could be improved for all adults. Nevertheless, focusing on improving the system for young adults is important because their access to and utilization of the health care system will be carried forward throughout their lives.

CONCLUSIONS AND RECOMMENDATIONS

From among the many topics discussed in this chapter, the committee selected three areas in which action would make a particular difference for young adults: improving the transition process from pediatric to adult health care, improving preventive care, and developing evidence-based practices. Health insurance coverage for young adults also is very important but, as the discussion above makes clear, extensive action is already occurring in this area. Improving behavioral and medical health care for young adults would improve their health, safety, and well-being, as well as their educational and employment outcomes. Young adults with chronic health conditions, including mental health and substance use disorders, often have lower educational attainment and less successful employment experiences and outcomes, as described in Chapter 4.

Improving the Transition Process

The transition from pediatric to adult health care—including both medical and behavioral health care—is associated with poor outcomes for young adults. Structural barriers, such as funding streams and eligibility requirements, as well as age limits set by health systems, impose artificial boundaries between the two systems. These barriers negatively impact the transition process by creating discontinuities in care and associated poor outcomes. Other challenges arise because of adult health care providers'

BOX 7-5
Characteristics of Two Frameworks for Delivering Health Care Services

Two general frameworks for delivering health care services may be applied to young adults' health care as follows:

Framework for Delivering Young Adult-Friendly Health Services (WHO, 2001, 2009)

- *Accessible*—Policies and procedures ensure that services are broadly accessible for young adults.
- *Acceptable*—Policies and procedures consider culture and relationships and the climate of engagement for young adults.
- *Appropriate*—Health services fulfill the needs of all young adults.
- *Effective*—Health services reflect evidence-based standards of care and professional guidelines.
- *Equitable*—Policies and procedures enable the provision of and eligibility for services for all young adults.

Institute of Medicine Framework for Delivering Quality Health Care Services (IOM, 2001)

- *Safe*—Protocols are in place to reduce medical errors and foster quality assurance.
- *Effective*—Services reflect accepted standards of clinical care.
- *Patient-centered*—Services are sensitive to the needs and preferences of the patient.
- *Timely*—Waiting times between assessment and treatment are reduced.
- *Equitable*—Services do not reflect disparities within the young adult population.
- *Incorporating consumer perspectives*—Services reflect young adults' perspectives on their health care needs (stay healthy, get better, live with illness or disability, or cope with the end of life).
- *Efficient*—Services are designed to reduce unnecessary time and costs.

lack of familiarity with disease processes and developmental issues among young adults.

Transitions of care have long been identified as an important problem in health care, as described in the IOM report *To Err Is Human: Building a Safer Health System* (IOM, 2000). As reported more recently,

> An expanding evidence base demonstrates that serious quality problems exist for patients undergoing transitions across sites of care. Qualitative

> studies performed in the United States as well as Canada, Europe, and Australia, have produced remarkably consistent results. These studies have shown that patients are often unprepared for their self-management role in the next care setting, receive conflicting advice regarding chronic illness management, are often unable to reach an appropriate health care practitioner who has access to their care plan when questions arise, have minimal input into their care plan, and are annoyed by having to repeatedly provide the same information to each new set of practitioners. Family caregivers voice feelings of frustration that they are often excluded from care planning meetings, despite their central role in the execution of this care plan. They are also dissatisfied with having to perform tasks that their health care practitioners have left undone. (Coleman, 2006, p. 254)

The ACA includes several provisions that impose penalties for poorly managed care transitions and offer financial incentives for improving transition care (Burton, 2012). Examples of these provisions include reduced payments for readmission rates that exceed particular targets and payment for transition care services in medical homes. State Medicaid agencies also can provide reimbursement for transition care that occurs in "health home" practices, which provide physical, behavioral, and long-term care services.

This recent movement has an associated focus on developing measures for and improving care transitions/handoffs. The transition to adult care is included in the National Committee for Quality Assurance's (NCQA's) 2014 Standards and Guidelines for NCQA's Patient-Centered Medical Home (NCQA, 2014). Transition of care for youth with special health care needs also is included as a *Healthy People 2020* indicator (HHS, 2014c). With these exceptions, however, the focus on measuring transitions generally has not included the transition between pediatric and adult systems. For example, the following transitions are considered by the National Transitions of Care Coalition Measures Working Group:

- "Within settings; e.g., primary care to specialty care, or intensive care unit (ICU) to ward.
- Between settings; e.g., hospital to sub-acute care, or ambulatory clinic to senior center.
- Across health states; e.g., curative care to palliative care or hospice, or personal residence to assisted living.
- Between providers; e.g., generalist to a specialist practitioner, or acute care provider to a palliative care specialist." (NTOCC, 2008, p. 1)

Rather than developing a separate approach for improving the transition to adult health care, we propose drawing attention to this transition and incorporating it in the current movement to improve transitions generally. Thus we propose that health care delivery systems develop a process for the transition from pediatric to adult care. The recommendations developed by AAP, AAFP, and ACP (AAP et al., 2011; see also Box 7-3) and the six core elements developed by the Got Transition initiative provide an appropriate guide for the develoment of this process, although additional research and evaluation are needed to support these recommendations. We also propose that health care delivery systems include metrics on this transition among their quality performance metrics. Since metrics for this transition do not yet exist, we suggest that AHRQ develop them.

Recommendation 7-1: Health care delivery systems and provider organizations serving young adults (e.g., medical homes, accountable care organizations)—with input from the Agency for Healthcare Research and Quality (AHRQ) and the Centers for Medicare & Medicaid Services (CMS)—should improve the transition process for young adults moving from pediatric to adult medical and behavioral health care.

To implement this recommendation, the committee recommends the following specific actions:

- AHRQ should develop quality performance metrics on the transition-of-care process to ensure continuity of care for young adults making this transition.
- CMS should encourage greater attention to this transition within the innovation models that it solicits and funds, such as those from the Center for Medicare & Medicaid Innovation.
- Health care delivery systems and provider organizations serving young adults should develop a coordinated pediatric-to-adult transition-of-care process within their organizations.
- Pediatric-to-adult transition-of-care performance metrics should be incorporated into quality measurement and reporting frameworks by the National Committee for Quality Assurance, the National Quality Forum, and other quality measurement entities for all health care delivery models serving young adults, such as medical homes, accountable care organizations, and integrated delivery systems.
- The Office of the National Coordinator for Health Information Technology should ensure that meaningful use criteria enable the capture of relevant data elements for this reporting.
- CMS, health insurers, and purchasing entities such as employer coalitions should incorporate young adult transition-of-care met-

rics into pay-for-performance initiatives, contracting, and other provider assessments.
- The Maternal and Child Health Bureau in the HRSA should expand its work on transition-of-care metrics for youth with special health care needs to include all youth and young adults, incorporate such metrics in Title V program requirements, and support related capacity development and training in states.

Careful design of these metrics is important so as not to generate perverse incentives for health systems to exclude young adults with special health care needs. Comprehensive coordinated health care delivery systems should give substantial weight to performance metrics for such patients to help ensure that they meet performance requirements by applying better practices to populations similar to those they have served in the past rather than by excluding more unhealthy patients.

The transition from pediatric to adult health care is a lengthier process than some of the other health care transition processes, such as transfers from primary to intensive care. When done well, the transition to adult health care begins several years prior to the actual transfer time and includes patient education and engagement. However, many of the issues related to discontinuities for this transition are analogous to those entailed in other types of transitions. Placing greater emphasis on this transition by including it in transition metrics is likely to have benefits for other aspects of the transition process from pediatric to adult care as well.

Improving Preventive Care for Young Adults

As described in Chapters 2 and 6, young adults are less healthy than commonly perceived, the majority of the health problems they face are preventable, and the health habits developed during these years have lifelong implications. Knowledge about the use and delivery of preventive services for young adults is limited, but the available evidence suggests that young adults receive little preventive care. As discussed earlier, for example, during visits with physicians, including primary care and obstetrics-gynecology providers, most young adults receive no preventive counseling on such critical issues for this age group as injury, smoking, exercise, weight reduction, mental health, and STIs/HIV. Various sets of recommendations (e.g., from USPSTF, ACOG, and Bright Futures) can inform the care of young adults aged 18-26, but there is no consolidated set of guidelines for preventive medical, behavioral, and oral health care specifically focused on the young adult population. Furthermore, the efficacy of these guidelines for young adults is unclear because the age ranges are broad, and young adults are grouped with adults overall. Because young adults' burden of disease is different from that of older adults and because other issues, such as fertility, may be of greater concern for this age group, it is important to have evidence-based recommendations assessed specifically for efficacy with young adults.

In addition to recommendations for adults in general, USPSTF provides a special focus on children and adolescents and older adults (USPSTF, 2011, 2013), and convenes workgroups and makes evidence-based recommendations specifically for these populations. USPSTF is the preferred body to develop a consolidated package of evidence-based recommendations for young adults because its existing model could be extended to provide a special focus on the health problems that most affect young adults.

Recommendation 7-2: The U.S. Preventive Services Task Force should develop a consolidated set of standardized evidence-based recommendations for clinical preventive services such as screenings, counseling services, and preventive medications specifically for young adults aged 18-26. Behavioral and oral health should be included in these recommendations.

Once these recommendations have been developed, they will need to be implemented. Federal, state, and local governmental entities that fund or provide physical or behavioral health services—including the U.S. Department of Defense, HHS (through AHRQ, CMS, HRSA, the Indian Health Service, and SAMHSA), the U.S. Department of Veterans Affairs, and corresponding state and local agencies—in partnership with commercial insurers and employer-sponsored health plans, should be involved in improving preventive care for young adults, including increased access to care and content of care that emphasizes preventive visits as part of an array of integrated, comprehensive services.

Recommendation 7-3: Federal, state, and local governments, commercial insurers, employer-sponsored health plans, and medical and behavioral health systems should adopt the clinical preventive services recommended by the U.S. Preventive Services Task Force, include the delivery of those services in quality performance metrics used for pay-for-performance and other health care provider assessments, and require public reporting of compliance.

To improve preventive care for young adults, it will be critically important to drive provider interest in engaging young adults in receiving preventive care, as well as monitor the delivery of these services. Given the broad variety of entities—both governmental and private—involved in providing preventive care to young adults, we do not recommend specific approaches to driving provider interest and ensuring appropriate monitoring. Rather, we focus on outcomes that should be measured and leave it to organizations to develop their own processes and implementation approaches.

Developing Evidence-Based Practices for Young Adults

Most prevention approaches are targeted at children and adolescents, and some are targeted at college students. With the exception of interventions for treating early psychosis, there are few behavioral health interventions developed specifically for young adults, all of which are in early stages of development, and few interventions with demonstrated efficacy specifically in this age group. Although pharmacological treatments should be as effective in young adults as in older adults, psychosocial treatments and interventions need to be explicitly tested in this age group. Because of the psychosocial nature of nonpharmacological interventions, including preventive interventions, psychotherapy, and other related approaches, such interventions can be influenced by many of the factors that are changing or less mature in young compared with older adults, such as responsibility taking, response to authoritative figures, changing roles within the family, and responses to behavioral contingencies.

Recommendation 7-4: The National Institutes of Health should support research aimed at developing a set of evidence-based practices for medical and behavioral health care, including prevention, for young adults. This research should build on the existing and established evidence-based practices (EBPs) for populations that are older (i.e., adults in general) or younger (i.e., adolescents) to

- **identify those EBPs that hold promise for being effective in this age group and test them for efficacy;**
- **identify EBPs that are likely to be effective with modification for this age group and test the efficacy of the modified versions; and**
- **identify behavioral and medical health care needs that are unlikely to be addressed by existing or modified EBPs and conduct research to develop and establish new EBPs for young adults in these areas.**

In developing methodologies for implementing this recommendation, it will be important to take into account socioeconomic position and racial, ethnic, and geographic disparities and differences, as well as differences according to immigrant and refugee status, across the full spectrum of the social, behavioral, and health indicators under discussion.

Research Priorities

As described throughout this chapter, further research is needed to help improve medical and behavioral health care for young adults. We identified four research needs of particular importance:

- Develop preventive care guidelines for young adults (see Recommendation 7-2).
- Develop a set of evidence-based practices for young adults for medical and behavioral health care encompassing prevention and effective processes for the transition from pediatric to adult care (see Recommendations 7-1, 7-2, 7-3, and 7-4).
- Examine the efficacy of integrating behavioral and physical health care for improving health outcomes for young adults.
- Develop a comprehensive behavioral health screen. (Note that other efforts also are needed to ensure that treatment can be offered if concerns are identified during screening.)

REFERENCES

AAFP (American Academy of Family Physicians), AAP (American Academy of Pediatrics), ACP (American College of Physicians), and AOA (American Osteopathic Association). 2007. *Joint principles of the patient-centered medical home.* http://www.pcpcc.net/content/joint-principles-patient-centered-medical-home (accessed September 11, 2014).

AAP. 1996. Transition of care provided for adolescents with special health care needs. *Pediatrics* 98:1203-1206.

AAP. 2012. Health care of youth aging out of foster care. *Pediatrics* 130(6):1170-1173.

AAP, AAFP, and ACP. 2002. A consensus statement on health care transitions for young adults with special health care needs. *Pediatrics* 110(Suppl. 3):1304-1306.

AAP, AAFP, and ACP. 2011. Supporting the health care transition from adolescence to adulthood in the medical home. *Pediatrics* 128(1):182-200.

AAPD (American Academy of Pediatric Dentistry). 2013. Guideline on periodicity of examination, preventive dental services, anticipatory guidance/counseling, and oral treatment for infants, children, and adolescents. *Clinical Guidelines* 35(6):114-122.

Abbott, R. A., R. Whear, L. R. Rodgers, A. Bethel, J. Thompson Coon, W. Kuyken, K. Stein, and C. Dickens. 2014. Effectiveness of mindfulness-based stress reduction and mindfulness based cognitive therapy in vascular disease: A systematic review and meta-analysis of randomised controlled trials. *Journal of Psychosomatic Research* 76(5):341-351.

ABP (American Board of Pediatrics). 2010. *Content outline: Adolescent medicine subspecialty in-training, certification, and maintenance of certification examinations.* https://www.abp.org/abpwebsite/takeexam/subspecialtycertifyingexam/contentpdfs/adol2010.pdf (accessed March 28, 2014).

ACGME (Accreditation Council for Graduate Medical Education). 2007. *ACGME program requirements for graduate medical education in child and adolescent psychiatry.* https://www.acgme.org/acgmeweb/Portals/0/PFAssets/ProgramRequirements/405_child_and_adolescent_psych_07012014.pdf (accessed July 25, 2014).

ACGME. 2008a. *ACGME program requirements for graduate medical education in hospice and palliative medicine.* http://www.acgme.org/acgmeweb/Portals/0/PFAssets/ProgramRequirements/540_hospice_and_palliative_medicine_02122008.pdf (accessed March 28, 2014).

ACGME. 2008b. *ACGME program requirements for graduate medical education in obstetrics and gynecology.* https://www.acgme.org/acgmeweb/Portals/0/PFAssets/ProgramRequirements/220_obstetrics_and_gynecology_07012014.pdf (accessed July 25, 2014).

ACGME. 2009. *ACGME program requirements for graduate medical education in internal medicine.* https://www.acgme.org/acgmeweb/Portals/0/PFAssets/2013-PR-FAQ-PIF/140_internal_medicine_07012013.pdf (accessed July 25, 2014).

ACGME. 2012. *ACGME program requirements for graduate medical education in pediatrics.* http://www.acgme.org/acgmeweb/Portals/0/PFAssets/2013-PR-FAQ-PIF/320_pediatrics_07012013.pdf (accessed March 28 2014).

ACGME. 2013. *ACGME program requirements for graduate medical education in family medicine.* https://www.acgme.org/acgmeweb/Portals/0/PFAssets/ProgramRequirements/120_family_medicine_07012014.pdf (accessed July 25, 2014).

ADA (American Dental Association). 2013. *Affordable Care Act, dental benefits examined.* http://www.ada.org/en/publications/ada-news/2013-archive/august/affordable-care-act-dental-benefits-examined (accessed July 24, 2014).

Adams, S. H., P. W. Newacheck, M. J. Park, C. D. Brindis, and C. E. Irwin, Jr. 2013. Medical home for adolescents: Low attainment rates for those with mental health problems and other vulnerable groups. *Academic Pediatrics* 13(2):113-121.

Agorastos, A., C. R. Marmar, and C. Otte. 2011. Immediate and early behavioral interventions for the prevention of acute and posttraumatic stress disorder. *Current Opinion in Psychiatry* 24(6):526-532.

AHRQ (Agency for Healthcare Research and Quality). 2014. *Medical Expenditure Panel Survey.* http://meps.ahrq.gov/mepsweb (accessed July 24, 2014).

Álvarez-Jiménez, M., A. G. Parker, S. E. Hetrick, P. D. McGorry, and J. F. Gleeson. 2011. Preventing the second episode: A systematic review and meta-analysis of psychosocial and pharmacological trials in first-episode psychosis. *Schizophrenia Bulletin* 37(3):619-630.

American Board of Clinical Child and Adolescent Psychology. 2013. *Examination manual for board certification in clinical child and adolescent psychology.* http://www.abpp.org/files/page-specific/3352%20Clinical%20Child/16_Examination_Manual.pdf (accessed March 28, 2014).

Archer, J., P. Bower, S. Gilbody, K. Lovell, D. Richards, L. Gask, C. Dickens, and P. Coventry. 2012. *Collaborative care for people with depression and anxiety.* http://summaries.cochrane.org/CD006525/DEPRESSN_collaborative-care-for-people-with-depression-and-anxiety (accessed July 24, 2014).

Armstrong, E. 2012a. *NHeLP breaks down preventive health services standards & contraceptive coverage under the ACA.* Washington, DC: National Health Law Program.

Armstrong, E. 2012b. *Q&A on preventive services for women coverage requirements.* Washington, DC: National Health Law Program.

ASPE (Assistant Secretary for Planning and Evaluation). 2014. *Health insurance marketplace: Summary enrollment report for the initial annual open enrollment period.* Washington, DC: HHS.

ASWB (Association of Social Work Boards). 2014. *Content outlines and KSAs: Social work licensing examinations.* http://www.aswb.org/wp-content/uploads/2014/02/BachelorsKSAs.pdf (accessed July 25, 2014).

Baillargeon, J., S. Contreras, J. J. Grady, S. A. Black, and O. Murray. 2000. Compliance with antidepressant medication among prison inmates with depressive disorders. *Psychiatric Services* 51(11):1444-1446.

Beardslee, W. R., D. A. Brent, V. R. Weersing, G. N. Clarke, G. Porta, S. D. Hollon, T. R. Gladstone, R. Gallop, F. L. Lynch, and S. Iyengar. 2013. Prevention of depression in at-risk adolescents: Longer-term effects. *JAMA Psychiatry* 70(11):1161-1170.

Benson, R., D. Steidtmann, and Y. Valks. 2014. *A triple aim approach to transition from pediatric adult health care for youth with special health care needs.* http://cshcn.wpengine.netdna-cdn.com/wp-content/uploads/2014/05/A-Triple-Aim-Approach-to-Transition.pdf (accessed September 26, 2014).

Berwick D. M., T. W. Nolan, and J. Whittington. 2008. The triple aim: Care, health, and cost. *Health Affairs* 27(3):759-769.

Bleyer, A., and R. Barr. 2009. Cancer in young adults 20 to 39 years of age: Overview. *Seminars in Oncology* 36(3):194-206.

Bleyer, A., R. Barr, B. Hayes-Lattin, D. Thomas, C. Ellis, and B. Anderson. 2008. The distinctive biology of cancer in adolescents and young adults. *Nature Reviews Cancer* 8(4):288-298.

Blount, A. 2003. Integrated primary care: Organizing the evidence. *Families, Systems, & Health* 21(2):121.

Blum, A., A. Giordano, M. J. Park, S. Rosenbaum, and C. D. Brindis. in press. Implementing health reform in an era of semi-cooperative federalism: Lessons from the age 26 expansion. *Journal of Health and Biomedical Law.*

Blum, R. W., D. Garell, C. H. Hodgman, T. W. Jorissen, N. A. Okinow, D. P. Orr, and G. B. Slap. 1993. Transition from child-centered to adult health-care systems for adolescents with chronic conditions: A position paper of the Society for Adolescent Medicine. *Journal of Adolescent Health* 14(7):570-576.

Blumenthal, D., and S. R. Collins. 2014. Health care coverage under the Affordable Care Act—a progress report. *New England Journal of Medicine* 371:275-281.

Bodenlos, J. S., M. Noonan, and S. Y. Wells. 2013. Mindfulness and alcohol problems in college students: The mediating effects of stress. *Journal of American College Health* 61(6):371-378.

Boekeloo, B. O., and M. A. Griffin. 2007. Review of clinical trials testing the effectiveness of physician approaches to improving alcohol education and counseling in adolescent outpatients. *Current Pediatric Reviews* 3(1):93-101.

Boekeloo, B. O., M. P. Bobbin, W. I. Lee, K. D. Worrell, E. K. Hamburger, and E. Russek-Cohen. 2003. Effect of patient priming and primary care provider prompting on adolescent-provider communication about alcohol. *Archives of Pediatrics & Adolescent Medicine* 157(5):433-439.

Bond, G. R. 1998. Principles of the individual placement and support model: Empirical support. *Psychiatric Rehabilitation Journal* 22(1):11.

Bower, P. 2002. Primary care mental health workers: Models of working and evidence of effectiveness. *British Journal of General Practice* 52(484):926-933.

Bower, P., E. Garralda, T. Kramer, R. Harrington, and B. Sibbald. 2001. The treatment of child and adolescent mental health problems in primary care: A systematic review. *Family Practice* 18(4):373-382.

Bradley, G., B. Sparks, and D. Nesdale. 2001. Doctor communication style and patient outcomes: Gender and age as moderators. *Journal of Applied Social Psychology* 31(8): 1749-1773.

Braithwaite, S. R., and F. D. Fincham. 2007. ePREP: Computer based prevention of relationship dysfunction, depression and anxiety. *Journal of Social and Clinical Psychology* 26(5):609-622.

Brindis, C. D., M. Hadler, K. Jacobs, N. Pourat, M. Raymond-Flesch, R. Siemons, and E. Talamantes. 2014. *Realizing the dream for Californians eligible for deferred action for childhood arrivals (DACA): Health needs and access to health care.* San Francisco, CA: Philip R. Lee Institute for Health Policy Studies, University of California, San Francisco.

Brousseau, D. C., P. L. Owens, A. L. Mosso, J. A. Panepito, and C. A. Steiner. 2010. Acute care utilization and rehospitalizations for sickle cell disease. *Journal of the American Medical Association* 303:1288-1294.

Burke-Miller, J., L. A. Razzano, D. D. Grey, C. R. Blyler, and J. A. Cook. 2012. Supported employment outcomes for transition age youth and young adults. *Psychiatric Rehabilitation Journal* 35(3):171.

Burton, L. 2012. Health policy brief: Improving care transitions. *Health Affairs* September 12.

Callahan, S. T., and W. O. Cooper. 2010. Changes in ambulatory health care use during the transition to young adulthood. *Journal of Adolescent Health* 46(5):407-413.

Capoccia, V., C. Croze, M. Cohen, and J. P. O'Brien. 2013. Sustaining enrollment in health insurance for vulnerable populations: Lessons from Massachusetts. *Psychiatric Services* 64(4):360-365.

CDC (Centers for Disease Control and Prevention). 2014a. *Ambulatory health care data.* http://www.cdc.gov/nchs/ahcd.htm (accessed July 24, 2014).

CDC. 2014b. *Behavioral Risk Factor Surveillance System.* http://www.cdc.gov/brfss (accessed July 24, 2014).

CDC. 2014c. *National Health Interview Survey.* http://www.cdc.gov/nchs/nhis.htm (accessed August 7, 2014).

Center for Health Care Transition Improvement. 2012. *Guardianship and alternatives for decision-making support.* http://www.gottransition.org/resourceGet.cfm?id=17 (accessed September 25, 2014).

CFF (Cystic Fibrosis Foundation). 2012. *Patient registry annual data report 2012.* Bethesda, MD: CFF.

Chiesa, A., and A. Serretti. 2014. Are mindfulness-based interventions effective for substance use disorders? A systematic review of the evidence. *Substance Use & Misuse* 49(5):492-512.

Children's Bureau. 2013. *The AFCARS report.* Rockville, MD: HHS.

Children's Bureau Training and Technical Assistance Network. 2008. *Implementing the Fostering Connections Act: How the Children's Bureau national resource centers and implementation centers can help states and tribes.* https://www.ttaccportal.org/sites/www.ttaccportal.org/files/Implementing%20Fostering%20Connections%20Act%20Fact%20Sheet%20-%20Youth%20Transition%20D3%20ab%2011AUG08.pdf (accessed July 24, 2014).

Christensen, H., E. Pallister, S. Smale, I. B. Hickie, and A. L. Calear. 2010. Community-based prevention programs for anxiety and depression in youth: A systematic review. *Journal of Primary Prevention* 31(3):139-170.

Clarke, G. N., W. Hawkins, M. Murphy, L. B. Sheeber, P. M. Lewinsohn, and J. R. Seeley. 1995. Targeted prevention of unipolar depressive disorder in an at-risk sample of high school adolescents: A randomized trial of a group cognitive intervention. *Journal of the American Academy of Child & Adolescent Psychiatry* 34(3):312-321.

Clarke, G. N., M. Hornbrook, F. Lynch, M. Polen, J. Gale, W. Beardslee, E. O'Connor, and J. Seeley. 2001. A randomized trial of a group cognitive intervention for preventing depression in adolescent offspring of depressed parents. *Archives of General Psychiatry* 58(12):1127-1134.

Clarke, G., C. Kelleher, M. Hornbrook, L. DeBar, J. Dickerson, and C. Gullion. 2009. Randomized effectiveness trial of an Internet, pure self-help, cognitive behavioral intervention for depressive symptoms in young adults. *Cognitive Behaviour Therapy* 38(4):222-234.

CMHS (Center for Mental Health Services) and CSAT (Center for Substance Abuse Treatment). 2013. *Diagnoses and health care utilization of children who are in foster care and covered by Medicaid.* Rockville, MD: CMHS and CSAT, SAMHSA.

CMS (Center for Medicare & Medicaid Services). 2014a. *The Center for Consumer Information & Insurance Oversight: Additional information on proposed state essential health benefits benchmark plans.* http://www.cms.gov/CCIIO/Resources/Data-Resources/ehb.html (accessed August 4, 2014).

CMS. 2014b. *Student health insurance final rule.* http://www.regulations.gov/#!documentDetail;D=CMS-2011-0016-0108 (accessed July 24, 2014).

CMS. 2014c. *Catastrophic health insurance plans.* https://www.healthcare.gov/can-i-buy-a-catastrophic-plan (accessed September 27, 2014).

CMS. 2014d. *Young adults and the Affordable Care Act: Protecting young adults and eliminating burdens on families and businesses.* http://www.cms.gov/CCIIO/Resources/Files/adult_child_fact_sheet.html (accessed July 24, 2014).

CMS. 2014e. *2014 core set of health care quality measures for adults enrolled in Medicaid.* http://www.medicaid.gov/Medicaid-CHIP-Program-Information/By-Topics/Quality-of-Care/Downloads/AdultCoreMeasures.pdf (accessed July 24, 2014).

CMS. 2014f. *Student health plans.* http://www.cms.gov/CCIIO/Programs-and-Initiatives/Health-Insurance-Market-Reforms/Student-Health-Plans.html (accessed September 26, 2014).

Coleman, E. 2006. Transitional care performance measurement. Paper commissioned by the Institute of Medicine. In *Performance measurement: Accelerating improvement* (Appendix I). Washington, DC: The National Academies Press. Pp. 250-286.

Collins, S. R., and J. Nicholson. 2010. *Realizing health reform's potential: Young adults and the Affordable Care Act of 2010.* New York: The Commonwealth Fund.

Collins, S. R., R. Robertson, T. Garber, and M. M. Doty. 2012. *Young, uninsured, and in debt: Why young adults lack health insurance and how the Affordable Care Act is helping findings from The Commonwealth Fund Health Insurance Tracking Survey of Young Adults, 2011.* Washington, DC: The Commonwealth Fund.

Collins, S. R., P. Rasmussen, T. Garber, and M. M. Doty. 2013. *Covering young adults under the Affordable Care Act: The importance of outreach and Medicaid expansion.* New York: The Commonwealth Fund.

Colorado Consumer Health Initiative and ProgressNow Colorado Education. 2014. *Got insurance?* http://doyougotinsurance.com/index.php?id=2 (accessed July 24, 2014).

Copeland, W., L. Shanahan, E. J. Costello, and A. Angold. 2011. Cumulative prevalence of psychiatric disorders by young adulthood: A prospective cohort analysis from the Great Smoky Mountains Study. *Journal of the American Academy of Child and Adolescent Psychiatry* 50(3):252-261.

Copeland, W. E., L. S. Shanahan, M. Davis, B. J. Burns, A. Angold and E. J. Costello. in press. Untreated psychiatric cases increase during the transition to adulthood. *Psychiatric Services.*

Cruess, D. G., M. H. Antoni, M. Kumar, G. Ironson, P. McCabe, J. B. Fernandez, M. Fletcher, and N. Schneiderman. 1999. Cognitive-behavioral stress management buffers decreases in dehydroepiandrosterone sulfate (DHEA-S) and increases in the cortisol/DHEA-S ratio and reduces mood disturbance and perceived stress among HIV-seropositive men. *Psychoneuroendocrinology* 24(5):537-549.

Cukrowicz, K. C., and T. E. Joiner, Jr. 2007. Computer-based intervention for anxious and depressive symptoms in a non-clinical population. *Cognitive Therapy and Research* 31(5):677-693.

Cunningham, C. E., J. R. Walker, J. D. Eastwood, H. Westra, H. Rimas, Y. Chen, and M. Marcus. 2014. Modeling mental health information preferences during the early adult years: A discrete choice conjoint experiment. *Journal of Health Communication: Internatonal Perspectives* 19(4):413-440.

Cutcliffe, J. R., and B. Saadeh. 2014. Grounded in evidence or a puritanical legacy: A critique of twenty-first-century U.S. drug policy. *Mental Health and Substance Use* 7(3):195-206.

Davis, M. 2003. Addressing the needs of youth in transition to adulthood. *Administration and Policy in Mental Health and Mental Health Services Research* 30(6):495-509.

Davis, M. 2013. *Young adult mental health*. Presentation at IOM/NRC Workshop on Improving the Health, Safety, and Well-Being of Young Adults, Washington, DC. http://www.iom.edu/~/media/Files/Activity%20Files/Children/ImprovingYoungAdultsHealth/Davis%20Presentation.pdf (accessed September 27, 2014).

Davis, M., and N. Koroloff. 2006. The great divide: How public mental health policy fail young adults. *Community Based Mental Health Services for Children and Adolescents* 14:53-74.

Davis, M., J. Geller, and B. Hunt. 2006. Within-state availability of transition-to-adulthood services for youths with serious mental health conditions. *Psychiatric Services* 57(11):1594-1599.

Davis, M., M. Green, and C. Hoffman. 2009. The service system obstacle course for transition-age youth and young adults. In *Transition of youth and young adults with emotional or behavioral difficulties: An evidence-based handbook*, edited by H. B. Clark and D. Unruh. Baltimore, MD: Paul H. Brookes Publishing Company. Pp. 25-46.

Davis, M., N. Koroloff, and M. L. Ellison. 2012a. Between adolescence and adulthood: Rehabilitation research to improve services for youth and young adults. *Psychiatric Rehabilitation Journal* 35(3):167-170.

Davis, M., N. Koroloff, and M. Johnsen. 2012b. Social network analysis of child and adult interorganizational connections. *Psychiatric Rehabilitation Journal* 35(3):265-272.

Davis, M., M. Abrams, L. Wissow, and E. Slade. 2014. Imminent Medicaid enrollment lapses after inpatient mental health treatment in young adults. *Psychiatric Services* 65(4):461-468.

De Bont, J., B. Van Der Holt, and A. Dekker. 2004. Significant difference in outcome for adolescents with acute lymphoblastic leukemia treated on pediatric vs. adult protocols in the Netherlands. *Leukemia* 18(12):2032-2035.

DeBaun, M. R., and J. Telfair. 2012. Transition and sickle cell disease. *Pediatrics* 130(5): 926-935.

Delman, J. 2012. Young adults with mental illness: Their active participation in medication decisions and in research. Ph.D. dissertation, Boston University.

Drucker, E. 2012. Drugs: The third rail of U.S. politics. *Lancet* 380(9854):1626-1628.

Druss, B. G., L. Zhao, S. A. von Esenwein, J. R. Bona, L. Fricks, S. Jenkins-Tucker, E. Sterling, R. DiClemente, and K. Lorig. 2010. The Health and Recovery Peer (HARP) Program: A peer-led intervention to improve medical self-management for persons with serious mental illness. *Schizophrenia Research* 118(1):264-270.

Edlund, M. J., P. S. Wang, P. A. Berglund, S. J. Katz, E. Lin, and R. C. Kessler. 2002. Dropping out of mental health treatment: Patterns and predictors among epidemiological survey respondents in the United States and Ontario. *American Journal of Psychiatry* 159(5):845-851.

Elster, A., and N. Kuznets. 1994. *Guidelines for Adolescent Preventive Services (GAPS): Recommendations and rationale*. Baltimore, MD: American Medical Association.

Emans, S. J., S. B. Austin, E. Goodman, D. P. Orr, R. Freeman, D. Stoff, I. F. Litt, M. A. Schuster, R. Haggerty, and R. Granger. 2010. Improving adolescent and young adult health—training the next generation of physician scientists in transdisciplinary research. *Journal of Adolescent Health* 46(2):100-109.

English, A., and M. Park. 2012. *The Supreme Court ACA decision: What happens now for adolescents and young adults.* Chapel Hill, NC: Center for Adolescent Health and the Law National Adolescent and Young Adult Health Information Center.

English, A., A. Stinnett, and E. Dunn-Georgiou. 2006. *Health care for adolescents and young adults leaving foster care: Policy options for improving access.* Chapel Hill, NC: Center for Adolescent Health and the Law.

English, A., J. Scott, and M. Park. 2014. *Implementing the Affordable Care Act: How much will it help vulnerable adolescents and young adults?* Chapel Hill, NC: Center for Adolescent Health and the Law.

EuTEACH. 2014. *About EuTEACH.* http://www.unil.ch/euteach/home/menuinst/about-euteach.html (accessed March 28, 2014).

Fagan, J., and F. E. Zimring. 2000. *The changing borders of juvenile justice: Transfer of adolescents to the criminal court.* Chicago, IL: University of Chicago Press.

FamiliesUSA. 2014. *Federal poverty guidelines.* http://familiesusa.org/product/federal-poverty-guidelines (accessed July 25, 2014).

Ford, C., A. English, and G. Sigman. 2004. Confidential health care for adolescents: Position paper of the society for adolescent medicine. *Journal of Adolescent Health* 35(2):160-167.

Fordham, B., C. E. Griffiths, and C. Bundy. 2013. Can stress reduction interventions improve psoriasis?: A review. *Psychology, Health and Medicine* 18(5):501-514.

Fortuna, R. J., B. W. Robbins, and J. S. Halterman. 2009. Ambulatory care among young adults in the United States. *Annals of Internal Medicine* 151(6):379-385.

Fortuna, R. J., B. W. Robbins, N. Mani, and J. S. Halterman. 2010. Dependence on emergency care among young adults in the United States. *Journal of General Internal Medicine* 25(7):663-669.

Fox, H. B., M. A. McManus, J. D. Klein, A. Diaz, A. B. Elster, M. E. Felice, D. W. Kaplan, C. J. Wibbelsman, and J. E. Wilson. 2010. Adolescent medicine training in pediatric residency programs. *Pediatrics* 125(1):165-172.

Fox, S., and M. Duggan. 2013. *Tracking for health.* Washington, DC: Pew Research Center's Internet and American Life Project.

GAO (U.S. Government Accountability Office). 2008. *Young adults with serious mental illness: Some states and federal agencies are taking steps to address their transition challenges.* Washington, DC: GAO.

Garrett, C. C., J. Hocking, M. Y. Chen, C. K. Fairley, and M. Kirkman. 2011. Young people's views on the potential use of telemedicine consultations for sexual health: Results of a national survey. *BMC Infectious Diseases* 11:285.

Georgetown University Center for Child and Human Development. 2014. *Emerging adults initiative.* http://gucchdtacenter.georgetown.edu/transitions.html (accessed July 26, 2014).

Gettens, J., M. Mitra, A. D. Henry, and J. Himmelstein. 2011. Have working-age people with disabilities shared in the gains of Massachussetts health reform? *INQUIRY: The Journal of Health Care Organization, Provision, and Financing* 48(3):183-196.

Gilmer, T. P., V. D. Ojeda, K. Fawley-King, B. Larson, and P. Garcia. 2012. Change in mental health service use after offering youth-specific versus adult programs to transition-age youths. *Psychiatric Services* 63(6):592-596.

Gleeson, J., S. M. Cotton, M. Álvarez-Jiménez, D. Wade, D. Gee, K. Crisp, T. Pearce, B. Newman, D. Spiliotacopoulos, and D. Castle. 2009. A randomized controlled trial of relapse prevention therapy for first-episode psychosis patients. *Journal of Clinical Psychiatry* 70(4):477-486.

Glied, S., and D. Oellerich. 2014. Two-generation programs and health. *The Future of Children* 24(1):79-98.

GPO (U.S. Government Printing Office). 2012. Medicaid program: Initial core set of health care quality measures for Medicaid-eligible adults. *Federal Register* 77(2):286-291.

GPO. 2013. Patient Protection and Affordable Care Act; health insurance market rules; rate review. *Federal Register* 78(39):13406-13442.

Green, M. 1994. *Bright Futures: Guidelines for health supervision of infants, children, and adolescents.* Arlington, VA: National Center for Education in Maternal and Child Health.

Gudeman, R. 2013. *The Affordable Care Act and adolescent health.* http://www.youthlaw.org/publications/yln/2013/jul_sep_2013/affordable_care_act_adolescent_health (accessed July 26, 2014).

Gupta, A. A., K. Edelstein, A. Albert-Green, and N. D'Agostino. 2013. Assessing information and service needs of young adults with cancer at a single institution: The importance of information on cancer diagnosis, fertility preservation, diet, and exercise. *Support Care Cancer* 21(9):2477-2484.

Gurvitz, M., A. M. Valente, C. Broberg, S. Cook, K. Stout, J. Kay, J. Ting, K. Kuehl, M. Earing, and G. Webb. 2013. Prevalence and predictors of gaps in care among adult congenital heart disease patients: HEART-ACHD (The Health, Education, and Access Research Trial). *Journal of the American College of Cardiology* 61(21):2180-2184.

Gusmano, M. 2012. *Undocumented immigrants in the United States: U.S. health policy and access to care.* http://www.undocumentedpatients.org/issuebrief/health-policy-and-access-to-care (accessed July 24, 2014).

GW (George Washington) Cancer Institute). 2014. *Thriving after cancer.* http://smhs.gwu.edu/gwci/patient-care/survivors/tac (accessed September 24, 2014).

Haddock, G., S. Lewis, R. Bentall, G. Dunn, R. Drake, and N. Tarrier. 2006. Influence of age on outcome of psychological treatments in first-episode psychosis. *The British Journal of Psychiatry* 188(3):250-254.

Hagan, J. F., J. S. Shaw, and P. M. Duncan. 2008. *Bright futures: Guidelines for health supervision of infants, children, and adolescents.* Elk Grove Village, IL: AAP.

Halfon, N., A. Mendonca, and G. Berkowitz. 1995. Health status of children in foster care: The experience of the Center for the Vulnerable Child. *Archives of Pediatrics & Adolescent Medicine* 149(4):386-392.

Hall, K. S., C. Moreau, and J. Trussell. 2012. Continuing social disparities despite upward trends in sexual and reproductive health service use among young women in the United States. *Contraception* 86(6):681-686.

Hayes-Lattin, B., B. Mathews-Bradshaw, and S. Siegel. 2010. Adolescent and young adult oncology training for health professionals: A position statement. *Journal of Clinical Oncology* 28(32):4858-4861.

HealthSource RI. 2014. *HealthSource RI launches "nag tool kit" Facebook campaign for young invincibles and their moms.* http://www.healthsourceri.com/press-releases/healthsource-ri-launches-nag-tool-kit-facebook-campaign-for-young-invincibles-and-their-moms (accessed July 24, 2014).

Heberlein, M., T. Brooks, J. Guyer, S. Artiga, and J. Stephens. 2012. *Performing under pressure: Annual findings of a 50-state survey of eligibility, enrollment, renewal, and cost-sharing policies in Medicaid and CHIP, 2011-2012.* Washington, DC: KFF.

Hemmeter, J. 2012. Research and statistics note no. 2012-04. http://www.socialsecurity.gov/policy/docs/rsnotes/rsn2012-04.html (accessed July 28, 2014).

Henggeler, S. W., S. K. Schoenwald, C. M. Borduin, M. D. Rowland, and P. B. Cunningham. 1998. *Multisystemic treatment of antisocial behavior in children and adolescents.* New York: Guilford Press.

Hergenroeder, A. C., P. A. Benson, M. T. Britto, M. Catallozzi, L. J. D'Angelo, J. C. Edman, S. J. Emans, E. C. Kish, R. H. Pasternak, and G. B. Slap. 2010. Adolescent medicine: Workforce trends and recommendations. *Archives of Pediatrics & Adolescent Medicine* 164(12):1086-1090.

Hernandez-Boussard, T., C. S. Burns, N. Ewen Wang, L. C. Baker, and B. A. Goldstein. 2014. The Affordable Care Act reduces emergency department use by young adults: Evidence from three states. *Health Affairs* 33(9):1648-1654.

HHS (U.S. Department of Health and Human Services). 1999. *Mental health: A report of the Surgeon General.* Washington, DC: U.S. Department of Health and Human Services, Substance Abuse and Mental Health Services Administration, Center for Mental Health Services, National Institutes of Health, National Institute of Mental Health.

HHS. 2012. *Preventive services covered under the Affordable Care Act.* http://www.hhs.gov/healthcare/facts/factsheets/2010/07/preventive-services-list.html (accessed July 24, 2014).

HHS. 2014a. *Deferred action for childhood arrivals.* http://www.dhs.gov/deferred-action-childhood-arrivals (accessed August 12, 2014).

HHS. 2014b. *mHealth initiative.* http://www.hhs.gov/open/initiatives/mhealth (accessed July 26, 2014).

HHS. 2014c. *Healthy People 2020 DH-5 data details.* http://www.healthypeople.gov/2020/topicsobjectives2020/DataDetails.aspx?hp2020id=DH-5 (accessed September 26, 2014).

Hoge, C. W., and C. A. Castro. 2012. Preventing suicides in U.S. service members and veterans: Concerns after a decade of war. *Journal of the American Medical Association* 308(7):671-672.

Hourani, L. L., C. L. Council, R. C. Hubal, and L. B. Strange. 2011. Approaches to the primary prevention of posttraumatic stress disorder in the military: A review of the stress control literature. *Military Medicine* 176(7):721-730.

Hower, H., B. G. Case, B. Hoeppner, S. Yen, T. Goldstein, B. Goldstein, B. Birmaher, L. Weinstock, D. Topor, and J. Hunt. 2013. Use of mental health services in transition age youth with bipolar disorder. *Journal of Psychiatric Practice* 19(6):464-476.

HRSA (Health Resources and Services Administration). 2014. *Women's preventive services guidelines.* http://hrsa.gov/womensguidelines (accessed July 24, 2014).

Hughes, J. W., D. M. Fresco, R. Myerscough, M. H. van Dulmen, L. E. Carlson, and R. Josephson. 2013. Randomized controlled trial of mindfulness-based stress reduction for prehypertension. *Psychosomatic Medicine* 75(8):721-728.

IHI (Institute for Healthcare Improvement). 2014. *The Triple Aim Initiative.* http://www.ihi.org/Engage/Initiatives/TripleAim/pages/default.aspx (accessed September 29, 2014).

Insel, T. 2014. *Director's blog: The paradox of parity.* http://www.nimh.nih.gov/about/director/2014/the-paradox-of-parity.shtml (accessed July 28, 2014).

IOM (Institute of Medicine). 1994. *Reducing risks for mental disorders: Frontiers for preventive intervention research.* Washington, DC: National Academy Press.

IOM. 2000. *To err is human: Building a safer health system.* Washington, DC: National Academy Press.

IOM. 2001. *Envisioning the National Health Care Quality Report.* Washington, DC: National Academy Press.

IOM. 2009. *America's uninsured crisis: Consequences for health and health care.* Washington, DC: The National Academies Press.

IOM. 2011. *Clinical preventive services for women: Closing the gaps.* Washington, DC: The National Academies Press.

IOM. 2013a. *Best care at lower cost: The path to continuously learning health care in America.* Washington, DC: The National Academies Press.

IOM. 2013b. *Identifying and addressing the needs of adolescents and young adults with cancer: Workshop summary.* Washington, DC: The National Academies Press.

IOM. 2014. *Developing evidence-based standards for psychosocial interventions for mental disorders.* http://iom.edu/Activities/MentalHealth/PsychosocialInterventions.aspx (accessed July 28, 2014).

Irwin, Jr., C. E. 2010. Young adults are worse off than adolescents. *Journal of Adolescent Health* 46(5):405-406.

Jan, S., G. Slap, K. Smith-Whitley, D. Dai, R. Keren, and D. M. Rubin. 2013. Association of hospital and provider types on sickle cell disease outcomes. *Pediatrics* 132(5):854-861.

Jones, S. P., V. Patel, S. Saxena, N. Radcliffe, S. Ali Al-Marri, and A. Darzi. 2014. How Google's "ten things we know to be true" could guide the development of mental health mobile apps. *Health Affairs* 33(9):1603-1611.

Joseph-William, N., G. Elwyn, and A. Edwards. 2014. Knowledge is not power for patients: A systematic review and thematic synthesis of patient-reported barriers and facilitators to shared decision making. *Patient Education and Counseling* 94(3):291-309.

Kaplan, K., M. S. Salzer, and E. Brusilovskiy. 2012. Community participation as a predictor of recovery-oriented outcomes among emerging and mature adults with mental illnesses. *Psychiatric Rehabilitation Journal* 35(3):219-229.

Kaufman, L., W. Brooks, M. Steinley-Bumgarner, and S. Stevens-Manser. 2012. *Peer specialist training and certification programs: A national overview.* Austin: University of Texas at Austin Center for Social Work Research.

Kenyon, R. V., and J. Leigh. 2011. Human augmentics: Augmenting human evolution. *Conference Proceedings: Annual International Conference of the IEEE Engineering in Medicine and Biology Society* 2011:6758-6761.

Kessing, L. V., L. Søndergård, K. Kvist, and P. K. Andersen. 2007. Adherence to lithium in naturalistic settings: Results from a nationwide pharmacoepidemiological study. *Bipolar Disorders* 9(7):730-736.

KFF (The Henry J. Kaiser Family Foundation). 2013. *Establishing health insurance exchanges: An overview of state efforts.* http://kff.org/health-reform/issue-brief/establishing-health-insurance-exchanges-an-overview-of (accessed July 25, 2014).

KFF. 2014a. *Status of state action on the Medicaid expansion decision, 2014.* http://kff.org/health-reform/state-indicator/state-activity-around-expanding-medicaid-under-the-affordable-care-act (accessed July 28, 2014).

KFF. 2014b. *The coverage gap: Uninsured poor adults in states that do not expand Medicaid.* Washington, DC: KFF. http://kff.org/medicaid/issue-brief/analyzing-the-impact-of-state-medicaid-expansion-decisions (accessed October 13, 2014).

KFF. 2014c. *How will the uninsured fare under the Affordable Care Act?* http://kff.org/health-reform/fact-sheet/how-will-the-uninsured-fare-under-the-affordable-care-act (accessed September 28, 2014).

Khoury, B., T. Lecomte, B. A. Gaudiano, and K. Paquin. 2013. Mindfulness interventions for psychosis: A meta-analysis. *Schizophrenia Research* 150(1):176-184.

Killackey, E., H. J. Jackson, and P. D. McGorry. 2008. Vocational intervention in first-episode psychosis: Individual placement and support v. Treatment as usual. *The British Journal of Psychiatry* 193(2):114-120.

Klein, J. D., T. S. Sesselberg, B. Gawronski, L. Handwerker, F. Gesten, and A. Schettine. 2003. Improving adolescent preventive services through state, managed care, and community partnerships. *Journal of Adolescent Health* 32(6):91-97.

Knopik, V. S. 2009. Maternal smoking during pregnancy and child outcomes: Real or spurious effect? *Developmental Neuropsychology* 34(1):1-36.

Kotogal, M., A. C. Carle, L. G. Kessler, and D. R. Flum. 2014. Limited impact on health and access to care for 19- to 25-year olds following the Patient Protection and Affordable Care Act. *JAMA Pediatrics* [Epub ahead of print].

Kovacs, A. H., and B. W. McCrindle. 2014. So hard to say goodbye: Transition from paediatric to adult cardiology care. *Nature Reviews Cardiology* 11:51-62.

Koyanagi, K., and E. Alfano. 2013. *Promise for the future: How federal programs can improve the career outcomes for youth and young adults with serious mental health conditions.* Worcester, MA: University of Massachusetts Medical School and Washington, DC: Bazelon Center for Mental Health Law.

Kramer, T., and M. E. Garralda. 2000. Child and adolescent mental health problems in primary care. *Advances in Psychiatric Treatment* 6(4):287-294.

Kulesza, M., M. A. McVay, M. E. Larimer, and A. L. Copeland. 2013. A randomized clinical trial comparing the efficacy of two active conditions of a brief intervention for heavy college drinkers. *Addictive Behavior* 38(4):2094-2101.

Labacher, L., and C. Mitchell. 2013. Talk or text to tell? How young adults in Canada and South Africa prefer to receive STI results, counseling, and treatment updates in a wireless world. *Journal of Health Communication* 18(12):1465-1476.

Lau, J. S., S. H. Adams, W. J. Boscardin, C. E. Irwin, Jr. 2013a. Health care utilization and expenditures among young adults prior to the Affordable Care Act 2010. *Journal of Adolescent Health* 52(2 Suppl 1):S1-121.

Lau, J. S., S. H. Adams, C. E. Irwin, Jr., and E. M. Ozer. 2013b. Receipt of preventive health services in young adults. *Journal of Adolescent Health* 52(1):42-49.

Lau, J. S., S. H. Adams, W. J. Boscardin, and C. E. Irwin, Jr. 2014a. Young adults' health care utilization and expenditures prior to the Affordable Care Act. *Journal of Adolescent Health* 54(6):663-671.

Lau, J., S. Adams, M. Park, J. Boscardin, and C. E. Irwin, Jr. 2014b. Improvement in preventive care of young adults after the Affordable Care Act: The Affordable Care Act is helping. *JAMA Pediatrics*. Published online October 27, 2014. doi:10.1001/jamapediatrics.2014.1691.

Lauche, R., H. Cramer, G. Dobos, J. Langhorst, and S. Schmidt. 2013. A systematic review and meta-analysis of mindfulness-based stress reduction for the fibromyalgia syndrome. *Journal of Psychosomatic Research* 75(6):500-510.

Lehmann, B., J. Guyer, and K. Lewandowski. 2012. *Child welfare and the Affordable Care Act: Key provisions for foster care children and youth.* Washington, DC: Georgetown University Health Policy Institute.

Lehrer, J. A., R. Pantell, K. Tebb, and M.-A. Shafer. 2007. Forgone health care among U.S. adolescents: Associations between risk characteristics and confidentiality concern. *Journal of Adolescent Health* 40(3):218-226.

Lindstrom Johnson, S., S. D. Tandon, M. Trent, V. Jones, and T. L. Cheng. 2012. Use of technology with health care providers: Perspectives from urban youth. *Journal of Pediatrics* 160(6):997-1002.

Lloyd-Evans, B., E. Mayo-Wilson, B. Harrison, H. Istead, E. Brown, S. Pilling, S. Johnson, and T. Kendall. 2014. A systematic review and meta-analysis of randomised controlled trials of peer support for people with severe mental illness. *BMC Psychiatry* 14(1):39.

Long, S. K., A. Yemane, and K. Stockley. 2010. Disentangling the effects of health reform in Massachusetts: How important are the special provisions for young adults? *The American Economic Review* 297-302.

Lorig, K., P. L. Ritter, F. J. Villa, and J. Armas. 2009. Community-based peer-led diabetes self-management a randomized trial. *The Diabetes Educator* 35(4):641-651.

Lotstein, D. S., M. Seid, G. Klingensmith, D. Case, J. M. Lawrence, C. Pihoker, D. Dabelea, E. J. Mayer-Davis, L. K. Gilliam, and S. Corathers. 2013. Transition from pediatric to adult care for youth diagnosed with type 1 diabetes in adolescence. *Pediatrics* 131(4):e1062-e1070.

Magrab, P., and H. Millar. 1989. *Growing up and getting medical care: Youth with special health care needs.* Surgeon General's Conference. Washington, DC: Georgetown University Child Development Center.

Major, B. S., M. F. Hinton, A. Flint, A. Chalmers-Brown, K. McLoughlin, and S. Johnson. 2010. Evidence of the effectiveness of a specialist vocational intervention following first episode psychosis: A naturalistic prospective cohort study. *Social Psychiatry and Psychiatric Epidemiology* 45(1):1-8.

Mammen, G., and G. Faulkner. 2013. Physical activity and the prevention of depression: A systematic review of prospective studies. *American Journal of Preventive Medicine* 45(5):649-657.

Mann, C. 2012. *CMCS informational bulletin.* http://www.medicaid.gov/Federal-Policy-Guidance/downloads/CIB-1-4-2012.pdf (accessed July 24, 2014).

Marwick, A. E. 2013. *Status update: Celebrity, publicity, and branding in the social media age.* New Haven, CT: Yale University Press.

MCH (Maternal and Child Health) Leadership Competencies Workgroup. 2009. *Maternal and Child Health leadership competencies. Version 3.0.* Rockville, MD: MCH, HRSA, HHS.

McManus, M. A., H. Fox, K. O'Connor, T. Chapman, and J. MacKinnon. 2008. *Pediatric perspectives and practices on transitioning adolescents with special needs to adult health care.* Washington, DC: National Alliance to Advance Adolescent Health.

McPheeters M., A. M Davis, J. L. Taylor, R. F. Brown, S. A. Potter, and R. A. Epstein. 2014. Transition care for children with special health needs. Technical brief no. 15. Rockville, MD: AHRQ.

MD Anderson Cancer Center. 2014. *Adolescent and Young Adult (AYA) Program.* http://www.mdanderson.org/patient-and-cancer-information/care-centers-and-clinics/childrens-cancer-hospital/support-programs/aya-program.html (accessed April 24, 2014).

mHealth Alliance. 2014. *mHealth Alliance.* http://mhealthalliance.org (accessed July 26, 2014).

mHealth Summit. 2014. *mHealth Alliance summit.* http://www.mhealthsummit.org (accessed July 26, 2014).

Minnes, S., A. Lang, and L. Singer. 2011. Prenatal tobacco, marijuana, stimulant, and opiate exposure: Outcomes and practice implications. *Addiction Science & Clinical Practice* 6(1):57-70.

NACo (National Association of Counties). 2012. *County jails and the Affordable Care Act: Enrolling eligible individuals in health coverage.* Washington, DC: NACo.

NAHIC (National Adolescent and Young Adult Health Information Center). 2014. *Summary of recommended guidelines for clinical preventive services for young adults ages 18-26.* San Francisco, CA: UCSF Division of Adolescent and Young Adult Medicine.

Narayanan, S., and P. J. Shami. 2012. Treatment of acute lymphoblastic leukemia in adults. *Critical Reviews in Oncology/Hematology* 81(1):94-102.

Nardi, B., S. Laurenzi, M. Di Nicolo, and C. Bellantuono. 2012. Is the cognitive-behavioral therapy an effective intervention to prevent the postnatal depression? A critical review. *International Journal of Psychiatry in Medicine* 43(3):211-225.

NASW (National Association of Social Workers). 1993. *NASW standards for the practice of social work with adolescents.* https://www.socialworkers.org/practice/standards/sw_adolescents.asp (accessed July 24, 2014).

The National Alliance to Advance Adolescent Health. 2014a. *About Got Transition.* http://www.gottransition.org/about/index.cfm (accessed August 4, 2014).

The National Alliance to Advance Adolescent Health. 2014b. *Six core elements of health care transition 2.0.* http://www.gottransition.org/resourceGet.cfm?id=206 (accessed September 24, 2014).

National Conference of State Legislatures. 2014. *Medicaid for juvenile justice-involved children: Juvenile justice guidebook for legislators*. Denver, CO: National Conference of State Legislatures.

NCCAP (National Certification Council for Activity Professionals). 2011. *National certification examination for addiction counselors, level 1 and level 2: Candidate handbook*. http://www.ptcny.com/pdf/NCC.pdf (accessed July 25, 2014).

NCI (National Cancer Institute). 2014. *Adolescents and young adults with cancer*. http://www.cancer.gov/cancertopics/aya (accessed July 28, 2014).

NCQA (National Committee for Quality Assurance). 2014. *Standards and guidelines for NCQA's Patient-Centered Medical Home (PCMH) 2014*. Washington, DC: NCQA.

Neinstein, L. S. 2014. *Adolescent health curriculum: Outline of curriculum*. http://www.usc.edu/student-affairs/Health_Center/adolhealth (accessed March 28, 2014).

NRC (National Research Council) and IOM. 2009. *Adolescent health services: Missing opportunities*. Washington, DC: The National Academies Press.

NTOCC (National Transitions of Care Coalition). 2008. *Transitions of care measures*. Washington, DC: NTOCC.

Okumura, M. J., M. Heisler, M. M. Davis, M. D. Cabana, S. Demonner, and E. A. Kerr. 2008. Comfort of general internists and general pediatricians in providing care for young adults with chronic illnesses of childhood. *Journal of General Internal Medicine* 23(10):1621-1627.

Okumura, M. J., E. A. Kerr, M. D. Cabana, M. M. Davis, S. Demonner, and M. Heisler. 2010. Physician views on barriers to primary care for young adults with childhood-onset chronic disease. *Pediatrics* 125(4):e748-e754.

Olson, A. L., C. A. Gaffney, V. A. Hedberg, and G. R. Gladstone. 2009. Use of inexpensive technology to enhance adolescent health screening and counseling. *Archives of Pediatrics & Adolescent Medicine* 163(2):172-177.

Ostrom, C. M. 2014. State using fake rappers, real patients in new health-insurance ad campaign. *The Seattle Times*, February 19.

Ozer, E. M. 2007. The adolescent primary care visit: Time to build on strengths. *Journal of Adolescent Health* 41(6):519-520.

Ozer, E. M., S. H. Adams, J. L. Lustig, S. Gee, A. K. Garber, L. R. Gardner, M. Rehbein, L. Addison, and C. E. Irwin. 2005. Increasing the screening and counseling of adolescents for risky health behaviors: A primary care intervention. *Pediatrics* 115(4):960-968.

Ozer, E. M., J. T. Urquhart, C. D. Brindis, M. J. Park, and C. E. Irwin. 2012. Young adult preventive health care guidelines: There but can't be found. *Archives of Pediatrics & Adolescent Medicine* 166(3):240-247.

Ozer, E. M., J. T. Scott, and C. D. Brindis. 2013. Seizing the opportunity: Improving young adult preventive health care. *Adolescent Medicine: State of the Art Reviews* 24:507-525.

Partnership for Male Youth. 2014. *Health provider toolkit for adolescent and young adult males*. http://www.ayamalehealth.org/index.php#sthash.qD9oPHAu.OO4iihBd.dpbs (accessed March 28, 2014).

Passel, J. S., and D. Cohn. 2009. *A portrait of unauthorized immigrants in the United States*. Washington, DC: Pew Hispanic Center.

Passel, J. S., and M. H. Lopez. 2012. *Up to 1.7 million unauthorized immigrant youth may benefit from new deportation rules*. Washington, DC: Pew Hispanic Center.

Passel, J. S., D. Cohn, and A. Gonazalez-Barrera. 2013. *Population decline of unauthorized immigrants stalls, may have reversed*. Washington, DC: Pew Hispanic Center.

Pauly, M. V., and J. A. Pagán. 2007. Spillovers and vulnerability: The case of community uninsurance. *Health Affairs* 26(5):1304-1314.

Peppercorn, J. M., J. C. Weeks, E. F. Cook, and S. Joffe. 2004. Comparison of outcomes in cancer patients treated within and outside clinical trials: Conceptual framework and structured review. *Lancet* 363(9405):263-270.

Perrin, E. C., and R. C. Sheldrick. 2012. The challenge of mental health care in pediatrics. *Archives of Pediatrics & Adolescent Medicine* 166(3):287-288.

Peter, N. G., C. M. Forke, K. R. Ginsburg, and D. F. Schwarz. 2009. Transition from pediatric to adult care: Internists' perspectives. *Pediatrics* 123(2):417-423.

Porteous, N., and G. Waghorn. 2007. Implementing evidence-based employment services in New Zealand for young adults with psychosis: Progress during the first five years. *The British Journal of Occupational Therapy* 70(12):521-526.

Pottick, K. J., S. Bilder, A. Vander Stoep, L. A. Warner, and M. F. Alvarez. 2008. U.S. patterns of mental health service utilization for transition-age youth and young adults. *The Journal of Behavioral Health Services & Research* 35(4):373-389.

Pottick, K. J., L. A. Warner, A. Vander Stoep, and N. M. Knight. 2014. Clinical characteristics and outpatient mental health service use of transition-age youth in the USA. *The Journal of Behavioral Health Services & Research* 41(2):230-243.

Pullmann, M. D., C. A. Heflinger, and L. S. Mayberry. 2010. Patterns of Medicaid disenrollment for youth with mental health problems. *Medical Care Research and Review* 67(6):657-675.

Querstret, D., and M. Cropley. 2013. Assessing treatments used to reduce rumination and/or worry: A systematic review. *Clinical Psychology Review* 33(8):996-1009.

Quinn, C. T., Z. R. Rogers, T. L. McCavit, and G. R. Buchanan. 2010. Improved survival of children and adolescents with sickle cell disease. *Blood* 115(17):3447-3452.

Ramanujachar, R., S. Richards, I. Hann, and D. Webb. 2006. Adolescents with acute lymphoblastic leukaemia: Emerging from the shadow of paediatric and adult treatment protocols. *Pediatric Blood & Cancer* 47(6):748-756.

Regier, D. A., W. E. Narrow, D. S. Rae, R. W. Manderscheid, B. Z. Locke, and F. K. Goodwin. 1993. The de facto U.S. mental and addictive disorders service system: Epidemiologic catchment area prospective 1-year prevalence rates of disorders and services. *Archives of General Psychiatry* 50(2):85-94.

Reid, G. J., M. J. Irvine, B. W. McCrindle, R. Sananes, P. G. Ritvo, S. C. Siu, and G. D. Webb. 2004. Prevalence and correlates of successful transfer from pediatric to adult health care among a cohort of young adults with complex congenital heart defects. *Pediatrics* 113(3):e197-e205.

Reiner, K., L. Tibi, and J. D. Lipsitz. 2013. Do mindfulness-based interventions reduce pain intensity? A critical review of the literature. *Pain Medicine* 14(2):230-242.

Reiss, J. G., R. W. Gibson, and L. R. Walker. 2005. Health care transition: Youth, family, and provider perspectives. *Pediatrics* 115(1):112-120.

Rice, C., R. Longabaugh, M. Beattie, and N. Noel. 1993. Age group differences in response to treatment for problematic alcohol use. *Addiction* 88(10):1369-1375.

Rihmer, Z., and X. Gonda. 2013. Pharmacological prevention of suicide in patients with major mood disorders. *Neuroscience and Biobehavioral Reviews* 37(10):2398-2403.

Ringeisen, H., C. Casanueva, M. Urato, and L. Stambaugh. 2009. Mental health service use during the transition to adulthood for adolescents reported to the child welfare system. *Psychiatric Services* 60(8):1084-1091.

Robison, L. L. 2011. Late effects of acute lymphoblastic leukemia therapy in patients diagnosed at 0-20 years of age. *ASH Education Program Book* 2011(1):238-242.

Rosenbach, M., K. Lewis, and B. Quinn. 2001. *Children in foster care: Challenges in meeting their health care needs through Medicaid.* Princeton, NJ: Mathematica.

SAHM (Society for Adolescent Health and Medicine). 2014. *Mission.* http://www.adolescenthealth.org/About-SAHM/Mission.aspx (accessed March 28, 2014).

SAMHSA (Substance Abuse and Mental Health Services Administration). 2011. *Leading change: A plan for SAMHSA's roles and actions 2011-2014*. Rockville, MD: HHS.

SAMHSA. 2013a. *Results from the 2012 National Survey on Drug Use and Health: Mental health findings and detailed tables*. http://www.samhsa.gov/data/NSDUH/2k12MH_FindingsandDetTables/MHDT/NSDUH-MHDetTabsTOC2012.htm (accessed September 26, 2014).

SAMHSA. 2013b. *Results from the 2012 National Survey on Drug Use and Health: Detailed tables*. http://www.samhsa.gov/data/NSDUH/2012SummNatFindDetTables/DetTabs/NSDUH-DetTabsTOC2012.htm (accessed September 26, 2014).

Sanci, L., B. Grabsch, P. Chondros, A. Shiell, J. Pirkis, S. Sawyer, K. Hegarty, E. Patterson, H. Cahill, and E. Ozer. 2012. The prevention access and risk taking in young people (PARTY) project protocol: A cluster randomised controlled trial of health risk screening and motivational interviewing for young people presenting to general practice. *BMC Public Health* 12(1):400.

Schoenbaum, M., J. Unützer, C. Sherbourne, N. Duan, L. V. Rubenstein, J. Miranda, L. S. Meredith, M. F. Carney, and K. Wells. 2001. Cost-effectiveness of practice-initiated quality improvement for depression: Results of a randomized controlled trial. *Journal of the American Medical Association* 286(11):1325-1330.

Schoenbaum, M., J. Unützer, D. McCaffrey, N. Duan, C. Sherbourne, and K. B. Wells. 2002. The effects of primary care depression treatment on patients' clinical status and employment. *Health Services Research* 37(5):1145-1158.

Schoenbaum, M., J. Miranda, C. Sherbourne, N. Duan, and K. Wells. 2004. Cost-effectiveness of interventions for depressed Latinos. *Journal of Mental Health Policy and Economics* 69-76.

Seattle Children's Hospital. 2014. *Adolescent and Young Adult (AYA) Cancer Program*. http://www.seattlechildrens.org/clinics-programs/cancer/services/adolescent-young-adult-program (accessed July 24, 2014).

Shah, L. B., P. Klainin-Yobas, S. Torres, and P. Kannusamy. 2014. Efficacy of psychoeducation and relaxation interventions on stress-related variables in people with mental disorders: A literature review. *Archives of Psychiatric Nursing* 28(2):94-101.

Shufelt, J. L., and J. J. Cocozza. 2006. *Youth with mental health disorders in the juvenile justice system: Results from a multi-state prevalence study*. Delmar, NY: National Center for Mental Health and Juvenile Justice.

Siegenthaler, E., T. Munder, and M. Egger. 2012. Effect of preventive interventions in mentally ill parents on the mental health of the offspring: Systematic review and meta-analysis. *Journal of the American Academy of Child & Adolescent Psychiatry* 51(1):8-17, e18.

Simon, G. E., W. J. Katon, M. VonKorff, J. Unützer, E. H. Lin, E. A. Walker, T. Bush, C. Rutter, and E. Ludman. 2001. Cost-effectiveness of a collaborative care program for primary care patients with persistent depression. *American Journal of Psychiatry* 158(10):1638-1644.

Simon, G. E., M. Von Korff, E. J. Ludman, W. J. Katon, C. Rutter, J. Unützer, E. H. Lin, T. Bush, and E. Walker. 2002. Cost-effectiveness of a program to prevent depression relapse in primary care. *Medical Care* 40(10):941-950.

Simon, T. D., S. Lamb, N. A. Murphy, B. Hom, M. L. Walker, and E. B. Clark. 2009. Who will care for me next? Transitioning to adulthood with hydrocephalus. *Pediatrics* 124(5):1431-1437.

Sinha, R., C. Easton, and K. Kemp. 2003. Substance abuse treatment characteristics of probation-referred young adults in a community-based outpatient program. *The American Journal of Drug and Alcohol Abuse* 29(3):585-597.

Slade, E., L. Wissow, M. Davis, M. Abrams, and L. Dixon. 2014. Medicaid lapses and low-income young adults' receipt of outpatient mental health care after an inpatient stay. *Psychiatric Services* 65(4):454-460.

Slive, L., and R. Cramer. 2012. Health reform and the preservation of confidential health care for young adults. *The Journal of Law, Medicine & Ethics* 40(2):383-390.

SSA (Social Security Administration). 2014. *Understanding Supplemental Security Income SSI and other government programs—2014 edition.* http://www.ssa.gov/ssi/text-other-ussi.htm (accessed September 12, 2014).

Stafford, M. R., H. Jackson, E. Mayo-Wilson, A. P. Morrison, and T. Kendall. 2013. Early interventions to prevent psychosis: Systematic review and meta-analysis. *British Medical Journal* 346.

Stevens, J., K. J. Kelleher, W. Gardner, D. Chisolm, J. McGeehan, K. Pajer, and L. Buchanan. 2008. Trial of computerized screening for adolescent behavioral concerns. *Pediatrics* 121(6):1099-1105.

Stice, E., H. Shaw, C. Bohon, C. N. Marti, and P. Rohde. 2009. A meta-analytic review of depression prevention programs for children and adolescents: Factors that predict magnitude of intervention effects. *Journal of Consulting and Clinical Psychology* 77(3):486.

Stroul, B. A. 2002. *Issue brief—system of care: A framework for system reform in children's mental health.* Washington, DC: Georgetown University Child Development Center, National Technical Assistance Center for Children's Mental Health.

Stroul, B. A., and R. M. Friedman. 1986. *A system of care for children and youth with severe emotional disturbances.* Washington, DC: CASSP Technical Assistance Center, Center for Child Health and Mental Health Policy, Georgetown University Child Development Center.

Tanis, C. 2012. Performance enhancement and stress reduction using biofeedback with women collegiate volleyball players. *Athletic Insight: The Online Journal of Sport Psychology* 4(2):127-140.

Tebb, K. P., E. Sedlander, G. Pica, A. Diaz, K. Peake, and C. D. Brindis. 2014. *Protecting adolescent confidentiality under health care reform: The special case regarding explanations of benefits (EOBs).* San Francisco: Philip R. Lee Institute of Health Policy and Division of Adolescent and Young Adult Medicine, Department of Pediatrics, University of California, San Francisco.

Tighe, E., and L. Saxe. 2006. Community-based substance abuse reduction and the gap between treatment need and treatment utilization: Analysis of data from the "fighting back" general population survey. *Journal of Drug Issues* 36(2):295-312.

Todd, S. R., and B. D. Sommers. 2012. *Overview of the uninsured in the United States: A summary of the 2012 Current Population Survey report.* Washington, DC: HHS Office of the Assistant Secretary for Planning and Evaluation.

Tuchman, L. K., and M. Schwartz. 2013. Health outcomes associated with transition from pediatric to adult cystic fibrosis care. *Pediatrics* 132(5):847-853.

Tuchman, L. K., L. A. Schwartz, G. S. Sawicki, and M. T. Britto. 2010. Cystic fibrosis and transition to adult medical care. *Pediatrics* 125(3):566-573.

Turrisi, R., J. Jaccard, R. Taki, H. Dunnam, and J. Grimes. 2001. Examination of the short-term efficacy of a parent intervention to reduce college student drinking tendencies. *Psychology of Addictive Behaviors* 15(4):366-372.

Tylee, A., D. M. Haller, T. Graham, R. Churchill, and L. A. Sanci. 2007. Youth-friendly primary-care services: How are we doing and what more needs to be done? *Lancet* 369(9572):1565-1573.

USPSTF (U.S. Preventive Services Task Force). 2011. *Focus on children and adolescents.* http://www.uspreventiveservicestaskforce.org/tfchfocus.htm (accessed July 26, 2014).

USPSTF. 2012. *Grade definitions.* http://www.uspreventiveservicestaskforce.org/uspstf/grades.htm (accessed September 26, 2014).

USPSTF. 2013. *Focus on older adults.* http://www.uspreventiveservicestaskforce.org/tfolderfocus.htm (accessed July 26, 2014).

van Hasselt, F., P. Krabbe, D. Ittersum, M. Postma, and A. Loonen. 2013. Evaluating interventions to improve somatic health in severe mental illness: A systematic review. *Acta Psychiatrica Scandinavica* 128(4):251-260.

Van Voorhees, B. W., N. Mahoney, R. Mazo, A. Z. Barrera, C. P. Siemer, T. R. Gladstone, and R. F. Muñoz. 2011. Internet-based depression prevention over the life course: A call for behavioral vaccines. *Psychiatric Clinics of North America* 34(1):167-183.

VanDenBerg, J. E., and E. M. Grealish. 1996. Individualized services and supports through the wraparound process: Philosophy and procedures. *Journal of Child and Family Studies* 5(1):7-21.

Vujicic, M., C. Yarbrough, and K. Nasseh. 2014. The effect of the Affordable Care Act's expanded coverage policy on access to dental care. *Medical Care* 52(8):715-719.

Wallace, S., J. Torres, T. Nobari, and N. Pourat. 2013. *Undocumented and uninsured: Barriers to affordable care for immigrant populations.* Washington, DC, and New York: The Commonwealth Fund and the UCLA Center for Health Policy Research.

Warner, C. H., G. N. Appenzeller, J. R. Parker, C. M. Warner, and C. W. Hoge. 2011. Effectiveness of mental health screening and coordination of in-theater care prior to deployment to Iraq: A cohort study. *American Journal of Psychiatry* 168(4):378-385.

Weissman, M. M., P. Wickramaratne, Y. Nomura, V. Warner, D. Pilowsky, and H. Verdeli. 2006. Offspring of depressive parents: 20 years later. *American Journal of Psychiatry* 163(6):1001-1008.

WHO (World Health Organization). 2001. *Global consultation on adolescent friendly health services: A consensus statement.* Geneva, Switzerland: WHO.

WHO. 2009. *Quality assessment guidebook: A guide to assessing health services for adolescent clients.* Geneva, Switzerland: WHO.

Young Invincibles. 2014. Health care. http://younginvincibles.org/issues/health-care (accessed July 22, 2014).

Zebrack, B. 2008. Information and service needs for young adult cancer patients. *Support Care Cancer* 16(12):1353-1360.

Zemel, S., and N. Kaye. 2009. *Medicaid eligibility, enrollment, and retention policies: Findings from a survey of juvenile justice and Medicaid policies affecting children in the juvenile justice system.* Portland, ME: National Academy for State Health Policy.

8

Government Investments in Marginalized Young Adults

Key Findings

- Marginalized young adults—such as those living in poverty, those aging out of foster care, those in the justice system, those with disabilities, and young parents—are much less likely than other young adults to experience a successful transition to adulthood, although many of these young people ultimately fare very well as adults, and their hopes and aspirations are similar to those of young people who have not been marginalized. Meeting the needs of marginalized young adults not only improves their lives, but also has the potential to help them become fully contributing members of society.
- Although marginalized young adults are a heterogeneous group, they often share a number of characteristics and experiences, such as low income and behavioral health problems. Similarly, there is considerable overlap in the populations targeted by the many programs that serve marginalized young adults.
- A comprehensive view of populations of marginalized young adults is lacking, which limits the development of policies and programs intended to reduce their marginalization.
- Fragmented programs have narrow and idiosyncratic eligibility criteria that pose obstacles to young adults' getting the help

they need, often create lapses in help when it is provided, and too often are stigmatizing. Major entitlement programs intended to help vulnerable populations provide limited support for young adults, and discretionary programs targeting these populations often fall far short of meeting demonstrable need.

- Variations in the categorization of marginalized young adults across programs result in a lack of accountability, with multiple distinct outputs and outcomes being associated with the plethora of programs. There is no collective accountability for improving the overall health and well-being of marginalized young adults.

While the transition to adulthood can be challenging for anyone, some young people are particularly vulnerable to experiencing difficulty during this period. This vulnerability can be manifest as individual or group characteristics that serve as risk factors for a poor transition to adulthood in one or more areas of health and well-being. For example, prior chapters of this report have illustrated how living in poverty, being a single parent, or having a disability all increase the likelihood that a young adult's health and well-being will suffer. Concern about the risks posed by these individual characteristics has led to the creation and evolution of various government-supported programs. Many of these programs are intended to serve populations perceived as needing help beyond what is available from their families and communities, while some are more focused on controlling the behavior of those perceived to be a threat to others. In many cases, these programs do not serve all of their target populations. Some, such as foster care or the corrections system, are what might be called custodial systems, but most are not.

"We need to encourage professionals to not only open doors for their children, but open doors for young people in marginalized communities."*

We refer to young people who exhibit characteristics that put them at risk for poor outcomes during young adulthood as marginalized young adults, whether or not they are currently served by government programs. Our use of this term is informed by the concept of social exclusion, a concept

* Quotations are from members of the young adult advisory group during their discussions with the committee.

denoting the economic, social, political, racial and ethnic, and cultural marginalization experienced by specific groups of people because of social forces such as poverty, discrimination, violence and trauma, disenfranchisement, and dislocation (Daly and Silver, 2008; Mathiesen et al., 2008; Sen, 2000). Commitment to social inclusion is based on the belief that a democratic society benefits when all its members participate fully in community affairs. Viewing marginalized populations through this lens helps shift the focus from individuals' difficulties or limitations to how society portrays and treats them. An emphasis on social inclusion calls for the identification of policies that exclude certain groups from full participation in society and the development of policies that enhance opportunities for full participation. We believe social exclusion is a useful lens through which to view how policies contribute to or ameliorate the relatively poor outcomes experienced by the groups of young people on which we focus here.

In this chapter, we describe selected programs that serve marginalized young adults and what is known about the populations they serve. We summarize evidence for the effectiveness of these programs and the services they fund and make recommendations regarding policies and research that could improve the prospects of marginalized young adults. In some cases (e.g., foster care, homeless youth programs), these programs explicitly target young adults as a distinct population in need of special assistance; other programs (e.g., Temporary Assistance for Needy Families [TANF], the criminal justice system) serve large numbers of young adults but generally do not distinguish them from older adults. Available evidence suggests that on average, marginalized young adults are much less likely than other young adults to experience a successful transition to adulthood. Nonetheless, it is important to keep in mind that many of these young people ultimately fare very well as adults. Moreover, their hopes and aspirations are similar to those of young people who have not been marginalized. We believe they should be seen as young people who could potentially benefit greatly from supportive policies, and that everyone would benefit from their full participation in society.

> "No longer depending on welfare, finding a job, and breaking through the system and living above it is what I define as success."

We do not attempt here to describe every population that might be considered vulnerable or to provide an exhaustive review of federal programs for young people likely to experience a challenging transition to adulthood. Most notably, while we do not focus explicitly here on poverty and racial discrimination, it should be clear from prior chapters of this report and from the demographic makeup of the populations described in this chapter that these factors are central to the marginalization of many young adults. Young adults with disabilities also are among the marginalized populations of young adults; they are discussed at length in Chapters 4 and 7, and therefore are not examined here in detail. Lesbian, gay, bisexual, and transgender (LGBT) young adults may also be marginalized in certain circumstances, but are not addressed in depth here because they are not targeted by any federal programs. Nevertheless, while it is difficult to obtain reliable estimates, research indicates that these young people likely are overrepresented in some of the programs discussed here (e.g., services for the homeless, the criminal justice system, and foster care) and experience poorer outcomes in these programs than heterosexual young adults (Courtney et al., 2011; Dworsky, 2013; Hanssens et al., 2014; Wilson et al., 2014).

> "Programs and services should provide help in a way that aims to understand the person, the whole person—their interests and strengths as well as areas for improvement."

Our choices for discussion in this chapter are intended to highlight the following kinds of populations and programs:

- marginalized populations that include a relatively large number of young adults;
- marginalized populations that are the target of relatively large government investments; and
- programs that help illustrate important between-program distinctions (e.g., between entitlement programs and those with annual appropriations, between federally administered programs and those left largely to state and local administration).

We focus on the following populations:

- young adults aging out of foster care,
- young adults in the justice system,
- homeless young adults,
- young parents, and
- young unauthorized immigrants.

For each of these populations, we describe their characteristics, programs intended to help address their needs, and available evidence for program effectiveness.

Next we examine common characteristics of the programs included in this review and the populations they serve, and the implications for improving the health and well-being of young adults. Of particular note is the overlap of populations served by these programs and the frequency with which the young people they serve exhibit characteristics that can imperil a successful transition to adulthood (e.g., poverty, early parenting, mental health conditions, limited education, poor social support). We then look at evidence for assisting marginalized young adults. The final section presents conclusions and recommendations.

YOUNG ADULTS AGING OUT OF FOSTER CARE

An understanding of the conditions of young people transitioning out of foster care to adulthood requires an understanding of the overall purposes of the foster care system.[1] State child welfare programs are operated under federal policies found in Titles IV-B and IV-E of the Social Security Act, with Title IV-E providing federal reimbursement to states for a significant portion of the costs for children in foster care (SSA, 2014).[2] Juvenile and family courts supervise state and local public child welfare agencies' care of children. Children enter foster care after determination from a public child welfare agency, generally with the approval of the court, that removal from the home will protect them from abuse, neglect, and/or dependency.[3]

The vast majority of children who enter foster care will exit into legally "permanent" placements; of the estimated 240,923 children leaving out-of-home care in the United States during fiscal year (FY) 2012, 87 percent left to live with family, were adopted, or were placed with a legal guardian (ACF, 2013c). Two percent of children were transferred to a different public agency (e.g., a probation or mental health department), and 1 percent ran away and were discharged from foster care.

Despite child welfare agencies' efforts to identify permanent homes for those in foster care, some become "emancipated" to "independent liv-

[1] Consistent with its use in federal policy, the term "foster care" is used here to describe out-of-home care provided by government for abused and neglected children and youth. Foster care includes family foster care, kinship foster care, and group care placement settings.

[2] States receive reimbursement for a portion of payments to foster care providers and allowable administrative costs.

[3] While short-term emergency placements can be made by child welfare agencies prior to court review, child welfare agencies must obtain court approval to place children against their parents' will for more than a few days.

ing," usually upon turning 18 or achieving a high school diploma.[4] This is known as as "aging out of foster care." Recent changes in federal law allow states to claim reimbursement for foster care up to age 21, but in most states youth may not remain in foster care much beyond their 18th birthday (NRCYD, 2014). Data provided to the federal government by states show that 23,396 youth (10 percent of all exits) were discharged from foster care to independent living in 2012, although it is unclear from the data how many youth entered independent living voluntarily versus those who were involuntarily discharged because of their age (ACF, 2013c). The data also do not include the number of youth who leave foster care without permission from the child welfare agency and court as they near the age of discharge (i.e., runaways). Anecdotal evidence suggests that some young people labeled as runaways exit foster care for this reason, and some approaching the age of discharge leave care without agency approval to live with members of their family of origin and are recorded in state data systems as "reunified" with their family rather than having aged out of foster care.

Relatively few young people who age out of foster care spent the majority of their childhood in care. A study that examined the placement experiences of youth in foster care on their 16th birthday found that the majority entered care after turning 15, and only 10 percent entered care at age 12 or younger (Wulczyn and Brunner Hislop, 2001); 47 percent of the youth in the study were returned to their families. More youth experienced "other" exits (21 percent, mainly transfers to other child-serving systems, e.g., the juvenile justice system) or ran away from care (19 percent), compared with the 12 percent who aged out.

In summary, the majority of older youth in foster care entered during adolescence, and comparatively few remain in care until officially aging out. Those who do age out generally have lived for many years in troubled homes before child welfare intervention.

Characteristics of Young Adults Aging Out of Foster Care

Research on the health and well-being of current and former foster youth during young adulthood is limited. Nevertheless, studies conducted over the past two decades provide a fairly consistent picture, offering somber evidence of the difficulty of transitioning to adulthood for former foster youth:

---

[4] The terms "emancipation" and "discharge to independent living" are not the same as "legally emancipated minor," which typically describes an individual under age 18 who has been rendered legally independent of control by parents and courts.

- Former foster youth are less likely to graduate from high school than their peers, and they have low rates of college attendance (Cook et al., 1991; Courtney and Dworsky, 2006; Courtney et al., 2001, 2011; Pecora et al., 2005).
- They have more problems with mental health than the general population (Courtney and Dworsky, 2006; Keller et al., 2010; McMillen et al., 2005; Pecora et al., 2005), often experience poorer physical health than other young adults (Ahrens et al., 2010; Courtney and Dworsky, 2006; Courtney et al., 2001), and have been found by most studies to have high rates of drug and alcohol abuse and dependence (Keller et al., 2010; Pecora et al., 2005).
- Compared with the general population, they have a much higher rate of criminal justice system involvement (Courtney and Dworsky, 2006; Courtney et al., 2001, 2011; Cusick et al., 2012).
- They have difficulties achieving financial independence. Compared with the general population, for example, former foster youth have a higher rate of public assistance dependency (Barth, 1990; Cook et al., 1991; Courtney and Dworsky, 2006; Courtney et al., 2001, 2011; Pecora et al., 2005), are more likely to be unemployed (Cook et al., 1991; Courtney and Dworsky, 2006; Courtney et al., 2011; Goerge et al., 2002), have lower wages (Barth, 1990; Cook et al., 1991; Courtney et al., 2011; Dworsky and Courtney, 2001; Goerge et al., 2002; Pecora et al., 2005), and are much more likely to report various economic hardships (Courtney et al., 2011). They also experience high levels of housing instability and homelessness (Cook et al., 1991; Courtney and Dworsky, 2006; Courtney et al., 2001; Dworsky et al., 2013; Pecora et al., 2005).
- They are less likely than their peers to marry or cohabitate (Courtney et al., 2010) but have higher rates of nonmarital parenting (Cook et al., 1991; Courtney and Dworsky, 2006; Courtney et al., 2011); more children (Courtney and Dworsky, 2006; Courtney et al., 2011); and more nonresident children, including those placed in foster care or for adoption (Courtney et al., 2011).

Programs for Young Adults Aging Out of Foster Care

Current federal policy provides several sources of support for youth transitioning to adulthood from foster care: funding for independent living services, education and training vouchers to support postsecondary education for foster youth up to age 23, health insurance through the Medicaid program up to age 26, and partial reimbursement to states for continuation of foster care up to age 21. Federal funding for services intended to help prepare young people in care for adulthood comes through the John H. Chafee Foster Care Independence Program (CFCIP), part of Title IV-E of the Social Security Act. Created in 1999 to address perceived limitations of its predecessor, the Independent Living Initiative of 1986, this program is intended to serve individuals who are likely to stay in care until they age out, those who leave foster care for kinship guardianship or adoption after their 16th birthday, and 18- to 21-year-olds who have aged out (SSA, 2014). The program provides states with $140 million annually in funding for independent living services, including outreach programs for eligible individuals, basic living skills training, education and employment assistance, counseling, case management, and transition planning. States can use up to 30 percent for room and board. The law creating the CFCIP also allowed states to extend eligibility for Medicaid to individuals up to age 21 who had been in foster care, but this policy has been superseded by a provision of the Patient Protection and Affordable Care Act (ACA) discussed below. The CFCIP was amended in 2002 to allow Congress to appropriate up to $60 million annually for vouchers of up to $5,000 per year for postsecondary education and training for individuals up to age 23. CFCIP-eligible youth are eligible for these vouchers. Approximately $44 million is the estimated appropriation for FY 2014 (GSA, 2014a).

The Department of Health and Human Services developed regulations for assessing state performance in managing independent living programs. These regulations established the National Youth in Transition Database (NYTD) and require that states collect data on (1) each youth receiving independent living services through the state agency that administers the CFCIP, and (2) transition outcomes from program-eligible foster youth cohorts at ages 17, 19, and 21. This data collection focuses on six outcome domains: financial self-sufficiency, experience with homelessness, educational attainment, positive connections with adults, high-risk behavior, and access to health insurance (ACF, 2012). States began collecting NYTD data in late 2010 and report data to the federal government semiannually. The NYTD has the potential to become a nationwide longitudinal database for former foster youth (at least through age 21) who are transitioning to adulthood in the United States. Furthermore, the 1999 law establishing the CFCIP sets aside 1.5 percent of funding for rigorous evaluations of promising independent living programs.[5]

The Fostering Connections Act of 2008 extends the foster care entitlement, providing states with the option to continue to provide foster care support until age 21 to individuals who are either "(1) completing secondary education or a program leading to an equivalent credential, (2) enrolled in an institution which provides postsecondary or vocational education,

[5] See p. 356 for a description of the first round of program evaluations conducted under this provision of the law, the Multi-Site Evaluation of Foster Youth Programs.

(3) participating in a program or activity designed to promote, or remove barriers to, employment, (4) employed for at least 80 hours per month, or (5) incapable of doing any of these activities . . . due to a medical condition." Young adults aged 18-21 can "be placed in a supervised setting in which they are living independently, as well as in a foster family home, kinship foster home, or group care facility" (Courtney, 2010, p. 123). States also can continue adoption assistance and/or payments to guardians on behalf of individuals through age 21 if the adoption or guardianship was arranged after the youth turned 16 (Courtney, 2010). In addition, the Fostering Connections Act requires child welfare agencies to help youth and young adults aged 18-21 develop a personalized transition plan during the 90 days immediately before they exit from care between ages 18 and 21. The new law does not alter the CFCIP; states still can use CFCIP funds for a variety of transition services (Courtney, 2010). As of spring 2014, 24 states had federally approved plans for providing foster care past age 18 (Jim Casey Youth Opportunities Initiative, 2014).

Lastly, the ACA requires states to provide, as of January 2014, the full Medicaid benefit available in their state until age 26 to all young adults who were in foster care on their 18th birthday (Emam and Golden, 2014). This provision of the ACA is not affected by the Supreme Court decision allowing states the option of extending Medicaid; in other words, all youth in foster care on their 18th birthday are now eligible for Medicaid in their state of origin up to age 26. States have the option of providing coverage to all foster youth regardless of which state system they have aged out of, but are not required to provide Medicaid benefits to foster youth who have aged out of care in other states.

Evidence for the Effectiveness of Programs for Young Adults Aging Out of Foster Care

Research provides some support for the policy option under the Fostering Connections Act allowing foster youth to remain in care past age 18. Studies relying on differences among states in the age at which youth are discharged from care have shown that extending care to age 21 is associated with increased educational attainment (Courtney et al., 2007), higher earnings (Hook and Courtney, 2011), delayed pregnancy (Dworsky and Courtney, 2010), reduced crime among females (Lee et al., 2012), and delayed homelessness (Dworsky et al., 2013). Studies also indicate that when youth age out of foster care, their health insurance may be discontinued, which contributes to decreases in utilization of physical and mental health services (Courtney et al., 2005b; Kushel et al., 2007; McMillen and Raghavan, 2009).

However, little evidence exists regarding the effectiveness of specific programs and practices targeting young adults aging out of care. Montgomery and colleagues (2006) reviewed evaluation research on the effectiveness of independent living services and found no experimental evaluations; they concluded that the validity of findings from prior nonexperimental evaluations was severely tempered by methodological limitations. More recently, the Administration for Children and Families (ACF) sponsored the Multi-Site Evaluation of Foster Youth Programs, which is part of the evaluation research on independent living programs funded by the CFCIP.[6] This study involved experimental evaluations of classroom-based life skills training, tutoring, employment support, and intensive case management programs for foster youth. Of the four programs evaluated, only the intensive case management program was found to have positive impacts, most notably on youths' enrollment and persistence in college. However, these impacts appeared to be mediated by the program's effect on the probability of youth remaining in care past age 18, implying that the program may have positive impacts only in jurisdictions that have opted to extend care.

Fortunately, the federally supported program of rigorous evaluation of interventions targeting youth aging out of foster care is ongoing. In addition, implementation of the NYTD provisions requiring tracking of transition outcomes by states for foster youth aged 17-21 may help identify strategies for improving foster youths' transitions to adulthood. The NYTD potentially provides data with which to analyze how variation among states in policies and service provision influences transition outcomes.

YOUNG ADULTS IN THE JUSTICE SYSTEM

Involvement in the criminal justice system is a clear marker of marginalization for young people in the United States. As noted in earlier chapters of this report, criminal convictions and incarceration negatively affect young adults' employment, educational attainment, and civic engagement. Moreover, the harm associated with incarceration is borne disproportionately by racial and ethnic minorities, groups likely to experience other forms of social exclusion (NRC, 2014). Unfortunately, high rates of incarceration are common in the United States. A recent National Research Council (NRC) report concludes that "the growth in incarceration rates in the United States over the past 40 years is historically unprecedented and internationally unique" (NRC, 2014, p. 2). That report further concludes that while penal policy over the past four decades may have contributed to a decrease in crime, the magnitude of that decrease is highly uncertain and unlikely to

[6] For more information about the Multi-Site Evaluation of Foster Youth Programs, see http://www.acf.hhs.gov/programs/opre/research/project/multi-site-evaluation-of-foster-youth-programs-chafee-independent-living (accessed October 22, 2014).

have been large, whereas the increase in incarceration is likely to have had a wide range of unwanted social costs. The report recommends that public policy be revised to reduce incarceration, particularly mandatory and long prison sentences, to improve the experience of incarceration and to reduce harm to the families and communities of those who are incarcerated. The recently issued recommendations of an NRC committee studying juvenile justice reform sound a similar note, calling for a shift away from harsh and costly containment and isolation of young people. Instead, that committee recommends that all levels of government contribute to the creation of developmentally appropriate strategies for holding young people accountable for their transgressions while reintegrating them into their families and communities (NRC, 2013).

Characteristics of Young Adults in the Justice System

Millions of young people encounter the criminal justice system each year. Fully 2.7 million young adults aged 18-24 were arrested in 2012 (29 percent of the total number of individuals arrested), along with 1.4 million aged 25-29 (15 percent of the total number arrested) (FBI, 2012). Approximately 410,900 young adults aged 18-24 and 368,800 aged 25-29 were in state or federal prisons or local jails in 2010 (Child Trends, 2012). In addition, 8,875 young adults aged 18-20 were in residential placements operated by the juvenile justice system in 2011 (Sickmund et al., 2013).

Gender, race, and ethnicity are strongly associated with incarceration (NRC, 2014). As noted earlier, young adult males are much more likely than females to be incarcerated; in 2010, among young people aged 18-19, males were almost 16 times more likely than females to be in jail or prison (1.5 percent versus 0.1 percent), and among young adults aged 20-24, the rate of incarceration was nearly 10 times higher for males (2.8 percent) than for females (0.3 percent) (Child Trends, 2012). Black and Hispanic young adults are more likely than their white counterparts to be incarcerated, and this is particularly true for young men. For example, among young men aged 18-19, 3.8 percent of non-Hispanic blacks, 1.5 of Hispanics, and 0.8 percent of non-Hispanic whites were in jail or prison in 2010. Among young men aged 20-24, 8 percent of non-Hispanic blacks, 3.3 percent of Hispanics, and 1.3 percent of whites were incarcerated in 2010. The net result of the association among gender, race, and incarceration is that young black males are particularly likely to be marginalized by incarceration.

Also as noted earlier, many incarcerated young adults are parents, which has implications for both the young adults and their children. In 2007, for example, an estimated 44.1 percent of adults aged 24 or younger in state prisons (43.5 percent of men, 55.4 percent of women) and 45.8 percent of that age group in federal prisons (45.7 percent of men, 47.5 percent of women) were parents (Glaze and Maruschak, 2008). Research on the impact of parental incarceration on parents and their children has not focused on incarcerated young adults. Nevertheless, research on the broader population has found that parental incarceration is associated with instability in male-female unions, family economic hardship, reductions in fathers' involvement in their children's lives, and increased child behavior problems (NRC, 2014).

Young adults involved with the justice system exhibit other characteristics that put them at risk of social marginalization, including mental health problems and drug use, dependence, and abuse. Research has consistently reported high rates (ranging from 20 to 64 percent) of later criminal offense for youth who received public mental health services (Pullmann, 2010). Moreover, studies of state and federal corrections facilities in 2004 and local jails in 2002 found that an estimated 62.6 percent of individuals in state prisons, 57.8 percent of those in federal prisons, and 70.3 percent of those in county jails had a mental health problem (James and Glaze, 2006). In those studies, mental health problems included a recent clinical diagnosis or treatment by a mental health professional and/or recent self-reported symptoms of depression, mania, or psychotic disorders based on the criteria in the *Diagnostic and Statistical Manual of Mental Disorders*, Fourth Edition (DSM-IV). Young adults were more likely than any other prisoner age group to report a mental health problem (James and Glaze, 2006).

Young adults also are more likely than older adults to report use of illegal drugs immediately prior to incarceration. In 2004, 66.2 percent of prisoners in state and federal prisons reported using illegal drugs in the month prior to the offense that led to their incarceration (Mumola and Karberg, 2006). Similarly, approximately 53 percent of state and 45 percent of federal prisoners reported meeting DSM-IV criteria for drug dependence or abuse during the 12 months prior to their admission to prison. While these data were not reported for specific age groups, given the higher rate of drug use by young adults relative to other age groups (see Chapters 2 and 6), it is likely that their rates of drug dependence and abuse are comparable to if not higher than those of the overall prison population.

Of course, one of the most important characteristics of young adults involved with the justice system is that, left on their own, most would soon desist from criminal behavior. Social and behavioral scientists have long acknowledged the "age-crime curve," which illustrates that various forms of antisocial behavior peak in late adolescence and decline rapidly in early adulthood (Farrington, 1986; Hirschi and Gottfredson, 1983; Loeber et al., 2012; Moffitt, 1993; Steinberg, 2013). Figure 8-1 provides some examples of the age-crime curve using Federal Bureau of Investigation arrest data (Steinberg, 2013). It shows a consistent relationship between age and crime; the shape of the curve is similar across time periods and different

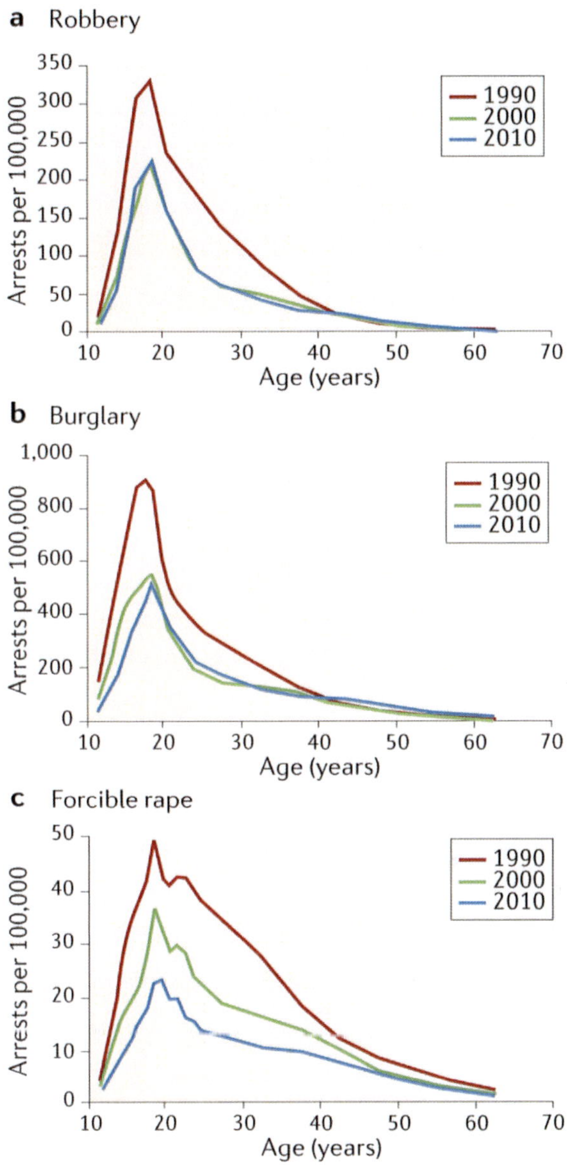

FIGURE 8-1 The age-crime curve.
SOURCE: Steinberg, 2013, reprinted with permission.

types of offence, including robbery, burglary, and forcible rape. Theories explaining this phenomenon have evolved over the past three decades, and recent research suggests that the age at which involvement in crime peaks is influenced by a variety of individual characteristics and conditions, varying to some extent across offenses (Loeber et al., 2012). Nevertheless, those adolescents who begin committing crimes when they are older generally desist from crime as they become adults, and social scientists attribute this pattern primarily to normative developmental processes regarding middle-adolescence peaks in deviancy and sensation seeking, as well as cognitive maturation. Thus, lengthy mandatory sentences and other long-lasting or permanent forms of punishment for criminal behavior by young people (e.g., ineligibility for public welfare benefits and for financial aid for post-secondary education) run counter to current understanding of the relationship between age and crime (NRC, 2013).

Jurisdictional Issues for Young Adults

Young adults who are age 18 and over when charged with a criminal law violation are under the authority of the adult criminal justice system in all states. However, young adults can in some states remain under the jurisdiction of the juvenile courts past the age of 18, and young people can in some places enter the adult criminal justice system as minors. In most states, for example, juvenile courts can retain authority over youth for dispositional purposes in delinquency matters until age 20, and in 4 states this authority extends through age 24 (OJJDP, 2013a). In addition, in certain states, juvenile courts have original authority over cases such as those involving status offenses, abuse, neglect, and dependency matters for those over 18, often through age 20 (OJJDP, 2012). While 39 states limit the original jurisdiction of juvenile courts in criminal matters to youth under age 18, in some states the original jurisdiction of the juvenile court is restricted to youth under age 16. In other words, in such states prosecutions for criminal offenses routinely occur in adult criminal courts rather than juvenile courts for defendants as young as 16. In addition, all states have laws that allow or require criminal prosecution in adult courts for some offenders who are younger than the juvenile side of the jurisdictional age line (Adams and Addie, 2014). Although the precise number of such transfers of juvenile offenders to adult courts is unknown, the practice has become more common in recent years (Griffin et al., 2011).

Recognition of the unique developmental needs of young adults has led some states to create policies and programs specifically for this age group. For example, some states have laws that treat individuals aged 18-21 within a special category that has various names, including "youthful offenders" and "young adult offenders." For a review of these laws, see Velázquez

(2013). In addition, some states, such as Pennsylvania, have created special corrections facilities for young adults (Loeber et al., 2013).

The U.S. Department of Justice sponsored a Study Group on the Transitions between Juvenile Delinquency and Adult Crime, which focused on ages approximately 15-29 (Loeber et al., 2013). The authors conclude that "young adult offenders aged 18-24 are more similar to juveniles than to adults with respect to their offending, maturation, and life circumstances" (p. 20).

Programs for Young Adults Involved in the Justice System

The federal role in the criminal justice system is limited. For example, federal prisons housed only 216,900 (9.7 percent) of the 2,228,400 inmates in state or federal prisons or in local jails in 2012 (Glaze and Herberman, 2013). Moreover, few federal programs specifically target young adults who are involved in the justice system. The majority of federal programs for justice-involved young adults serve them either alongside adolescents in the juvenile justice system or alongside the general adult population in the criminal justice system. In both of the latter cases, there are virtually no data on what proportion of the population served are young adults or on program effectiveness and outcomes specifically for this age group. We describe here selected federal programs that, among other things, are explicitly intended to assist young adults involved with the justice system.

Several programs of the U.S. Department of Justice's Office of Juvenile Justice and Delinquency Prevention (OJJDP) include a focus on key outcomes for young adults, such as employment; education; housing stability; safety; health, including avoidance of risk behaviors; connections to responsible adults; and effective parenting. These programs are more directly relevant to young adults than programs that target at-risk minors to prevent them from becoming involved in the juvenile justice system. OJJDP provides formula grants to support "efforts related to delinquency prevention and reduction, juvenile justice system improvement, research, evaluation, statistical analysis, and training and technical assistance in all 50 States, the District of Columbia, and the 5 U.S. territories" (OJJDP, 2009a, p. 1). States provide subgrants to local government and private agencies and to American Indian tribes. Program areas include mental health, substance abuse, education, and job training. In federal FY 2012, $33 million was obligated, with a 10 percent matching requirement; in federal FY 2013 and 2014, an estimated $41 million and $70 million was obligated, respectively (GSA, 2014c).

OJJDP also provides funding to states through the Juvenile Accountability Block Grant (JABG) program. The aim of this program is to "hold youth accountable for delinquent behavior through the imposition of graduated sanctions that are consistent with the severity of the offense" and "strengthen the juvenile justice system's capacity to process cases efficiently and work with community partners to keep youth from reoffending" (OJJDP, 2009b, p. 1). Target areas that are relevant to key outcomes for young adults include a variety of school-related behaviors, job skills and employment status, family relationships and functioning, and substance use (OJJDP, 2013c). In federal FY 2013, $23 million was obligated, with a 10 percent matching requirement; in federal FY 2014 and 2015, an estimated $30 million per year was obligated (GSA, 2014b).

Several components of the Title V Community Prevention Grants Program are directly relevant to key outcomes for young adults, including community-based programs that provide job training and mental health and substance abuse services (OJJDP, 2013d). In addition to the block and formula grants programs, various OJJDP discretionary programs are relevant, including the Second Chance Act Grant Program, mentoring programs, and programs for tribal youth.

Program data and performance measures collected on these programs through OJJDP's reporting system provide information on how many of the grantees serve young adults aged 18 and older (OJJDP, 2014). For the formula grants described above, data from the most recent reporting period indicate that 139 of 280 grantees served young adults over age 18 (OJJDP, 2013b). Data from the most recent reporting period of the JABG program indicate that 215 of 242 grantees served young adults over age 18 (OJJDP, 2013c). However, these data do not break out information on the number or characteristics of young adults served, nor do they break out performance measures by age group.

In addition to OJJDP-funded programs, several other federally funded programs include justice system-involved young adults among their target populations. The Reintegration of Ex-Offenders program, administered by the U.S. Department of Labor's Employment Training Administration (ETA), includes programs aimed at both youthful offenders and adults (DOL, 2014). The youthful offenders program targets youth and young adults aged 14-24 who have been involved in the juvenile justice system but not the adult criminal justice system, and in some cases limits participation to those aged 18-24. The adult program serves individuals aged 18 and older who have been convicted and imprisoned within the adult criminal justice system. This program is intended to reduce recidivism by supporting employment, vocational training and educational interventions, and mentoring. Housing and substance abuse treatment are not provided using ETA funds. Through a competitive grants process, ETA offers funding to community- and faith-based organizations that provide services to ex-offenders. The ultimate goal is to use effectiveness evaluations of these demonstration and pilot programs to inform the development of state and local programs that can improve ex-offenders' workforce outcomes. In federal FY 2013, $79 million was obligated; estimated amounts for federal FY 2014 and 2015 are $74 million and $78 million, respectively (GSA, 2014d). An experimental impact evaluation of this program is being conducted, focused exclusively on those over 18 who have been convicted and imprisoned as adults, but results have yet to be reported (Leshnick et al., 2012).

Job Corps, administered by the U.S. Department of Labor, offers high school education, vocational training, and health care to low-income, at-risk youth and young adults aged 16-24. In the 2011 program year, more than 43,000 young adults aged 18-24 participated, representing 79.2 percent of a total 55,000 participants (Job Corps, 2012). Job Corps does not explicitly target justice-involved young adults; in fact, a condition of eligibility is that the person not have face-to-face court or institutional supervision or court-imposed fines during the time he or she participates in the program (Job Corps, 2013). However, according to a review by Welsh and colleagues (2013) examining job training and education programs for at-risk youth, Job Corps has demonstrated modest benefits for participants in the areas of reduced criminal activity, improved educational attainment, and increased earnings (Schochet et al., 2008; Welsh et al., 2013).

YouthBuild is another program administered by the U.S. Department of Labor that includes young adults with justice system involvement as a target population (YouthBuild USA, 2014d). Participants work full-time for 6-24 months toward their General Educational Development (GED) credential or high school diploma in YouthBuild programs while learning job skills by building affordable housing. YouthBuild's program philosophy emphasizes leadership development, community service, and creation of a community of adults and youth committed to each other's success. The program is intended to place young people in college, jobs, or both at program exit. A participant must be aged 16-24 at entrance, and at least 75 percent of participants in a YouthBuild site must have dropped out of high school and belong to one of the program's target populations, which include

- youthful offenders,
- adult offenders,
- current and former foster youth,
- youth with disabilities,
- migrant farm worker youth,
- children with an incarcerated parent, and
- low-income youth.

While offenders are a target population for YouthBuild, only about one-third of program participants are court involved (YouthBuild USA, 2014a). In addition, the waiver of eligibility criteria for up to 25 percent of program participants and the imposition of additional optional program eligibility criteria, such as minimum reading level and drug testing, by some YouthBuild sites likely results in the exclusion of many difficult-to-serve young adults.

Currently there are 264 YouthBuild programs across 46 states, the District of Columbia, and the Virgin Islands (YouthBuild USA, 2014d). These programs engage approximately 10,000 participants per year (YouthBuild USA, 2014d), predominantly men (71 percent), and a large proportion (53 percent) are African American (YouthBuild USA, 2014a). In federal FY 2013, $72 million was obligated; estimated amounts for FY 2014 and 2015 are $75 million and $74 million, respectively (GSA, 2014f). YouthBuild program administrative data indicate that in 2010, 78 percent of participants completed the program, 63 percent of these obtained their GED credential or high school diploma, and three-fifths were placed in college or in jobs with an average wage of $9.20/hour (YouthBuild USA, 2014a). The Department of Labor commissioned an evaluation of YouthBuild in 2010; results are expected in 2017 (Mathematica Policy Research, 2014; MDRC, 2014).

In addition to its core program, YouthBuild is implementing an initiative aimed at young people aged 16-24 who have been in the juvenile justice system. The SMART (Start Making a Real Transformation) initiative enhances YouthBuild's core program model with additional program elements such as mentoring, flexible programming, alternative career tracks, and community-based crime and violence prevention activities (YouthBuild USA, 2014c). The U.S. Department of Labor has provided $8.5 million toward this demonstration program, which currently serves more than 550 youth across nine sites.

The National Forum on Youth Violence Prevention brings together communities and federal agencies—including the U.S. Departments of Justice, Education, Health and Human Services, Housing and Urban Development (HUD), and Labor and the Office of National Drug Control Policy—to address youth and gang violence in the United States. As of March 2014, 10 communities were involved in the forum: Boston, Camden, Chicago, Detroit, Memphis, Minneapolis, New Orleans, Philadelphia, Salinas, and San Jose (FindYouthInfo, 2014). The foundational strategy document for the forum states that "strategies should include prevention efforts spanning from early childhood into young adulthood, such as youth development, family support, school and community mentoring, and school-based and out-of-school recreational activities" (National Forum on Youth Violence Prevention, 2011, p. 7). However, the extent to which any or all of the participating communities have focused a significant part of their efforts on young adults is unclear.

Lastly, various federal programs serve adults in the criminal justice system and upon reentry into the community. These programs include the Reintegration of Ex-Offenders program, described above, and U.S. Department of Justice programs such as the Second Chance Act Prisoner Reentry Initiative and the Serious and Violent Offender Reentry Initiative. The Second Chance Act Prisoner Reentry Initiative provides funding for "state, tribal, and local reentry courts; family-based substance abuse treatment; evaluate and improve education at prisons, jails, and juvenile facilities; technology careers training demonstration grants; offender reentry substance abuse and criminal justice collaboration; adult and juvenile demonstration; [and] mentoring grants to nonprofit organizations" (GSA, 2014e, p. 1). In federal FY 2013, $63 million was obligated; in federal FY 2014 and 2015, an estimated $68 and $115 million was obligated, respectively (GSA, 2014e).

This overview reveals that justice-involved young adults are eligible for many programs—juvenile and adult—that provide services relevant to the key outcomes for this age group, such as avoidance of further justice system involvement, employment skills, and education. With the exception of a small number of programs that target young adults, however, little is known about the size of the young adult population served by these programs and how much of the program funding is spent on this population. Even less is known about whether these programs improve outcomes for young adults. Moreover, some of these programs apply eligibility criteria that exclude many young adults in the greatest need of assistance.

Evidence for the Effectiveness of Programs for Young Adults in the Justice System

With the exception of Job Corps, evidence for the impact of the major federally supported programs described above on the health and well-being of young adults is sparse. However, since the programs have yet to be subjected to rigorous evaluation, and available program data seldom distinguish young adults from other populations served, this lack of evidence should not lead one to conclude that these government investments have had no impact on young adults. Moreover, a variety of interventions other than those currently funded by the federal government may improve the health and well-being of young adults. A recent review of the effectiveness of prevention and intervention programs was conducted for the National Institute of Justice Study Group on the Transitions between Juvenile Delinquency and Adult Crime to assess the impact of these programs on individuals in the transitional period between adolescence and young adulthood (Welsh et al., 2013). The primary focus of the review was on serious offending in young adulthood, but it included other outcomes as well, focusing on

- "Programs implemented during the later juvenile years (ages 15-17) that have measured the impact on offending in early adulthood (ages 18-29)
- Programs implemented in early adulthood that have measured the impact on offending up to age 29
- Programs implemented in early childhood that have measured the impact on offending in early adulthood." (Welsh et al., 2013, pp. 4-5)

The review assessed the impacts of prevention and intervention programs focused on family, peers and community, school, the labor market, and the individual. The authors conclude that "there is a paucity of high-quality evaluations of programs that have measured the impact on offending in early adulthood" (Welsh et al., 2013, p. 33). They identified certain promising early prevention programs in preschools and schools that appear to impact offending and other important outcomes into the young adult years. They also found some promising family-based interventions for adjudicated delinquents (but operating in an environment outside of the juvenile justice system) that reduce offending in young adulthood. With the exception of the Job Corps study described above, Welsh and colleagues did not identify programs implemented exclusively in young adulthood that impact offending up to age 29. However, they did find that "the available evidence about intervention modalities used with both juvenile and adult offenders indicates that their effects are substantially similar. This generality across the major age divide in juvenile and criminal justice implies that such programs should be effective with young adult offenders as well" (Welsh et al., 2013, p. 34). The four broad intervention modalities they identified that had positive effects were (1) cognitive-behavioral therapy; (2) educational, vocational, and employment programs; (3) drug treatment; and (4) treatment for sex offenders. They also found that for both adolescents and adults, "sanctions and incarceration appear to have essentially negligible or slightly undesirable effects" (Welsh et al., 2013, p. 29).

HOMELESS YOUNG ADULTS

Many young adults spend time with no stable residence, living on the streets or "couch surfing" from one unstable living arrangement to another. Unfortunately, no reasonably current and reliable data are available regarding the size and characteristics of the homeless young adult population nationally. Moreover, studies of local populations vary in their definition of homelessness and often include adolescents and older adults, making it difficult to draw conclusions about the size and needs of the population of homeless young adults.

Characteristics of Homeless Young Adults

Estimates of the size of the population of homeless young adults range widely; for example, estimates of the number of young adults aged 18-24 who experience a homelessness episode each year vary from about 750,000 to 2 million (Ammerman et al., 2004). However, most estimates are based on extrapolations from studies of local populations and the number of individuals who come into contact with providers of homeless services. The most recent national estimate based on data from service providers comes from the 2013 Annual Homeless Assessment Report to Congress from the HUD (2013). This estimate is based on a point-in-time count of the number of sheltered and unsheltered homeless people derived from reports from Continuums of Care, local planning bodies responsible for coordinating homelessness services within HUD-defined geographic areas. According to HUD, there were 610,042 homeless individuals on a given night in January 2013, 65 percent of whom were living in emergency shelters or transitional housing and 35 percent of whom were living in unsheltered locations. Ten percent of these individuals (61,541) were aged 18-24. About two-thirds of these young adults (40,727) were unaccompanied youth (i.e., they were not a part of a family during their homeless spell), half of whom were unsheltered at the time (HUD, 2013). Using HUD data on young adults reported in adult emergency shelter or transitional housing programs (i.e., excluding unsheltered youth), the National Alliance to End Homelessness estimated that approximately 150,000 youth aged 18-24 utilized these services at some point during 2011 (National Alliance to End Homelessness, 2012).

Although many studies of homeless youth include both minors and young adults and rely on convenience samples or samples drawn from local populations of service recipients, the available research supports the following general conclusions regarding the vulnerability experienced by homeless young people (see, e.g., Burt et al., 1999; Hagan and McCarthy, 2005; Toro et al., 2007; Whitbeck, 2009):

- They are likely to have grown up in a low-income family.
- Their family relationships are likely to be strained or nonexistent.
- They are likely to have experienced childhood maltreatment and trauma.
- Many experience physical and sexual victimization into adulthood.
- They experience high rates of mental and behavioral health problems.

- They are likely to engage in risky sexual behavior.
- Many become parents at an early age.
- They are likely to be unemployed and work outside of the legal economy.
- They lag behind their peers in educational attainment.

Not surprisingly, these young people also are likely to have come into contact with other systems that serve vulnerable young adults (e.g., the foster care and criminal justice systems).

Programs for Homeless Young Adults

The Runaway and Homeless Youth Act (RHYA) is the primary source of federal support for services to homeless young adults, although some of the programs funded by the act focus primarily on homeless minors (Fernandes-Alcantara, 2013). The Runaway and Homeless Youth Program,[7] administered by the Family and Youth Services Bureau within the U.S. Department of Health and Human Services' ACF, supports street outreach, emergency shelters, and transitional living and maternity group home programs for young people at risk of or experiencing homelessness. These programs are operated by public and private social service agencies and federally recognized tribes. The RHYA programs received approximately $110 million in FY 2013 (National Alliance to End Homelessness, 2013). Each of these programs is described below.

Basic Center Program (BCP)

The BCP provides youth and their families with short-term shelter and services. In FY 2013, a total of $45.1 million was allocated to 303 BCP-funded centers—about $150,000 per center (ACF, 2014b). The centers provide emergency shelter, food, clothing, counseling, and referrals to health care providers for youth up to age 18. The majority of centers provide up to 20 youth with 21 days of shelter. BCP-funded centers focus on reuniting young people with their families or locating appropriate alternative placements when reunification is not possible. Some centers offer street-based services, home-based services, and substance abuse education and prevention services for homeless young adults older than 18 (Fernandes-Alcantara, 2013). BCP centers were designed to offer these services outside of the law

---

[7] For more information about the Runaway and Homeless Youth Program, see the ACF program website: http://www.acf.hhs.gov/programs/fysb/programs/runaway-homeless-youth/about (accessed October 22, 2014).

enforcement, juvenile justice, child welfare, and mental health systems, although centers conduct outreach to these systems to identify eligible youth.

In 2011, BCP centers reported serving 38,758 youth with preventive or shelter services (ACF, 2013a). Slightly more than half of these youth were female. African Americans and Native Americans were overrepresented among the youth served relative to their proportions of the general population. According to data from the Runaway and Homeless Youth Management Information System, or RHYMIS, lesbian, gay, bisexual, and questioning youth make up about 6-7 percent of BCP-served youth, although program providers believe these figures may understate the prevalence of sexual minority youth served by their programs (ACF, 2013a).

Transitional Living Program (TLP)

The TLP supports programs that provide long-term (up to 21 months) residential services to homeless youth aged 16-22. Youth who are pregnant or parenting are eligible for TLP services (see the description of the Maternity Group Home [MGH] Program below). In FY 2013, 206 programs received a total of $37.2 million—about $180,000 per program (ACF, 2014c). TLP grantees may shelter up to 20 youth in a variety of settings, including host family homes, maternity homes, apartments supervised and owned by a social service agency, or apartments rented with agency assistance (ACF, 2013a). TLP providers are required to provide young people with the following services: safe and stable living accommodations, basic life-skills building, interpersonal skills building, education and employment services, substance abuse counseling, mental health care, and physical health care. In 2011, the TLP served a total of 4,104 young people (ACF, 2013a). More than half of the youth served are 18 or 19 when they enter a shelter. About 60 percent of program participants are female, while African Americans, Native Americans, and Native Hawaiians and Pacific Islanders are overrepresented relative to their proportions of the general population. Based on RHYMIS data, lesbian, gay, bisexual, and questioning youth make up about one-tenth of the young people served by TLP providers. About 30 percent of youth served, both male and female, were pregnant or parenting when they entered the program.

The MGH Program, funded by ACF through the TLP, provides services for up to 21 months to homeless young people aged 16-22 who are pregnant or parenting and their dependent children (ACF, 2013a). In addition to standard TLP services, the MGH Program offers services designed to help young people improve their parenting skills, knowledge of child development, family budgeting, and health and nutrition, as well as access affordable child care and early childhood education services.

Street Outreach Program (SOP)

The SOP targets runaway and homeless young people living on the streets or in areas that increase their risk of being subjected to sexual abuse or exploitation. The program is intended to help youth transition to safe and appropriate living arrangements (ACF, 2013b). Services include street-based education and outreach, crisis intervention, access to emergency shelter, needs assessments, treatment and counseling, information and referrals to other services, prevention and education activities, and follow-up. In FY 2013, 107 SOPs received a total of $14.8 million—about $138,000 per program (ACF, 2013b). Outreach workers do not collect detailed information about the demographic characteristics of youth served, and the program cannot provide unduplicated counts of the number of youth served, but the 155 grantees funded through the program in 2011 reported making 693,270 contacts with youth that year (ACF, 2013a).

Other Programs Providing Assistance to Homeless Young Adults

A variety of other federal programs that do not specifically target young people undoubtedly provide assistance to homeless young adults. Federally funded programs for which at least some homeless young adults are eligible include Continuum of Care programs; the Emergency Shelter Grants program; the Housing Opportunities for Persons with AIDS program; Veterans Affairs Supportive Housing; the Community Development Block Grants program; the Housing Choice Voucher program (Section 8, for which youth aging out of foster care are a targeted population under the Family Unification Program); the Public Housing program; and Section 811 Supportive Housing for Persons with Disabilities. With the exception of the annual point-in-time survey conducted by Continuum of Care providers described above, however, data are not readily available on the numbers of young adults served by these programs. States and localities also fund a variety of programs that provide assistance to young adults, but the size of the populations served and the amount of funding for such services are unknown.

In summary, while no reliable data exist regarding the size of the homeless young adult population, available data on service receipt indicate that at least several hundred thousand homeless young people come to the attention of federally funded service providers each year. Moreover, service providers report turning away many homeless youth in need of assistance, and studies of homeless youth populations indicate that many of these youth do not access services, suggesting that the number of homeless young adults is much higher than counts of service recipients would indicate (Fernandes-Alcantara, 2013; Toro et al., 2007). Homeless young adults also exhibit many indicators of marginality beyond their lack of residential stability. Lastly, while the exact amount spent on federally and state-funded services for homeless young adults is unknown, it is certainly in the tens of millions of dollars per year.

Evidence for the Effectiveness of Programs for Homeless Young Adults

Little is known about the effectiveness of federally funded programs for homeless young adults. While ACF is in the process of establishing performance standards for RHYA programs and improving its data collection system to monitor key program outcomes, there are as yet no reliable data on postprogram participation outcomes for young people served by these programs. Nor are data available on outcomes for young adults served by other federal programs.

Moreover, research on the effectiveness of interventions targeting homeless youth,[8] while identifying promising programs, has failed to establish the effectiveness of programs in improving outcomes for young adults. Reviews of the evaluation literature conclude that rigorous evaluation of services for homeless youth is sorely needed (see, e.g., Altena et al., 2010; Slesnick et al., 2009; Toro et al., 2007). Knowledge of the effectiveness of these services is limited by the poor quality and small number of intervention studies and the heterogeneity of interventions, participants, research methods, and outcomes assessed.

YOUNG PARENTS

As noted in Chapter 3, given that about half of all first births are to women aged 26 or younger, it is not at all unusual for young adults to be parents (Martin et al., 2013). Nevertheless, while many young parents thrive personally and are able to parent their children effectively, having children early is a marker of vulnerability for many young adults, as well as their children.

Characteristics of Young Parents

On average, young parents are more likely than older parents to be raising children under circumstances that pose risks to themselves and to the future of their children, as described below. About two-thirds of parents under age 25 are single parents, making them more than twice as likely as older parents to be leading a single-parent household (Vespa et al., 2013).

---

[8] Almost all evaluation research on homeless youth has focused exclusively or primarily on homeless minors rather than homeless young adults.

And of course, by virtue of their place in the life course, they are more likely than older parents to be parenting young children.

Being a parent and having young children both are associated with an increased likelihood of living in poverty during early adulthood, particularly for single parents. For example, families headed by young adults aged 18-24, especially single-mother families,[9] have higher rates of poverty than families headed by individuals 25 and older (Redd et al., 2011). The poverty rate for families with single mothers aged 18-24 as the head of household was 67 percent in 2010, compared with 27.9 percent among married-couple families of the same age (Redd et al., 2011). Moreover, single mothers aged 18-24 were much more likely to live in poverty than single mothers aged 25-34 (48.7 percent), 35-44 (33.8 percent), or 45-54 (30.1 percent). Having young children also is associated with living in poverty (Redd et al., 2011). Higher rates of poverty have been found in families with children under age 6 compared with all families with children under age 18. This is especially true for families headed by single mothers; in 2010, 54 percent of families headed by single mothers with children under age 6 lived in poverty, compared with 40.7 percent of families headed by single mothers with children under age 18 (Redd et al., 2011).

Programs for Young Parents

While young parents are served by a wide variety of government programs, we focus here on three federally supported programs: TANF, the Supplemental Nutrition Assistance Program (SNAP), and the Special Supplemental Nutrition Program for Women, Infants, and Children (WIC). These programs, while not targeting young adults, nevertheless serve a large number of low-income young parents. Moreover, young parents make up a significant proportion of the service population of each.

TANF

TANF is intended to help needy families achieve economic self-sufficiency. The TANF block grant provides states funding with which to design and operate programs that accomplish one of the following four purposes:

- provide assistance to needy families so children can be cared for in their own homes;
- reduce the reliance of needy parents on public aid by promoting job preparation, work, and marriage;

[9] Single mothers accounted for 95 percent of all single parents under age 25 in 2012 (Vespa et al., 2013).

- prevent and reduce nonmarital pregnancies; and
- encourage the formation and maintenance of two-parent families (ACF, 2014a).

The TANF block grant was funded at $16.5 billion in FY 2013 (Falk, 2013). To receive federal TANF funds, states must contribute at least $10.4 billion of their own funds under a maintenance-of-effort (MOE) requirement.

TANF funds may be used broadly for the purposes described above. In FY 2012, $31.4 billion of both federal TANF and state MOE funds was either expended for TANF program purposes or transferred to other block grant programs (e.g., the Child Care and Development Block Grant or Social Services Block Grant) (Falk, 2013). In contrast with its predecessor Aid to Families with Dependent Children (AFDC) program, most TANF funds are not used for cash assistance to low-income parents and their children (Falk, 2013). Funding for basic assistance, which most closely reflects cash assistance, was $9 billion in FY 2012, or 28.6 percent of total TANF and MOE dollars. TANF is a major source of funding for child care for low-income parents. In FY 2012, 16.0 percent of TANF funds was spent on child care or transferred to the child care block grant (Falk, 2013). TANF also is a major source of funding for state child welfare systems, although the TANF accounting system is poor at capturing expenditures that are associated with child welfare services. States use TANF funds for foster care, kinship foster care, adoption assistance, and services to families with children who have been maltreated or are at risk of maltreatment. Most TANF funding for child welfare programs is subsumed in the "other" spending category, which accounted for 31 percent of TANF and state MOE spending in FY 2012 (Falk, 2013). A survey of state child welfare agencies found that TANF funds accounted for 20 percent of total federal, state, and local expenditures on child welfare programs in FY 2004 (Scarcella et al., 2006). The remainder of TANF and MOE funds expended in FY 2012 went to "other work supports" (9.6 percent), administration (7.2 percent), and "work expenditures" (6.9 percent) (Falk, 2013). Because TANF is a fixed block grant, its value has declined considerably over time; the inflation-adjusted value of the TANF block grant declined by 30.1 percent between 1997, its first full year of operation, and 2012 (Falk, 2013).

Individuals living in a household that receives TANF support are either considered "work-eligible" or exempted from the work requirements of the law. The latter group includes primarily adult nonrecipients who are non-parental caregivers of TANF-eligible children (e.g., a grandparent, aunt, or uncle). TANF provides assistance to some of the most disadvantaged American families (Falk, 2012). In FY 2009, for example, two-thirds of families with work-eligible individuals that received TANF cash assistance reported no other source of cash income. Even including their TANF benefits, more than three-quarters of these families had incomes below 50 percent of the federal poverty level (Falk, 2012).

Although data are unavailable on the ages of all TANF recipients who are not work eligible, states provide the federal government with some demographic information on work-eligible program participants (Falk, 2012). A large proportion of adult TANF program participants are young adults; in FY 2009 nearly one-third (32.2 percent) of work-eligible individuals receiving TANF were under age 25, and more than half (54 percent) were under 30 (Falk, 2012). In FY 2009, 85 percent of work-eligible individuals were women, 73 percent of whom had never been married. Racial and ethnic minorities (African Americans and Hispanics) made up a majority of TANF work-eligible individuals. More than two-fifths (43 percent) of work-eligible TANF participants lacked a high school diploma or equivalent.

SNAP

SNAP provides food-purchasing assistance for low-income people. Formerly known as the Food Stamp program, it is an entitlement program administered by the U.S. Department of Agriculture (USDA), although benefits are distributed by state government agencies. SNAP is the nation's largest nutrition assistance program, having served an average of 47.6 million people per month in 2013 and providing a total of $76 billion in benefits over the course of the fiscal year (USDA, 2014b). The average monthly benefit per individual in FY 2013 was $133.07. Actual food stamps were phased out starting in the late 1990s, and today states provide SNAP benefits through the Electronic Benefit Transfer (EBT) debit card system (USDA, 2013a). Households may use the benefits, which are deposited directly into their accounts, to pay for food at eligible food retailers.

A household's size, income, and expenses help determine the amount of assistance the household receives (USDA, 2014a). In addition, able-bodied working adults aged 18-50 without dependents only receive SNAP benefits for 3 months in a 36-month period if they do not work or take part in a workfare or employment and training program. States currently are allowed to waive this requirement for unemployed working-age adults without children in specific areas with high unemployment rates. In general, able-bodied individuals aged 16-60 must register for work, accept reasonable employment, and take part in employment and training programs they are referred to by local SNAP offices or risk disqualification from the program.

Despite the work requirements that limit SNAP assistance for adults without children, young adults make up a significant proportion of SNAP beneficiaries. In 2011, an average of 4.3 million low-income young adults aged 18-24 received SNAP benefits each month (Lower-Basch, 2013). Approximately 2.7 million of these young adults were living in households with minor children.

WIC

Like SNAP, WIC is administered by USDA, although unlike SNAP it is not an entitlement program. WIC provides benefits to eligible pregnant, breastfeeding, and postpartum women; infants; and children up to age 5 (USDA, 2013b). To be eligible, individuals must be at nutritional risk and have a family income of less than 185 percent of the federal poverty level. Participants in other benefit programs, including SNAP, Medicaid, and TANF, automatically meet the WIC income eligibility requirement. WIC is intended to improve fetal development and reduce the incidence of low birth weight, short gestation, and anemia during the prenatal period for pregnant women and their unborn children. It also is intended to provide nutritious foods during critical times of growth and development for infants and young children to improve their health and prevent health problems. WIC benefits include supplemental foods, nutrition education and counseling (including breastfeeding promotion and support), and referrals to health and social service providers. Eligible applicants can purchase specific types of food (for example, milk, juice, and cereal) from participating retail vendors at no charge using vouchers, checks, or EBT cards. WIC expenditures in FY 2012 totaled $6.8 billion (Johnson et al., 2013); 9.7 million participants were enrolled in WIC in April 2012 (Johnson et al., 2013). Available program data do not provide estimates of the young adult population participating in WIC, but 85.9 percent of all women participants were aged 18-34.

Evidence for the Effectiveness of Programs for Young Parents

Estimating the effects of TANF on young parents is complicated by several factors. First, nearly all studies of the employment and antipoverty effects of TANF are quite dated. This means that outcomes generally were measured when the employment rate of young adults was quite different from what it has been in recent years and before the program's federal work requirements were significantly revised. Second, much of the research on TANF considers how replacing the individual entitlement to cash assistance in place prior to 1996 with today's work-based welfare program has influenced such outcomes as parental employment, earnings and poverty, material hardship, and child well-being. While those studies help inform debates over the wisdom of the fundamental change in the social safety net occasioned by welfare reform, they provide little or no information about whether the current TANF program helps the families it serves gain employment or otherwise improve their well-being. Nor do data collected by state TANF programs provide this information, if for no other reason than that TANF administrative data provide no information on postprogram outcomes. Third, the federal government gives states such discretion in operating TANF that it is more a flexible funding stream than a distinct program whose outcomes can be evaluated. Lastly, even the few studies that have sought to evaluate approaches to TANF provision do not provide information about young adults as a distinct population.

For these and other reasons, research has shed little light on whether the TANF program improves the employment and economic well-being of young parents, but its impact is likely minimal. While there have been many studies of the labor supply disincentive effects of the old cash assistance program (Danziger et al., 1981; Moffitt, 1992), TANF differs from a classic means-tested cash assistance program because of the potential work incentives provided by its work requirements and time limits. Unfortunately, there have been no studies of the labor supply effects of the current TANF program in terms of its impact on the hours current recipients would work in the program's absence (Ben-Shalom et al., 2011). And while analyses of the effects of TANF on poverty have not distinguished young adults from the broader population of parents, the estimated effects for low-income parents in general are small (Ben-Shalom et al., 2011).

The reduction in the size of the TANF caseload also has implications for the program's likely impact on young adults. Because state TANF caseloads have declined considerably since AFDC was replaced by TANF, fewer low-income families have been in a position to benefit from TANF as time has passed. For example, approximately 68 percent of families in the United States with children living in poverty received cash assistance through AFDC in 1996, but by 2010 only 27 percent of such families were receiving cash assistance through TANF (Trisi and Pavetti, 2012). Moreover, as the TANF caseload has declined, it appears to have increasingly comprised parents with significant obstacles to obtaining and maintaining employment, including low educational attainment, health problems, learning disabilities, histories of domestic violence, mental health disorders, substance abuse, and involvement with child protection authorities (Blank, 2007; Courtney et al., 2005a; Dworsky et al., 2007). Whether TANF is optimally designed for such needy populations is questionable, but many young adult parents exhibit these obstacles to employment.

An important measure of the effectiveness of SNAP is its ability to reduce food insecurity, defined by USDA as a household-level economic and social condition of limited or uncertain access to adequate food.[10] While the magnitude of the effects varies, studies of SNAP generally have concluded that program participation reduces food insecurity among the adults and children served (Mabli et al., 2013; Mykerezi and Mills, 2010; Ratcliffe et al., 2011). For example, one study found that SNAP benefits reduce the incidence of food insecurity by approximately 30 percent (Ratcliffe et al., 2011).

WIC is intended primarily to help low-income children, not their parents, although young parents arguably benefit from improvements in the well-being of their children. Although the range of estimated benefits is large, research on the effects of WIC participation generally has concluded that the program improves low-income children's health at birth (Bitler and Currie, 2005; Chatterji et al., 2002; Figlio et al., 2009; Joyce et al., 2008; Lee and Mackey-Bilaver, 2007; Rossin-Slater, 2013).

In Chapter 3, we review research on the benefits of two-generation programs that use strategies addressing the developmental needs of both young parents and their children. These programs target marginalized young parents, who need the increased social capital and connections to the workforce promoted by many of these programs (Chase-Lansdale and Brooks-Gunn, 2014; King et al., 2009).

In addition, while not a government program per se, the federal Earned Income Tax Credit (EITC) undoubtedly provides significant benefits to young low-income parents. In 2013, the EITC provided more than 27 million eligible individuals and families with more than $63 billion (IRS, 2014). The EITC is a tax credit for low- and moderate-income individuals and couples that is intended primarily for families with children. Taxpayers must have earnings from a job to claim the credit. The credit is refundable, which means that if it exceeds a worker's federal income tax liability, the Internal Revenue Service refunds the balance. Eligibility for and the amount of the EITC for families with children depend on the size of the family. In 2013, for example, a single parent with one child could earn up to $37,870 and a married couple with three or more children could earn up to $51,567 before becoming ineligible for a credit (IRS, 2014). Individual workers at least 25 years of age without children and with incomes below about $14,340 were eligible for a very small EITC benefit.

The EITC has been shown to dramatically increase the labor market participation of single women while having a modestly negative impact on married taxpayers' employment (Hotz and Scholz, 2003; Meyer, 2010).

[10] For a more thorough explanation of how USDA defines food insecurity and its relationship to hunger, visit the USDA website: http://www.ers.usda.gov/topics/food-nutrition-assistance/food-security-in-the-us/definitions-of-food-security.aspx#.U17TW4FdWSo (accessed October 22, 2014).

It also is associated with reduced reliance on cash assistance and reduced poverty among families with children (Grogger, 2003; Marr et al., 2014). In addition, through its impact on family income, the EITC has been shown to improve educational outcomes for young children (Dahl and Lochner, 2012; Duncan et al., 2011). However, its effects on young parents have not been directly examined, and its benefit for taxpayers without children is not currently available to young adults under age 25. Interest in expanding the EITC for childless workers, including those as young as 21 years old, is found in President Obama's most recent proposed budget and in current legislative proposals, although there is as yet no agreement on the nature of the expansion or how it would be funded (see, e.g., Executive Office of the President and U.S. Department of the Treasury, 2014; Marr and Huang, 2014; Vinik, 2014). Moreover, because the credit for individuals without children has been very small and has not been available to those under 25, little research is available on the likely effects of an enhanced EITC on young adult employment, poverty, and cash assistance utilization.

YOUNG UNAUTHORIZED IMMIGRANTS

In 2010, 11.3 million young people—approximately one-quarter of the U.S. population aged 16-26—were youth of immigrant origin (Batalova and Fix, 2011).[11] Members of first and second generations accounted for half of the population growth in the nation's youth and young adults aged 16-26 between 1995 and 2010 and accounted for 30 percent of all low-income youth in that age group in 2010 (Batalova and Fix, 2011). First-generation youth accounted for 10.3 percent and second-generation youth for 14.1 percent of young people aged 16-26 in 2010. This is a highly heterogeneous group, differing in age at arrival, language, legal status, race, ethnicity, and gender, all of which can contribute to their health and well-being as young adults (Rumbaut, 2004; Suárez-Orozco et al., 2010). Given the size of the population and its growth, youth of immigrant origin are of great importance to the nation's future.

Among youth of immigrant origin, first-generation immigrants are at particular risk of marginalization. For example, they are much more likely than the second generation to have entered the country during late adolescence and early adulthood, with 44 percent of first-generation youth having entered the country after age 16 (Portes and Rumbaut, 2006). Entering the country at a later age puts young people at risk during the transition to adulthood. Immigrants who enter the country at a later age generally are

---

[11] In this report, we use "first generation" to describe persons with no U.S. citizenship at birth and "second generation" to describe those born in the United States to immigrant parents. First and second generations make up youth of immigrant origin.

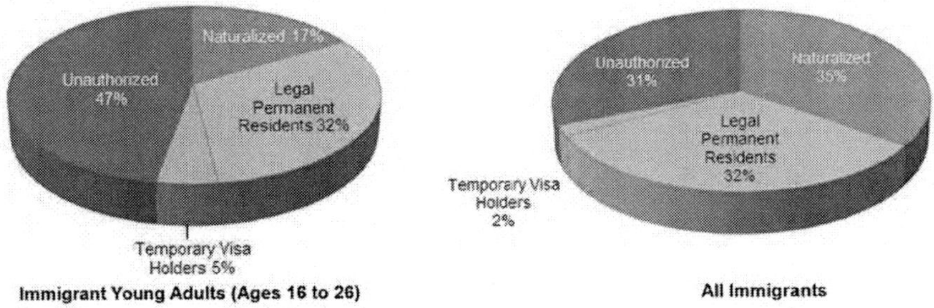

FIGURE 8-2 Citizenship and legal status of young adult and overall immigrant populations, 2007.
SOURCE: Batalova and Fix, 2011, reprinted with permission.

less likely than those who enter as children to master English or to enroll in and graduate from schools in the United States (Portes and Rumbaut, 2001). They also are less likely than the second generation to be living with their parents and have access to parental support during early adulthood and more likely than the second generation to have low incomes (Batalova and Fix, 2011). It is important to keep in mind, however, that research has shown that first-generation youth are healthier in many ways than second-generation and native-born youth, highlighting the strengths that many of these young people bring with them to the United States as well as the risks associated with their immigration (Perreira and Ornelas, 2011).

Most important, the legal status of many first-generation young adults puts them at high risk of marginalization since they are unlikely to have citizenship or lawfully permanent resident status, making them unauthorized immigrants.[12] Figure 8-2 shows that young adult immigrants are only about half as likely to be naturalized citizens relative to immigrants as a whole, but they are half again as likely as other immigrants to be unauthorized. Nearly half (47 percent) of young immigrants, accounting for about 1 in 20 young people aged 16-26 in the United States, are unauthorized.

Nearly half of all youth of immigrant origin are concentrated in just three states—California (28 percent), Texas (11 percent), and New York (10 percent) (Batalova and Fix, 2011). Ten states account for approximately three-quarters of immigrant-origin youth in the United States. In some states, immigrant youth make up a large percentage of all youth. For

[12] The legal status of refugees and asylees varies depending on where they are in the process of seeking refugee or asylum status. For a description of these processes and populations, see Burt and Batalova (2014).

example, first and second generations make up 53 percent of youth aged 16-26 in California, 38 percent in New Jersey, and 37 percent in New York (Batalova and Fix, 2011). Thus, a handful of states are responsible for providing whatever support young adult immigrants receive in the United States. This responsibility can be a significant fiscal burden for these states, but it also means they are the most important laboratories for exploring potential strategies for improving the health and well-being of immigrant youth.

Unlike other marginalized youth populations discussed in this chapter, unauthorized immigrants are distinguished from other young adults more by the benefits and programs from which they are excluded than by programs for which they are categorically eligible. While some states operate programs for unauthorized immigrants, these young adults are ineligible for major means-tested public benefit programs, including TANF, SNAP, and Medicaid, and virtually all other federally supported benefits, except for K-12 education, free and reduced-price lunches, and emergency health care (Fix, 2009; Fortuny and Chaudry, 2011). In addition, since unauthorized immigrants are not allowed to be legally employed, they are vulnerable to labor market exploitation. They also are ineligible for federal financial aid if they seek to obtain postsecondary education, although 18 states do provide some form of in-state tuition benefit to unauthorized students (NCSL, 2014).

Unauthorized immigrants are not the only immigrant young adults who are marginalized with respect to U.S. social and health policy. Pursuant to the 1996 welfare reform law, even lawfully permanent residents are eligible for major federally supported programs only after they have resided in the country for 5 years (Batalova and Fix, 2011). This means that many lawfully permanent immigrants spend much of their early adulthood ineligible for government assistance. In addition, immigrants who are eligible for various forms of assistance, including those with refugee and lawfully permanent status, often find it difficult to obtain help because of the complexity of application and eligibility processes, administrative burdens faced by program case managers, immigrants' limited literacy, language and cultural differences between immigrants and program providers, and climates of fear and mistrust (Perreira et al., 2012).

CHARACTERISTICS COMMON TO MARGINALIZED YOUNG ADULTS AND THE PROGRAMS THAT SERVE THEM

Our description of selected marginalized populations and other reviews of the research on these young adults show that, while they are a heterogeneous group, they nevertheless share a number of characteristics and experiences (Osgood et al., 2005, 2010):

> "I experienced a lot of trauma growing up, and a lot of programs in the system were not catered to my specific age group. The staff didn't know how to address young people, and how to deal with the issues they have lived through."

- They are very likely to have low incomes and experience economic hardships.
- They are disproportionately likely to be disadvantaged racial and ethnic minorities.
- Many of them are parents, quite often raising their children without another parent.
- They are likely to have disabilities, trauma histories, and mental health and substance abuse problems; to engage in risky behaviors; and to become victims of physical and/or sexual violence.
- Most enter adulthood with limited education and work experience.
- Many are estranged from their families or have problematic family relationships and few positive adult connections on which to rely.
- They often face the consequences of stigma and discrimination.
- Many, particularly those with a history of justice system involvement and unauthorized immigrants, are ineligible to receive assistance that is routinely available to similarly situated young people.

Our review of the programs that serve marginalized young people leads to the following conclusions:

- There is considerable population overlap across these programs. For example, young people in the corrections system often spent time in foster care, young people in the corrections system frequently have mental health disorders, many former foster youth have disabilities and/or receive Supplemental Security Income (SSI), young TANF recipients often have contact with child protective services, many homeless young adults have had experience with the child welfare and corrections systems, and many homeless youth are parents.
- Despite this overlap, program eligibility criteria create obstacles to collaboration across programs and gaps in marginalized young adults' access to needed help.
- Most programs either do not explicitly acknowledge young adults as having needs distinct from those of older adults and children or have not adapted well to those unique needs. Moreover, program age restrictions, generally imposed at the age of majority, often re-

sult in loss of services (e.g., foster care and some homeless services) as young people transition to adulthood.

- Most of these programs are not held accountable for improving the health or well-being of marginalized young adults; program data generally focus on eligibility determination and service provision at the expense of data on young adults' outcomes.
- With few exceptions, when programs are held accountable for outcomes, each program focuses on one or a few outcomes specific to that program (e.g., corrections programs focus on avoidance of reentry to jail and prison, TANF on employment, and homeless programs on housing stability). This is true even though these distinct outcomes arguably are inextricably linked.
- For a variety of reasons, most programs that serve marginalized young adults fall far short of serving the entire population eligible for assistance. In some cases (e.g., homeless youth services), programs are funded on a competitive basis through federal grants to local public or private agencies, leaving many jurisdictions with no services at all. In other cases, variation between state and local governments in the implementation of federal programs (e.g., extended foster care, TANF) means that some young adults receive assistance, while those across a state or county line do not. In many cases, the chronicity of inadequate funding means that there is always a long list of young people waiting for help, even where programs do nominally exist.

The distinction between entitlement and nonentitlement programs that serve marginalized young adults deserves special attention, since it reflects and helps illustrate the nature of social exclusion for these young people. While entitlement programs are rare in the United States, they are particularly rare for young adults. With relatively few exceptions, the elderly are entitled to Medicare, and if their incomes are low enough and they are in need of long-term care, Medicaid. Seniors also are eligible for Social Security, the nation's largest social insurance program. Similarly, minors living in low-income families generally are covered by Medicaid and SNAP, without regard to whether they or their parents are working.

In contrast, the entitlement programs that routinely serve young adults reach a much smaller and more narrowly defined segment of the population. The extension of foster care to age 21 is an option for states, but most states have not taken it up. Moreover, this entitlement reaches a miniscule population: only about 17,000 young adults aged 18 or over were in care in 2012, the last year for which these data are available (ACF, 2013c). SSI, the only other entitlement program routinely available to young adults without dependent children, serves only those with a relatively narrow range of disabilities; in December 2012, there were approximately 717,000 SSI recipients aged 18-25 (SSA, 2013). Other entitlement programs serving young adults (e.g., SNAP) impose restrictions on eligibility that significantly limit access. Nonentitlement programs serving young adults typically have complex and restrictive eligibility requirements and are severely underfunded. Put simply, few young adults arguably in need of government assistance are deemed worthy of an entitlement to that assistance; most who seek help will face obstacles that send an unmistakable message that assistance will be provided grudgingly, if at all.

Viewing the experiences of marginalized young adults in terms of the ways they are socially excluded can help inform public policy. From the social inclusion perspective, meeting the needs of marginalized groups will improve their lives and also help them contribute fully to society, thereby benefiting everyone. Marginalized youth may have a good opportunity to make a successful transition to adulthood if they are provided with the supports that match their strengths and needs. Unfortunately, although there are some bright spots, the evidence base for effective intervention on behalf of marginalized young adults remains weak.

THE EVIDENCE BASE FOR ASSISTING MARGINALIZED YOUNG ADULTS

Policies intended to improve the transition to adulthood for marginalized young adults should be based on sound knowledge of the strengths and needs of these populations, as well as interventions found to be effective in improving their health and well-being. The review provided in this chapter makes clear that existing evidence provides neither a comprehensive view of these populations nor a clear sense of how to help them. To be sure, available research provides glimpses of subpopulations and conveys both a general sense of the challenges they face and the resilience they often exhibit in the face of those challenges. Some programs (e.g., SNAP) are known to have positive effects on the general population and can reasonably be expected to benefit young adults, but program effects often are modest, and many marginalized youth are not eligible for these programs. A few programs have been shown to have positive impacts on some important outcomes for some subpopulations, but evidence is as yet inadequate to support large-scale expansion of interventions likely to benefit a wide range of marginalized young adults.

Nevertheless, prior research does provide some guidance regarding the characteristics of programs that have potential to improve the health and well-being of a broad range of marginalized young adults (Osgood et al., 2005, 2010). Such programs

- take into account the extreme poverty and economic hardships frequently experienced by marginalized young adults (e.g., homelessness and food insecurity);
- facilitate the participation of parents, including single parents, and support them in their parenting role;
- do not exclude young people based on their citizenship status;
- are accepting of LGBT young adults;
- are designed to include young people with a wide range of disabilities and behavioral health problems;
- focus on assisting young people in acquiring work experience and maintaining employment; and
- support young adults in completing secondary education and acquiring postsecondary credentials.

We now turn to recommendations for future research and government investments to help increase the likelihood that all young adults will participate fully in society.

CONCLUSIONS AND RECOMMENDATIONS

We recommend a series of interrelated actions by federal, state, and local governments to help develop understanding of the characteristics of marginalized young adults and improve policies and programs intended to reduce their marginalization. These recommendations reflect our belief that the heretofore categorical approach to assisting marginalized young adults is inefficient and contributes to their marginalization. However, while we believe that a more flexible and integrated approach to assisting these young people will ultimately be more effective than the current approach, we recognize that the available evidence does not yet provide a clear path forward. Only active and ongoing partnership across all levels of government to develop and evaluate new approaches will clearly identify the policies and programs needed to reduce the marginalization of young adults.

Research

Gaining better knowledge of how marginalized young adults fare is complicated by the fact that the character of their marginalization often changes over time, and many subpopulations make up a very small portion of the overall population of young adults. For example, homelessness is one serious form of marginalization, but it is often a transient experience, more a symptom of economic hardship and estrangement from family than a persistent state (Toro et al., 2007). Thus, the kinds of point-in-time data on homelessness gleaned from service providers are inherently limited for gauging the well-being of young adults who happen to come into contact with such services. Similarly, young people move into and out of the foster care and corrections systems, and these systems generally collect little or no information about what happens when a young person is not "in" the system.

Integration of information across the systems serving marginalized young adults and over time can provide a more complex, longitudinal perspective on their health and well-being.[13] While legal and operational concerns have in the past limited the extent to which federal agencies share data for the purposes described here, the Office of Management and Budget (OMB, 2014) recently issued a memorandum providing guidance to federal agencies for improving the provision and use of administrative data. This guidance is intended to help program and statistical agencies, including evaluation and policy analysis units, make greater use of administrative data while respecting individuals' privacy and protecting confidentiality. Maximizing the use of administrative data to better understand marginalized youth populations ultimately will require collaboration between state and local government agencies since many programs serving marginalized young adults are operated at these two levels. Researchers have for many years made one-off efforts to integrate administrative data for specific research projects, but those projects seldom have led to ongoing integration of data across systems for the purposes of research and evaluation. However, the past two decades have seen the development of a few integrated databases at the state and local levels, often funded by philanthropy (Advisory Panel on Research Uses of Administrative Data, 1998; Culhane et al., 2010). Examples include the Integrated Database on Child and Family Programs in Illinois,

> "When a young person goes into the foster care system and ends up in the criminal justice system, it is hell to get all the data that was in the foster care system to that other system so that they understand what the young person went through, the services he needed, and whether or not he needs them again."

[13] Prior reports by the Institute of Medicine have recognized the need for better coordination and integration of national data on the health and well-being of the U.S. population. For example, the Committee on Public Health Strategies to Improve Health recommended that the Secretary of Health and Human Services transform the mission of the National Center for Health Statistics to provide leadership for a population health information system through enhanced coordination and better integration of data on the determinants of health (IOM, 2011).

operated by Chapin Hall at the University of Chicago, and the network of local initiatives supported by Actionable Intelligence for Social Policy (AISP) at the University of Pennsylvania.[14]

Population-based longitudinal studies, such as the National Longitudinal Survey of Youth and the National Longitudinal Study of Adolescent Health, also could enhance knowledge of marginalized young adults' health and well-being by describing youths' trajectories in and out of various marginalized statuses over time. However, while some marginalized populations, such as young parents, are large enough to show up reasonably reliably in population-based longitudinal studies, many others are too small to study using these data sources or are otherwise poorly captured by them.

Recommendation 8-1: Federal and state government agencies—including the U.S. Departments of Health and Human Services, Labor, Justice, Housing and Urban Development, and Education and the corresponding state agencies—should incorporate a greater focus on marginalized young adults in ongoing and new population-based cross-sectional and longitudinal studies of young adults.

To implement this recommendation, the committee recommends the following specific actions:

- In conducting ongoing studies and developing new studies, agencies should actively involve planning and advisory groups comprising researchers and program managers familiar with the various marginalized populations, as well as representatives from these populations who have experienced such life events. Doing so would help ensure that study designs, including sampling and recruitment strategies and survey items, will better capture the experiences of these populations.
- Agencies should consider oversampling of marginalized populations to better distinguish their experiences from those of other young adults.

Recommendation 8-2: Federal and state governments should continue encouraging programs that serve marginalized populations to make better use of administrative data for describing the overlap of populations across service systems and young adults' trajectories into and out

[14] For a description of the Chapin Hall database, see http://www.chapinhall.org/about/looking-across-systems-need-collaboration (accessed October 22, 2014). For a description of the AISP network, see http://www.aisp.upenn.edu/about-us (accessed October 22, 2014).

of these systems, and for evaluating policies and programs affecting young adults.

To implement this recommendation, the committee recommends the following specific actions:

- Federal agencies operating programs that affect young adults should aggressively implement the recent Office of Management and Budget "Guidance for Providing and Using Administrative Data for Statistical Purposes."
- Federal agencies serving young adults—including the U.S. Departments of Health and Human Services, Labor, Justice, Housing and Urban Development, and Education—and philanthropic funders should fund demonstration projects at the state level to support states in integrating program administrative data to better understand marginalized young adults and evaluate programs serving them.
- State government agencies serving marginalized young adults should expand on existing state and local efforts to integrate and use administrative data to better understand and serve these young adults.

Given the prevalence of behavioral health problems among marginalized young adults, agencies responsible for the provision and coordination of behavioral health services (e.g., the Substance Abuse and Mental Health Services Administration, the Health Resources and Services Administration) should actively engage in implementing these recommendations.

Policy

Our recommendations for policy initiatives to reduce the marginalization of young adults are influenced by our concern about the consequences of the highly categorical nature of most current federal programs and our recognition of how federalism influences the provision of services in the United States. While states and localities have over the years initiated many attempts to serve vulnerable youth and young adults more efficiently and effectively (e.g., by reorganizing government departments charged with serving youth), they are hard pressed to do so without tailoring their efforts to maximize the receipt of federal funds. As described above, with few exceptions these federal programs have narrow and idiosyncratic eligibility criteria that create obstacles to young people's getting the help they need, often create gaps in help when it is provided, and too often are stigmatizing. Simply put, programs for marginalized young adults categorize them in counterproductive ways. Moreover, a troubling legacy of this categorization is the myriad distinct outputs and outcomes associated with attempts to hold the resulting plethora of programs accountable. Each program operates in its silo, understandably reluctant to be held accountable for any outcome that is not completely within its control. As a consequence, many programs are held accountable only for outputs, not outcomes, and there is no collective accountability for improving the overall health and well-being of marginalized young adults.

> "A huge problem is we still have many systems that address one aspect of an individual, so at one time the individual will get mental health services, and then when that is done, the individual will get academic services, and then financial. But we need all of those services at the same time in order to have our basic needs met. Then we can move forward to reaching our full potential."

There is a long history of efforts to overcome this program fragmentation and lack of shared accountability. For example, the 2003 *White House Task Force Report for Disadvantaged Youth* led to the creation of the Shared Youth Vision Federal Partnership (Abt Associates, 2009). Shared Youth Vision, which involved the U.S. Department of Defense, the U.S. Department of Education, the U.S. Department of Health and Human Services, the U.S. Department of Housing and Urban Development, the U.S. Department of Justice, the U.S. Department of Labor, the Social Security Administration, the U.S. Department of Transportation, and the Corporation for National and Community Service, was intended to "serve as a catalyst at the national, state, and local levels to strengthen coordination, communication, and collaboration among youth-serving agencies to support the neediest youth and their healthy transition to successful adult roles and responsibilities" (Abt Associates, 2009, p. 7). The Shared Youth Vision Partnership facilitated the development of model program coordination strategies, youth assessment tools, and outcome indicators, as well as several pilot state and local planning efforts, but none of these were rigorously evaluated in a manner that could identify their impact on youth outcomes (Abt Associates, 2009).

More recent recognition of program fragmentation and a lack of accountability can be seen in the creation of Performance Partnerships for

Disconnected Youth.[15] The Consolidated Appropriations Act of 2014 gives the U.S. Departments of Labor, Health and Human Services, and Education and the Corporation for National and Community Service authority to establish up to 10 state and local pilot initiatives to pool a portion of discretionary funds they receive through several federal streams while measuring and monitoring specified cross-program outcomes for "disconnected youth." The state and local pilot sites are expected to achieve significant improvements in educational, employment, and other key outcomes for disconnected youth, defined as low-income youth and young adults aged 14-24 who are homeless, in foster care, involved in the criminal justice system, not working, or not enrolled in (or at risk of dropping out of) an educational institution. To facilitate the pooling of funds and various forms of flexibility expected of the pilots, full or partial waivers may be granted by federal agencies for statutory, regulatory, and administrative requirements. This is a promising development, and important lessons may be learned from these pilots. Because of statutory limitations, however, only discretionary funds from the federal agencies involved may be used for the pilots; use of mandatory and entitlement funds is prohibited. This restriction illustrates the limited headway the federal government can currently make toward addressing the needs of marginalized young adults more comprehensively.

Federalism arguably contributes to the lack of accountability. With few exceptions, states (and often localities) are given substantial leeway in how they choose to implement federally supported social programs. In some cases, they are free to decide whether to provide a service at all. While the legal foundation for this latitude is found in the U.S. Constitution, federalism often is justified based on the belief that it results in services that reflect local needs more appropriately. In addition, federalism is believed to facilitate experimentation by states, helping to identify innovative and effective approaches to promoting the general welfare, while in the process providing examples other states can follow. In other words, federalism is supposed to result in improvement over time in government's ability to meet the needs of the people.

Unfortunately, these purported benefits of federalism have not been realized with respect to services for marginalized young adults. The lack of evidence supporting the effectiveness of programs for these young people is a testament to the failure to learn from state and local variations in service provision. U.S. society has long used social programs to experiment with the lives of marginalized young adults, but little has been learned from

---

[15] For more information about the Performance Partnerships for Disconnected Youth, see http://www.ed.gov/blog/wp-content/uploads/2014/03/2014-PPPs-Fact-Sheet.pdf (accessed October 22, 2014).

this experimentation. While states certainly can and should do more to rigorously evaluate their own program innovations, we believe the federal government is best positioned to create the conditions needed to learn from the experimentation spawned by federalism. That the evidence needed to justify major government investments in programs for marginalized young adults is lacking is likely more the result of a failure to rigorously evaluate the impacts of current investments than proof of the futility of trying to help these young people.

The following steps should be taken by the federal and state governments to improve the coordination and effectiveness of services for marginalized young adults.

Recommendation 8-3: Congress and the Executive Branch should amend federal laws and regulations to allow for more flexible and efficient eligibility determination and service provision across marginalized young adult populations.

Given the large number of programs involved, implementing this recommendation is likely to require a significant reworking of regulations, and potentially statutes, affecting multiple federal agencies. Major improvements in the flexibility and efficiency of program operations will require restructuring the fragmented federal funding streams currently supporting services for marginalized populations. Two general approaches to funding reform appear most likely to ultimately achieve the needed fundamental restructuring of programs:

- Combine some or all of the funds currently allocated to relevant federal programs into an integrated funding stream supporting state programs for marginalized young adults (i.e., a block grant). The proportion of funds initially transferred to this new block grant from an existing program would reflect the size of the marginalized young adult populations currently served by that program. This approach would essentially result in the creation of a new federal program, the elimination of some existing programs, and reductions in funding for other federal programs.
- Alternatively, the federal government could expand the use of waivers to allow some states to ignore or modify program rules that impede a more integrated and efficient approach to serving marginalized young adults. This approach is being used in the new Performance Partnerships for Disconnected Youth. It has also been used extensively with entitlement programs in creating innovation in welfare, Medicaid, and child welfare policy. Such waivers could ultimately be used to offer interested states the option of receiving

federal funds for programs serving marginalized young adults in a block grant, as described above.

Either of these strategies for better organizing federal programs for marginalized young adults could result in efficiencies in program administration at both the federal and state levels. Some of the programs affected are currently entitlements, and any recommendation for collapsing funding streams in the interest of flexibility should be balanced by concern for ensuring that resources grow with need. One means to this end would be to tie block grant funding, or funding provided to states through waivers, to increases in the cost of living. The population of young adults is expected to grow only modestly over the next two decades, so increases in the unit cost of providing services to marginalized young adults rather than increases in the size of the population are likely to be the primary driver of increases in overall program costs. Still, adjusting block grant and waiver funding to changes in the size of the young adult population would further minimize the likelihood that funding would decline over time relative to need.

Recommendation 8-4: Congress and the Executive Branch at the federal level and state legislatures and governors at the state level should amend laws and regulations to create accountability for achieving improvement on a limited set of key outcomes for marginalized young adults (e.g., employment, education, housing stability, safety, health, connections to responsible adults, and effective parenting).

This accountability would look different in the context of the creation of a new federal program from the way it would look if the federal government simply allowed states to ignore or modify the requirements of existing programs. In the former case, the federal government would create a set of outcomes that states serving marginalized young adults would be required to measure to receive federal support. In the latter case, the federal government would negotiate with states a set of outcomes to be monitored by states that sought waivers to provide services to marginalized young adults more flexibly and efficiently.

Either approach would represent a shift away from costly, disjointed, and ineffective collection of data on the outputs of multiple programs toward an information infrastructure capable of measuring the effects of government investments on the health and well-being of marginalized young adults. Comparable data on key outcomes would be collected across all marginalized young adults served. Over time, the federal government would be in a position to compare outcomes among states with dissimilar approaches to serving young adults, which in turn would help in identifying more effective policies and programs. Data sharing across public systems serving young adults, referenced above, would be essential to the success of this endeavor.

Recommendation 8-5: In funding evaluations of programs for marginalized young adults, the federal government and philanthropic funders should emphasize evaluation of programs aimed at improving outcomes across multiple marginalized populations while remaining sensitive to differences across subpopulations.

If government funding has tended to create narrowly categorical programs, so, too, has evaluation funding tended to steer evaluators toward programs that serve narrowly defined populations. Even when a program shows a positive impact on the population served, too often there is good reason to be skeptical that the same impact will result for populations experiencing other forms of marginalization. Of course, one-size-fits-all programs are unlikely to maximally meet the needs of all marginalized young people; program developers and evaluators should always pay attention to the distinct needs of subgroups. Nevertheless, given the characteristics shared across these populations, programs designed to be open to serving young people who exhibit many of these characteristics are most likely to benefit a large number of marginalized young adults.

REFERENCES

Abt Associates. 2009. *Common sense, uncommon commitment: A progress report on the shared youth vision partnership*. Washington, DC: U.S. Department of Labor.

ACF (Administration for Children and Families). 2012. *FY 2012 online performance appendix*. http://www.acf.hhs.gov/sites/default/files/opre/2012_appendix.pdf (accessed October 10, 2014).

ACF. 2013a. *Report to Congress on the runaway and homeless youth programs: Fiscal years 2010 and 2011*. Washington, DC: U.S. Department of Health and Human Services.

ACF. 2013b. *Street outreach program*. http://www.acf.hhs.gov/programs/fysb/resource/sop-fact-sheet (accessed October 20, 2014).

ACF. 2013c. *The AFCARS report: Preliminary FY 2012 estimates as of November 2013 (No. 20)*. http://www.acf.hhs.gov/sites/default/files/cb/afcarsreport20.pdf (accessed March 7, 2014).

ACF. 2014a. *About TANF*. http://www.acf.hhs.gov/programs/ofa/programs/tanf/about (accessed October 16, 2014).

ACF. 2014b. *Basic center program fact sheet*. http://www.acf.hhs.gov/programs/fysb/resource/bcp-fact-sheet (accessed October 20, 2014).

ACF. 2014c. *Transitional living program fact sheet*. http://www.acf.hhs.gov/programs/fysb/resource/tlp-fact-sheet (accessed October 20, 2014).

Adams, B., and S. Addie. 2014. Juveniles tried as adults. In *The encyclopedia of criminology and criminal justice*. Oxford, UK: Blackwell Publishing Ltd.

Advisory Panel on Research Uses of Administrative Data. 1998. *Administrative data for policy-relevant research: Assessment of current utility and recommendations for development*. http://public.econ.duke.edu/~vjh3/working_papers/adm_data.pdf (accessed September 5, 2014).

Ahrens, K. R., L. P. Richardson, M. E. Courtney, C. McCarty, J. Simoni, and W. Katon. 2010. Laboratory-diagnosed sexually transmitted infections in former foster youth compared with peers. *Pediatrics* 126(1):e97-e103.

Altena, A. M., S. N. Brilleslijper-Kater, and J. R. Wolf. 2010. Effective interventions for homeless youth: A systematic review. *American Journal of Preventive Medicine* 38(6):637-645.

Ammerman, S. D., J. Ensign, R. Kirzner, E. T. Meininger, M. Tornabene, C. W. Warf, S. Zerger, and P. Post. 2004. *Homeless young adults ages 18-24: Examining service delivery adaptations*. Nashville, TN: National Health Care for the Homeless Council.

Barth, R. P. 1990. On their own: The experiences of youth after foster care. *Child and Adolescent Social Work Journal* 7(5):419-440.

Batalova, J., and M. Fix. 2011. *Up for grabs: The gains and prospects of first- and second-generation young adults*. Washington, DC: Migration Policy Institute.

Ben-Shalom, Y., R. A. Moffitt, and J. K. Scholz. 2011. *An assessment of the effectiveness of anti-poverty programs in the United States*. Cambridge, MA: National Bureau of Economic Research.

Bitler, M. P., and J. Currie. 2005. Does WIC work? The effects of WIC on pregnancy and birth outcomes. *Journal of Policy Analysis and Management* 24(1):73-91.

Blank, R. M. 2007. Improving the safety net for single mothers who face serious barriers to work. *The Future of Children* 17(2):183-197.

Burt, L., and J. Batalova. 2014. *Refugees and Asylees in the United States*. Washington, DC: Migration Policy Institute. http://www.migrationpolicy.org/article/refugees-and-asylees-united-states (accessed September 15, 2014).

Burt, M. R., L. Y. Aron, T. Douglas, J. Valente, E. Lee, and B. Iwen. 1999. *Homelessness: Programs and the people they serve. Findings of the National Survey of Homeless Assistance Providers and Clients*. Washington, DC: Urban Institute.

Chase-Lansdale, P. L., and J. Brooks-Gunn. 2014. Two-generation programs in the twenty-first century. *The Future of Children* 24:13-40.

Chatterji, P., K. Bonuck, S. Dhawan, and N. Deb. 2002. *WIC participation and the initiation and duration of breastfeeding*. Madison, WI: Institute for Research on Poverty, University of Wisconsin.

Child Trends. 2012. *Young adults in jail or prison*. http://www.childtrends.org/wp-content/uploads/2012/04/89_Young_Adults_In_Prison.pdf (accessed September 5, 2014).

Cook, R., E. Fleischman, and V. Grimes. 1991. *A national evaluation of Title IV-E foster care independent living programs for youth. Phase 2 final report*. Vol. 1. Rockville, MD: Westat, Inc.

Courtney, M. E. 2010. Social policy and the transition to adulthood for foster youth in the US. In *From child welfare to child well-being: An international perspective on knowledge in the service of policy making*, edited by S. B. Kamerman, S. Phipps, and A. Ben-Arieh. New York: Dordrecht. Pp. 117-133.

Courtney, M. E., and A. Dworsky. 2006. Early outcomes for young adults transitioning from out-of-home care in the USA. *Child & Family Social Work* 11(3):209-219.

Courtney, M. E., I. Piliavin, A. Grogan-Kaylor, and A. Nesmith. 2001. Foster youth transitions to adulthood: A longitudinal view of youth leaving care. *Child Welfare, New York* 80(6):685-718.

Courtney, M. E., A. Dworsky, I. Piliavin, and A. Zinn. 2005a. Involvement of TANF applicant families with child welfare services. *Social Service Review* 79(1):119-157.

Courtney, M. E., A. Dworsky, G. Ruth, T. Keller, J. Havlicek, and N. Bost. 2005b. *Midwest evaluation of the adult functioning of former foster youth: Outcomes at 19*. Chicago, IL: Chapin Hall at the University of Chicago.

Courtney, M. E., A. Dworsky, and H. Pollack. 2007. *When should the state cease parenting? Evidence from the Midwest study*. Chicago, IL: Chapin Hall at the University of Chicago.

Courtney, M. E., A. L. Dworsky, J. Lee, and M. Raap. 2010. *Midwest evaluation of the adult functioning of former foster youth: Outcomes at age 23 and 24*. Chicago, IL: Chapin Hall at the University of Chicago.

Courtney, M. E., A. L. Dworsky, A. Brown, C. Cary, K. Love, and V. Vorhies. 2011. *Midwest evaluation of the adult functioning of former foster youth: Outcomes at age 26*. Chicago, IL: Chapin Hall at the University of Chicago.

Culhane, D. P., J. Fantuzzo, H. L. Rouse, V. Tam, and J. Lukens. 2010. *Connecting the dots: The promise of integrated data systems for policy analysis and systems reform*. Philadelphia: University of Pennsylvania.

Cusick, G. R., J. R. Havlicek, and M. E. Courtney. 2012. Risk for arrest: The role of social bonds in protecting foster youth making the transition to adulthood. *American Journal of Orthopsychiatry* 82(1):19-31.

Dahl, G. B., and L. Lochner. 2012. The impact of family income on child achievement: Evidence from the Earned Income Tax Credit. *American Economic Review* 102(5):1927-1956.

Daly, M., and H. Silver. 2008. Social exclusion and social capital: A comparison and critique. *Theory and Society* 37(6):537-566.

Danziger, S., R. Haveman, and R. Plotnick. 1981. How income transfer programs affect work, savings, and the income distribution: A critical review. *Journal of Economic Literature* 19(3):975-1028.

DOL (U.S. Department of Labor). 2014. *About RExO*. http://www.doleta.gov/RExO/about RExO.cfm (accessed March 18, 2014).

Duncan, G. J., P. A. Morris, and C. Rodrigues. 2011. Does money really matter? Estimating impacts of family income on young children's achievement with data from random-assignment experiments. *Developmental Psychology* 47(5):1263-1279.

Dworsky, A. 2013. *The economic well-being of lesbian, gay, and bisexual youth transitioning out of foster care*. Washington, DC: Mathematica Policy Research.

Dworsky, A., and M. E. Courtney. 2001. *Self-sufficiency of former foster youth in Wisconsin: Analysis of unemployment insurance, wage data and public assistance data*. Madison, WI: Institute for Research on Poverty.

Dworsky, A., and M. E. Courtney. 2010. The risk of teenage pregnancy among transitioning foster youth: Implications for extending state care beyond age 18. *Children and Youth Services Review* 32(10):1351-1356.

Dworsky, A., M. E. Courtney, and A. Zinn. 2007. Child, parent, and family predictors of child welfare services involvement among TANF applicant families. *Children and Youth Services Review* 29(6):802-820.

Dworsky, A., L. Napolitano, and M. Courtney. 2013. Homelessness during the transition from foster care to adulthood. *American Journal of Public Health* 103(Suppl. 2):S318-S323.

Emam, D., and O. Golden. 2014. *The Affordable Care Act and youth aging out of foster care: New opportunities and strategies for action*. http://www.clasp.org/resources-and-publications/publication-1/The-Affordable-Care-Act-and-Youth-Aging-Out-of-Foster-Care.pdf (accessed October 10, 2014).

Executive Office of the President and U.S. Department of the Treasury. 2014. *The President's Proposal to Expand the Earned Income Tax Credit, March 2014*. http://www.white house.gov/sites/default/files/docs/eitc_report_0.pdf (accessed September 14, 2014).

Falk, G. 2012. *Temporary Assistance for Needy Families (TANF): Welfare-to-work revisited*. Washington, DC: Congressional Research Service.

Falk, G. 2013. *The Temporary Assistance for Needy Families (TANF) block grant: Responses to frequently asked questions*. Washington, DC: Congressional Research Service.

Farrington, D. P. 1986. Age and crime. *Crime and Justice* 7:189-250.

FBI (Federal Bureau of Investigation). 2012. *Crime in the United States 2012: Table 28, arrests by age*. http://www.fbi.gov/about-us/cjis/ucr/crime-in-the-u.s/2012/crime-in-the-u.s.-2012/tables/38tabledatadecoverviewpdf (accessed March 18, 2014).

Fernandes-Alcantara, A. L. 2013. *Runaway and homeless youth: Demographics and programs*. Washington, DC: Congressional Research Service.

Figlio, D., S. Hamersma, and J. Roth. 2009. Does prenatal WIC participation improve birth outcomes? New evidence from Florida. *Journal of Public Economics* 93(1):235-245.

FindYouthInfo. 2014. *About the National Forum on Youth Violence Prevention*. http://findyouthinfo.gov/youth-topics/preventing-youth-violence/about-national-forum (accessed October 6, 2014)

Fix, M. E. 2009. *Immigrants and welfare: The impact of welfare reform on America's newcomers*. New York: Russell Sage Foundation.

Fortuny, K., and A. Chaudry. 2011. *A comprehensive review of immigrant access to health and human services*. Washington, DC: Urban Institute.

Glaze, L. E., and E. J. Herberman. 2013. *Correctional populations in the United States, 2011*. Washington, DC: U.S. Department of Justice.

Glaze, L. E., and L. M. Maruschak. 2008. *Parents in prison and their minor children*. Washington, DC: U.S. Department of Justice, Office of Justice Programs.

Goerge, R. M., L. Bilaver, B. J. Lee, B. Needell, A. Brookhart, and W. Jackman. 2002. *Employment outcomes for youth aging out of foster care*. Chicago, IL: Chapin Hall Center for Children, University of Chicago.

Griffin, P., S. Addie, B. Adams, and K. Firestine. 2011. *Trying juveniles as adults: An analysis of state transfer laws and reporting*. Washington, DC: U.S. Department of Justice, Office of Justice Programs, OJJDP.

Grogger, J. 2003. The effects of time limits, the EITC, and other policy changes on welfare use, work, and income among female-headed families. *Review of Economics and Statistics* 85(2):394-408.

GSA (General Services Administration). 2014a. *Catalog of federal domestic assistance: Chafee Education and Training Vouchers Program*. https://www.cfda.gov/index?s=program&mode=form&tab=core&id=ffbe8916a54f087ebdf147754111bf57 (accessed October 20, 2014).

GSA. 2014b. *Catalog of federal domestic assistance: Juvenile accountability block grants*. https://www.cfda.gov/index?s=program&mode=form&tab=step1&id=599c10e19547ea6d733425dc96438140 (accessed March 18, 2014).

GSA. 2014c. *Catalog of federal domestic assistance: Juvenile justice and delinquency prevention allocation to states*. https://www.cfda.gov/index?s=program&mode=form&tab=step1&id=79a02f0e29ab30706d1fb79487ecf28a (accessed March 18, 2014).

GSA. 2014d. *Catalog of federal domestic assistance: Reintegration of ex-offenders*. https://www.cfda.gov/index?s=program&mode=form&tab=step1&id=d69e451fa19934ebad489717f68f3b27 (accessed March 18, 2014).

GSA. 2014e. *Catalog of federal domestic assistance: Second Chance Act prisoner reentry initiative*. https://www.cfda.gov/index?s=program&mode=form&tab=step1&id=0f0083d29a6d817d18734debda07293a (accessed March 18, 2014).

GSA. 2014f. *Catalog of federal domestic assistance: YouthBuild*. https://www.cfda.gov/index?s=program&mode=form&tab=step1&id=f29cd846a50eb259f14c0b842c56efc8 (accessed March 18, 2014).

Hagan, J., and B. McCarthy. 2005. Homeless youth and the perilous passage to adulthood. In *On your own without a net*, edited by D. W. Osgood, E. M. Foster, C. Flanagan, and G. Ruth. Chicago, IL: The University of Chicago Press. Pp. 178-201.

Hanssens, C., A. C. Moodie-Mills, A. J. Ritchie, D. Spade, and U. Vaid. 2014. *A roadmap for change: Federal policy recommendations for addressing the criminalization of LGBT people and people living with HIV*. New York: Center for Gender & Sexuality Law at Columbia Law School.

Hirschi, T., and M. Gottfredson. 1983. Age and the explanation of crime. *American Journal of Sociology* 89(3):552-584.

Hook, J. L., and M. E. Courtney. 2011. Employment outcomes of former foster youth as young adults: The importance of human, personal, and social capital. *Children and Youth Services Review* 33(10):1855-1865.

Hotz, V. J., and J. K. Scholz. 2003. The earned income tax credit. In *Means-tested transfer programs in the United States*, edited by R. Moffitt. Chicago, IL: University of Chicago Press. Pp. 141-198.

HUD (U.S. Department of Housing and Urban Development). 2013. *The 2013 Annual Homeless Assessment Report (AHAR) to Congress: Part 1, point-in-time estimates of homelessness*. Washington, DC: HUD.

IOM (Institute of Medicine). 2011. *For the public's health: The role of measurement in action and accountability*. Washington, DC: The National Academies Press.

IRS (U.S. Internal Revenue Service). 2014. *Earned income tax credit; do I qualify?* http://www.irs.gov/uac/Newsroom/Earned-Income-Tax-Credit-Do-I-Qualify (accessed May 26, 2014).

James, D. J., and L. E. Glaze. 2006. *Mental health problems of prison and jail inmates*. Washington, DC: U.S. Department of Justice, Office of Justice Programs, Bureau of Justice Statistics.

Jim Casey Youth Opportunities Initiative. 2014. *Foster care extended to age 21*. http://jimcaseyyouth.org/foster-care-to-21(accessed October 10, 2014).

Job Corps. 2012. *Student outcomes/who Job Corps serves*. http://www.jobcorps.gov/Libraries/pdf/who_job_corps_serves.sflb (accessed March 20, 2014).

Job Corps. 2013. *Program administration*. http://www.jobcorps.gov/AboutJobCorps/program_admin.aspx (accessed March 20, 2014).

Johnson, B., B. Thom, B. McGill, A. Suchman, M. Mendelson, K. L. Patlan, B. Freeman, R. Gotlieb, and P. Connor. 2013. *WIC participant and program characteristics 2012*. Alexandria, VA: USDA.

Joyce, T., A. Racine, and C. Yunzal-Butler. 2008. Reassessing the WIC effect: Evidence from the Pregnancy Nutrition Surveillance System. *Journal of Policy Analysis and Management* 27(2):277-303.

Keller, T. E., A. M. Salazar, and M. E. Courtney. 2010. Prevalence and timing of diagnosable mental health, alcohol, and substance use problems among older adolescents in the child welfare system. *Children and Youth Services Review* 32(4):626-634.

King, C. T., R. W. Glover, T. C. Smith, R. Coffey, B. Levy, H. Yoshikawa, W. Beardslee, and M. Kordsmeier. 2009. *The CareerAdvance® pilot project: Recommended jobs strategy for families served by the Community Action Project of Tulsa County*. Austin, TX: Ray Marshall Center for the Study of Human Resources.

Kushel, M. B., I. H. Yen, L. Gee, and M. E. Courtney. 2007. Homelessness and health care access after emancipation: Results from the Midwest evaluation of adult functioning of former foster youth. *Archives of Pediatrics & Adolescent Medicine* 161(10):986-993.

Lee, B. J., and L. Mackey-Bilaver. 2007. Effects of WIC and food stamp program participation on child outcomes. *Children and Youth Services Review* 29(4):501-517.

Lee, J. S., M. E. Courtney, and J. L. Hook. 2012. Formal bonds during the transition to adulthood: Extended foster care support and criminal/legal involvement. *Journal of Public Child Welfare* 6(3):255-279.

Leshnick, S. S., C. Geckeler, A. Wiegand, B. Nicholson, and K. Foley. 2012. *Evaluation of the Re-integration of Ex-Offenders (RExO) Program: Interim report*. Washington, DC: DOL.

Loeber, R., B. Menting, D. R. Lynam, T. E. Moffitt, M. Stouthamer-Loeber, R. Stallings, D. P. Farrington, and D. Pardini. 2012. Findings from the Pittsburgh Youth Study: Cognitive impulsivity and intelligence as predictors of the age-crime curve. *Journal of the American Academy of Child and Adolescent Psychiatry* 51(11):1136-1149.

Loeber, R., D. P. Farrington, and D. Petechuk. 2013. *Bulletin 1: From juvenile delinquency to young adult offending (study group on the transitions between juvenile delinquency and adult crime)*. https://ncjrs.gov/pdffiles1/nij/grants/242931.pdf (accessed March 18, 2014).

Lower-Basch, E. 2013. *SNAP cuts put youth at risk*. Washington, DC: Center for Law and Social Policy.

Mabli, J., J. Ohls, L. Dragoset, L. Castner, and B. Santos. 2013. *Measuring the effect of Supplemental Nutrition Assistance Program (SNAP) participation on food security*. Cambridge, MA: Mathematica Policy Research.

Marr, C., and C.-C. Huang. 2014. *Strengthening the EITC for Childless Workers Would Promote Work and Reduce Poverty*. Washington, DC: Center on Budget and Policy Priorities.

Marr, C., C.-C. Huang, and A. Sherman. 2014. *Earned income tax credit promotes work, encourages children's success at school, research finds*. Washington, DC: Center on Budget and Policy Priorities.

Martin, J. A., B. E. Hamilton, J. K. Osterman, S. C. Curtin, and T. I. Mathews. 2013. *Births: Final data for 2012*. Washington, DC: HHS.

Mathematica Policy Research. 2014. *Evaluating the YouthBuild program: Helping high school dropouts*. http://www.mdrc.org/project/youthbuild-evaluation#featured_content (accessed October 20, 2014).

Mathiesen, J., J. Popay, E. Enoch, S. Escorel, M. Hernandez, H. Johnston, and L. Rispel. 2008. *Social exclusion: Meaning, measurement and experiences and links to health inequalities: A review of literature*. WHO Social Exclusion Knowledge Network Background Paper 1. http://www.who.int/social_determinants/media/sekn_meaning_measurement_experience_2008.pdf.pdf (accessed September 5, 2014).

McMillen, J. C., and R. Raghavan. 2009. Pediatric to adult mental health service use of young people leaving the foster care system. *Journal of Adolescent Health* 44(1):7-13.

McMillen, J. C., B. T. Zima, L. D. Scott, Jr., W. F. Auslander, M. R. Munson, M. T. Ollie, and E. L. Spitznagel. 2005. Prevalence of psychiatric disorders among older youths in the foster care system. *Journal of the American Academy of Child and Adolescent Psychiatry* 44(1):88-95.

MDRC. 2014. *YouthBuild evaluation*. http://www.mdrc.org/project/youthbuild-evaluation#featured_content (accessed March 18, 2014).

Meyer, B. D. 2010. The effects of the earned income tax credit and recent reforms. In *Tax policy and the economy*, Vol. 24, edited by J. R. Brown. Chicago, IL: The University of Chicago Press. Pp. 153-180.

Moffitt, R. 1992. Incentive effects of the US welfare system: A review. *Journal of Economic Literature* 30(1):1-61.

Moffitt, T. E. 1993. Adolescence-limited and life-course-persistent antisocial behavior: A developmental taxonomy. *Psychological Review* 100(4):674-701.

Montgomery, P., C. Donkoh, and K. Underhill. 2006. Independent living programs for young people leaving the care system: The state of the evidence. *Children and Youth Services Review* 28(12):1435-1448.

Mumola, C. J., and J. C. Karberg. 2006. *Drug use and dependence, state and federal prisoners, 2004*. Washington, DC: U.S. Department of Justice, Office of Justice Programs, Bureau of Justice Statistics.

Mykerezi, E., and B. Mills. 2010. The impact of food stamp program participation on household food insecurity. *American Journal of Agricultural Economics* 92(5):1379-1391.

National Alliance to End Homelessness. 2012. *An emerging framework for ending unaccompanied youth homelessness*. Washington, DC: National Alliance to End Homelessness.

National Alliance to End Homelessness. 2013. *FY2014 Appropriations: Runaway and homeless youth act*. http://homelessyouthnetwork.org/wp-content/uploads/2012/04/hyn_20130722041911.pdf (accessed October 7, 2014).

National Forum on Youth Violence Prevention. 2011. *National Forum on Youth Violence Prevention strategic plan: April 2011-April 2014*. http://www.findyouthinfo.gov/docs/Forum_Strategic_Plan_FINAL_10.27.11.pdf (accessed March 18, 2014).

NCSL (National Conference of State Legislatures). 2014. *Undocumented student tuition: State action*. www.ncsl.org/default.aspx?tabid=12846 (accessed October 9, 2014).

NRC (National Research Council). 2013. *Reforming juvenile justice: A developmental approach*. Washington, DC: The National Academies Press.

NRC. 2014. *The growth of incarceration in the United States: Exploring causes and consequences*. Washington, DC: The National Academies Press.

NRCYD (National Resource Center for Youth Development). 2014. *State by state facts*. http://www.nrcyd.ou.edu/state-pages (accessed October 20, 2014).

OJJDP (Department of Justice Office of Juvenile Justice and Delinquency Prevention). 2009a. *Formula Grants Program*. http://www.ojjdp.gov/programs/ProgSummary.asp?pi=16 (accessed March 18, 2014).

OJJDP. 2009b. *Juvenile Accountability Block Grant Program*. https://www.ncjrs.gov/pdffiles1/ojjdp/226357.pdf (accessed March 18, 2014).

OJJDP. 2012. *OJJDP statistical briefing book: Upper age of original court jurisdiction, 2011*. http://www.ojjdp.gov/ojstatbb/structure_process/qa04106.asp?qaDate=2012 (accessed March 18, 2014).

OJJDP. 2013a. *OJJDP statistical briefing book: Extended age of juvenile court jurisdiction, 2012*. http://www.ojjdp.gov/ojstatbb/structure_process/qa04106.asp?qaDate=2012 (accessed March 18, 2014).

OJJDP. 2013b. *Overview of the DCTAT data for formula grants*. https://www.ojjdp-dctat.org/help/FormulaFY2013.pdf (accessed March 18, 2014).

OJJDP. 2013c. *Overview of the DCTAT data for Juvenile Accountability Block Grants Program*. https://www.ojjdp-dctat.org/help/JABGApr2012Mar2013.pdf (accessed March 18, 2014).

OJJDP. 2013d. *Overview of the DCTAT data for Title V grants*. Washington, DC: OJJDP.

OJJDP. 2014. *Data Reporting Tool (DCTAT)*. https://www.ojjdp-dctat.org (accessed March 18, 2014).

OMB (Office of Management and Budget). 2014. *Guidance for providing and using administrative data for statistical purposes*. Washington, DC: OMB.

Osgood, D. W., E. M. Foster, C. Flanagan, and G. R. Ruth. 2005. *On your own without a net: The transition to adulthood for vulnerable populations*. Chicago, IL: University of Chicago Press.

Osgood, D. W., E. M. Foster, and M. E. Courtney. 2010. Vulnerable populations and the transition to adulthood. *The Future of Children* 20(1):209-229.

Pecora, P. J., R. C. Kessler, J. Williams, K. O'Brien, A. C. Downs, D. English, J. White, E. Hiripi, C. Roller White, T. Wiggins, and K. Holmes. 2005. *Improving family foster care: Findings from the Northwest Foster Care Alumni Study*. Washington, DC: Casey Family Programs.

Perreira, K. M., and I. J. Ornelas. 2011. The physical and psychological well-being of immigrant children. *The Future of Children* 21(1):195-218.

Perreira, K. M., R. Crosnoe, K. Fortuny, J. Pedroza, K. Ulvestad, C. Weiland, and H. Yoshikawa. 2012. *Barriers to immigrants' access to health and human services programs*. Washington, DC: Office of the Assistant Secretary for Planning and Evaluation.

Portes, A., and R. G. Rumbaut. 2001. *Legacies: The story of the immigrant second generation*. Oakland, CA: University of California Press.

Portes, A., and R. Rumbaut. 2006. *Immigrant America: A portrait*. Berkeley: University of California Press.

Pullmann, M. D. 2010. Predictors of criminal charges for youth in public mental health during the transition to adulthood. *Journal of Child and Family Studies* 19(4):483-491.

Ratcliffe, C., S.-M. McKernan, and S. Zhang. 2011. *How much does the Supplemental Nutrition Assistance Program reduce food insecurity?* Washington, DC: Urban Institute.

Redd, Z., T. S. Karver, D. Murphey, K. A. Moore, and D. Knewstub. 2011. *Two generations in poverty: Status and trends among parents and children in the United States, 2000-2010*. Washington, DC: Ascend at the Aspen Institute and Communications Consortium Media Center.

Rossin-Slater, M. 2013. WIC in your neighborhood: New evidence on the impacts of geographic access to clinics. *Journal of Public Economics* 102:51-69.

Rumbaut, R. G. 2004. Ages, life stages, and generational cohorts: Decomposing the immigrant first and second generations in the United States. *International Migration Review* 38(3):1160-1205.

Scarcella, C. A., R. Bess, E. H. Zielewski, and R. Geen. 2006. *The cost of protecting vulnerable children V: Understanding state variation in child welfare financing*. Washington, DC: Urban Institute.

Schochet, P. Z., J. Burghardt, and S. McConnell. 2008. Does Job Corps work? Impact findings from the National Job Corps Study. *The American Economic Review* 98(5):1864-1886.

Sen, A. K. 2000. *Social exclusion: Concept, application, and scrutiny*. Manila, Philippines: Office of Environment and Social Development, Asian Development Bank.

Sickmund, M., A. Sladky, and W. Kang. 2013. *Easy access to the census of juveniles in residential placement: 1997-2010*. Pittsburgh, PA: National Center for Juvenile Justice.

Slesnick, N., P. Dashora, A. Letcher, G. Erdem, and J. Serovich. 2009. A review of services and interventions for runaway and homeless youth: Moving forward. *Children and Youth Services Review* 31(7):732-742.

SSA (Social Services Administration). 2013. *SSI annual statistical report, 2012*. http://www.ssa.gov/policy/docs/statcomps/ssi_asr/2012/ssi_asr12.pdf (accessed June 23, 2014).

SSA. 2014. *Title IV grants to states for aid and services to needy families with children and for child-welfare services*. http://www.ssa.gov/OP_Home/ssact/title04/0400.htm (accessed August 11, 2014).

Steinberg, L. 2013. The influence of neuroscience on U.S. Supreme Court decisions about adolescents' criminal culpability. *Nature Reviews Neuroscience* 14(7):513-518.

Suárez-Orozco, M. M., C. Suárez-Orozco, and C. Sattin-Bajaj. 2010. Making migration work. *Peabody Journal of Education* 85(4):535-551.

Toro, P. A., A. Dworsky, and P. J. Fowler. 2007. *Homeless youth in the United States: Recent research findings and intervention approaches*. Paper read at National Symposium on Homelessness Research, Washington, DC.

Trisi, D., and L. Pavetti. 2012. *TANF weakening as a safety net for poor families*. Washington, DC: Center on Budget and Policy Priorities.

USDA (U.S. Department of Agriculture). 2013a. *A short history of SNAP.* http://www.fns.usda.gov/snap/short-history-snap (accessed October 7, 2014).

USDA. 2013b. *WIC participant and program characteristics 2012 final report*. Washington, DC: U.S. Department of Agriculture.

USDA. 2014a. *Supplemental Nutrition Assistance Program (SNAP) eligibility.* http://www.fns.usda.gov/snap/eligibility (accessed October 7, 2014).

USDA. 2014b. *Supplemental Nutrition Assistance Program participation and costs (data as of March 7, 2014)*. http://www.fns.usda.gov/pd/SNAPsummary.htm (accessed March 14, 2014).

Velázquez, T. 2013. *Young adult justice: A new frontier worth exploring*. https://chronicleofsocialchange.org/xpanel/wp-content/uploads/2013/05/Young-Adult-Justice-FINAL-revised.pdf (accessed March 18, 2014).

Vespa, J., J. M. Lewis, and R. M. Kreider. 2013. *America's families and living arrangements: 2012*. Washington, DC: U.S. Government Printing Office.

Vinik, D. 2014. The U.S. tax code drags millions of childless workers into poverty. *The New Republic*, April 14, 2014. http://www.newrepublic.com/article/117378/earned-income-tax-credit-offers-few-benefits-childless-workers (accessed, September 14, 2014).

Welsh, B. C., M. W. Lipsey, F. P. Rivara, J. D. Hawkins, S. Aos, M. E. Peel, and D. Petechuk. 2013. *Bulletin 6: Changing lives: Prevention and intervention to reduce serious offending (study group on the transitions between juvenile delinquency and adult crime)*. Washington, DC: U.S. Department of Justice.

Whitbeck, L. B. 2009. *Mental health and emerging adulthood among homeless young people*. New York: Psychology Press, Taylor & Francis Group.

Wilson, B. D., K. Cooper, A. Kastanis, and S. Nezhad. 2014. *Sexual and gender minority youth in foster care: Assessing disproportionality and disparities in Los Angeles*. Los Angeles, CA: Williams Institute.

Wulczyn, F., and K. Brunner Hislop. 2001. *Children in substitute care at age 16: Selected findings from the multistate data archive*. Chicago, IL: Chapin Hall at the University of Chicago.

YouthBuild USA. 2014a. *Demographics and outcomes*. https://youthbuild.org/youthbuild-demographics-and-outcomes (accessed March 18, 2014).

YouthBuild USA. 2014b. *Research*. https://youthbuild.org/research (accessed March 18, 2014).

YouthBuild USA. 2014c. *SMART initiative*. https://youthbuild.org/smart-initiative (accessed March 18, 2014).

YouthBuild USA. 2014d. *YouthBuild USA*. https://youthbuild.org (accessed March 18, 2014).

9

Next Steps

The committee was charged with reviewing current policies and programs pertaining to the health, safety, and well-being of young adults and offering recommendations for improvement. Previous chapters have fulfilled this assignment in six specific policy domains: relationships, education and employment, civic engagement and national service, public health, health care systems, and government programs for marginalized young adults. This chapter distills our conclusions and recommendations in these specific domains into a blueprint for moving forward. It begins by drawing several overall conclusions about current policies and programs for young adults across all six domains. Based on these conclusions, we then delineate key ingredients for moving forward and offer a broad, cross-cutting recommendation. Next, we organize the recommendations from previous chapters according to the entities to which they are directed—the federal government, state and local governments, and private entities that serve many young adults. Finally, we summarize our observations regarding the research needed to provide a stronger evidence base for the development of policies and programs that better support young adults.

OVERALL CONCLUSIONS ABOUT POLICIES AND PROGRAMS THAT SERVE YOUNG ADULTS

Three overall conclusions emerged from our review of public and private policies and programs pertaining to the domains of education and employment, civic engagement and national service, public health, health care systems, and government programs for marginalized young adults.

Current policies and programs serving the young adult population are often fragmented and uncoordinated.

With the exception of policies and programs that target exclusively either children and youth under 18 or older adults, young adults are among the population served by virtually every federal, state, and local program in the areas of education, employment, civic engagement and national service, and health and human services. For example, the United States currently has a wide array of policies to support higher education and workforce development services for both young and older adults at the federal, state, and local levels, as well as laws to protect the disabled. National service programs are supported and run by multiple entities, including the Corporation for National and Community Service and the U.S. Departments of Labor, Interior, and Housing and Urban Development at the federal level, and many more at the state and local levels, as well as private foundations and nonprofit organizations. Similarly, the wide range of policies and programs designed to support current members of the military serve many young adults.

In the realm of health, several major federal agencies and all state and local public health departments have programs that target many of the public health priorities for young adults identified in this report, including tobacco control, obesity prevention, injury prevention, and prevention of unprotected sexual activity. Health care coverage for young adults is fragmented across policies that guide employer-based insurance, insurance purchased through exchanges, student health coverage, and Medicaid.

Fragmentation is particularly noticeable in policies and programs aimed at supporting marginalized young adults. These include programs for young adults aging out of foster care, those in the justice system, those who are homeless, and young parents, as discussed in Chapter 8; education and employment programs for young adults neither in school nor working and those with disabilities, as discussed in Chapter 4; and policies and programs for young adults who experience particular difficulty accessing health care, as described in Chapter 7. Fragmented programs have narrow and idiosyncratic eligibility criteria that create obstacles to young people's getting the help they need, often create gaps in help when it is provided, and too often are stigmatizing. Major entitlement programs intended to help vulnerable populations provide limited support for young adults, and discretionary programs targeting these populations, often fall far short of meeting demonstrable need. The variable categorization of marginalized young adults across multiple programs results in a lack of accountability, with multiple distinct outputs and outcomes being associated with the plethora of programs. There is no collective accountability for improving the overall health and well-being of marginalized young adults.

Many states have recognized the importance of integration across different topic areas for adolescents. For example, many state public health agencies have created adolescent topic areas or have a designated state adolescent health coordinator. However, very few states have implemented a similar approach for young adults. Better coordination and, where possible, integration of services and supports and shared accountability are likely to achieve greater efficiency and effectiveness.

Policies and programs that serve young adults are often inadequately focused on their developmental needs and on specific interventions that would facilitate a successful transition to adulthood.

The majority of policies and programs that serve many young adults are not exclusively focused on this age group. A few exceptions include federal and state policies and programs that support young adults aging out of foster care and the young adult justice policies in several states. Some additional programs, such as YouthBuild, serve primarily young adults and older adolescents. However, it is much more common for young adults to be served along with all adults or, less frequently, adolescents.

Young adults cannot be treated like children because they are more mature and have more responsibilities, commitments, and expectations, as described in Chapter 2. However, general adult programs also are often inappropriate because young adults are still in the process of developing psychological and emotional maturity. Scaffolds such as mentoring, counseling, education and training, and specifically designed communication materials can help support young adults in the decisions and actions required of them as adults. Efforts to incorporate into programs for young adults parental support for their decision making and health care treatment also are worth exploring, whereas this would not be considered appropriate for general adult programs. Similarly, health care coordination approaches that are more common in pediatric than in adult systems could be helpful in supporting young adults, but with recognition of their decision-making ability and responsibilities. Although developmental research provides support for this general perspective on policies and programs for young adults, additional research and experimentation ultimately will be needed to support the development of effective interventions for young adults that appropriately strike this balance.

The evidence base on interventions, policies, programs, and service designs that are effective for young adults is limited.

Although gaps remain, much is known about the health, safety, and well-being of young adults as a group; about the factors associated with variations among them; and about trends over time. Much also is known about the changes that have occurred in the social and economic patterns that characterize the transition to adulthood. However, far less is known about the policies, programs, and service designs that will be effective in improving young adults' health, safety, and well-being and in facilitating their successful transition to adulthood.

One barrier to expanding the evidence base is that data often are not collected or reported by age, impeding evaluation of the effectiveness of interventions, policies, programs, and service designs for young adults. Program data and clinical trials that simply include this age group (e.g., studies of adults aged 18-55) are insufficient to establish efficacy in young adults. To do so, the sample size of young adults relative to that of older or younger age groups needs to be large enough to detect an age effect.

A second barrier is that the types of data collected may not cover key issues for young adults. For example, current adult health monitoring efforts do not encompass screening and counseling for many health concerns of particular relevance to young adults, such as obesity-related issues, substance use, mental health disorders, reproductive health issues, and dental diseases. This data gap impedes efforts to monitor adherence to guidelines in preventive care for young adults. Population-based studies and government programs also often fail to capture data that would help identify the presence and well-being of marginalized populations.

Third, although evidence is emerging on effective programs and interventions for young adults, many important gaps remain. For example, there is some evidence on successful workforce programs for young and older adults and youth with relatively strong basic skills, and limited evidence on programs designed to improve success rates for disadvantaged students who enroll in college. Research suggests that integrating useful labor market information or training into such developmental efforts holds promise. However, knowledge of exactly what works cost-effectively for the most difficult-to-serve populations who are already disconnected is limited. Similarly, research is sparse on how to assist high school students with disabilities in transitioning to postsecondary education or employment. Behavioral health interventions and preventive care practices also are important research gaps for this age group.

Fourth, even in areas in which there are evidence-based or promising interventions, the ability to replicate and scale the best programs remains limited. As noted above, for example, interventions with positive impacts on completion rates and on the alignment of education and the labor market have been developed and rigorously evaluated. However, these programs need to be replicated and scaled up at the county or state level.

Finally, a key problem we identified was fragmentation and lack of coordination among the multiple policies and programs that serve marginalized young adults. While we believe a more flexible and integrated approach to assisting these young people would ultimately be more effective than the current approach, the available evidence does not yet provide a clear path forward. Only active and ongoing partnership across all levels of government to develop and evaluate new approaches will clearly identify the policies and programs needed to reduce the marginalization of promising young adults.

A PLAN FOR MOVING FORWARD

Despite the challenges delineated above, it is important that the nation not find itself in the same position in 20 years, having failed to take advantage of opportunities to improve the trajectories of tens of millions of young adults. What is needed now is a coordinated effort by the public and private sectors to raise public awareness of the need to support and improve policies and programs focused on the needs of young adults, to engage young adults in the design and implementation of these policies and programs, and to further innovation and improvement by developing and experimentally evaluating new approaches. The key ingredients for such a concerted effort are delineated below.

Highlight Young Adulthood as a Distinct and Important Period of Development

An initial, critical ingredient for improving public policies and programs for young adults is for policy makers and program leaders to understand young adulthood as a distinct and important period of development that, under foreseeable social and economic circumstances, has significant implications for the future well-being of each cohort of young adults and of the nation as a whole. Heightened public understanding of this developmental period is needed to encourage appropriate public and private action.

Support Young Adults During the Critical Transitions They Face

A second key ingredient is public and private investment and a shared commitment to providing the training and tools needed to support young adults during the critical transitions they face, including obtaining education and entering the workforce. Investments in marginalized populations are particularly needed to reduce inequalities during the young adult years and increase the supply of skilled workers to serve the nation's needs. Investing in public health and clinical preventive services also will be crucial because health underlies young adults' ability to be successful in education, employment, and social relationships. Efforts to prevent and ameliorate the effects of behavioral health problems, including mood disorders, stress-related dysfunction, and substance use disorders, are particularly critical.

Engage Young Adults

The needs of young adults have been underresearched and underappreciated in policies and programs. Therefore, a third ingredient for action is to engage young adults themselves in the development of policies, programs, and services that impact them in the areas of education, social services, employment, and health care. It will be important to engage a range of young adults, not just high achievers. The powerful influence of young people with experience in foster care in developing federal and state child welfare policy over the past two decades illustrates the potential of engaging young adults in policy and program development.

Seek Developmentally Appropriate Outcomes

Government programs should identify and require outcomes that are appropriate for this age group and tailored to their developmental situation and their needs. The multiple programs serving marginalized young adults should be better coordinated, as discussed in the conclusions section above, and as part of this effort should share accountability for achieving developmentally appropriate outcomes for young adults. In an era of high-stakes accountability it is important to have program outcomes that are appropriate to the population(s) served.

Conduct Policy and Program Experimentation

While the need to invest in young adults is clear, the ideal nature of those investments is less so. As a result, we have generally avoided making recommendations for large-scale policy change. Instead, the current state of knowledge calls for *coordination* among federal, state, and local governments and philanthropies in policy and program *experimentation* to help identify the most effective approaches to improving the prospects of young adults. Promising interventions targeting the health, safety, and well-being of young adults, particularly those who have been socially excluded, should be rigorously evaluated. Government and private resources devoted to policy evaluation should be directed at learning from variations among and within states in current policies affecting young adults. In addition, demonstration projects should be developed, through coordination of government and private investments, to assess the costs and benefits of new policies intended to benefit young adults. Twenty years from now we will remain in the dark regarding how best to improve the health and well-being of young adults if we fail to make strategic investments in policy and program experimentation on their behalf.

CROSS-CUTTING RECOMMENDATION

Based on the findings and conclusions presented above, we first offer a cross-cutting recommendation that applies to all policies and programs addressing young adults, whether public or private and in all sectors of society. We then organize the specific recommendations made in previous chapters according to whether they are directed to the federal government, state and local governments, or the private sector.

Recommendation 9-1: Federal, state, and local governments and non-governmental entities that fund programs serving young adults or research affecting the health, safety, or well-being of this population should differentiate young adults from adolescents and older adults whenever permitted by law and programmatically appropriate.

To implement this recommendation, specific actions should be taken to

- modify reporting of data to identify young adults (aged 18-26) as a distinct age group in all reports, evaluations, and open data systems in which they are included;
- enhance new or existing surveys or experimental research focused on either adolescents or adults to advance knowledge regarding the health and well-being of young adults and healthy transitions into young adulthood;
- ensure that services provided to young adults are developmentally and culturally appropriate, recognizing that while adolescent or general adult services may sometimes be appropriate, modifications to existing services or entirely new approaches may be needed;
- engage diverse young adults in designing and implementing programs and services;
- support workforce training for health and human service providers to develop the skills and knowledge needed to work with young adults and their families;
- seek opportunities for coordinating services and, where possible, integrating them to achieve greater effectiveness and efficiency; and
- develop, implement, and evaluate systematic policy and program experiments to help identify the most effective approaches to improving the prospects of young adults.

It is important to note that this recommendation is not intended to imply the creation of an extensive set of new programs targeted only at young adults. Such an approach would have the potential to create new silos and generate concerns about discontinuities and lack of coordination similar to those that currently characterize programs for children/adolescents and adults. Rather, the intent is to increase focus on how policies and programs are working for young adults today. We recommend the adaptation or creation of new policies, programs, and practices *only when the evidence indicates that young adults' specific needs are not being met*, with an emphasis on first attempting to modify existing efforts to better suit young adults. Further, we emphasize the importance of considering the transitions into and out of young adulthood to avoid inadvertently creating new discontinuities.

ORGANIZATION OF DOMAIN-SPECIFIC RECOMMENDATIONS BY RESPONSIBLE ENTITIES

The recommendations presented in Chapters 3 through 8 of this report fall within the key domains of relationships, education and employment, civic engagement and national service, public health, health care systems, and government investments in marginalized young adults. Pursuant to the ambitious program of experimentation proposed above, these domain-specific recommendations include large-scale experimentation programs, such as demonstration projects, where initial evidence suggests promising approaches, and identify priorities for research where evidence on promising directions to pursue is currently lacking. Here we organize these recommendations according to the entities that would be responsible for their implementation. The original recommendation numbers are given in parentheses. Box 9-1 summarizes recommendations for the federal government, organized by branch and department. Box 9-2 summarizes recommendations for state and local governments; because states vary in the organization of their agencies, these recommendations are grouped by topic area and are targeted at whichever state or local agency covers that topic. Finally, Box 9-3 summarizes recommendations for various private entities, including philanthropic funders, private-sector entities such as health systems, and nonprofit organizations that serve young adults.

BOX 9-1
Recommendations for the Federal Government

In addition to Recommendation 9-1, above, the committee provides the following recommendations to assist the U.S. Congress and federal agencies in developing policies and programs designed to improve the health, safety, and well-being of young adults. Although young adults are not explicitly mentioned in each recommendation below, the committee recommends that they be engaged throughout the processes described. (Please note that recommendations directed at specific agencies include Recommendation 9-1; Recommendations 8-1 through 8-5, listed under "U.S. Departments of Education, Labor, Health and Human Services, Justice, and Housing and Urban Development, and Other Agencies Serving Large Numbers of Young Adults"; and applicable recommendations under the remaining headings in this box.)

U.S. Congress

- Amend federal laws to allow for more flexible and efficient eligibility determination and service provision across marginalized young adult populations. (8-3)

U.S. Departments of Education, Health and Human Services, Housing and Urban Development, Justice, and Labor, and Other Agencies Serving Large Numbers of Young Adults

- Incorporate a greater focus on marginalized young adults in ongoing and new population-based cross-sectional and longitudinal studies of young adults. (8-1)
- Implement the recent Office of Management and Budget "Guidance for Providing and Using Administrative Data for Statistical Purposes" to continue encouraging programs that serve marginalized populations to make better use of administrative data. (8-2)
- Fund demonstration projects at the state level to support states in integrating program administrative data to better understand marginalized young adults and to evaluate programs serving them. (8-2)
- Amend federal laws and regulations to allow for more flexible and efficient eligibility determination and service provision across marginalized young adult populations. (8-3)
- Amend laws and regulations to create accountability for achieving improvement on a limited set of key outcomes for marginalized young adults. (8-4)
- Emphasize evaluation of programs aimed at improving outcomes across multiple vulnerable populations while remaining sensitive to differences across subpopulations. (8-5)
- Actively monitor the outcomes of the young parent participants in addition to early childhood outcomes in the development, implementation, and evaluation of two-generation programs. Doing so would be valuable for programs that target primarily health and well-being (such as home visiting programs), as well as those that target primarily human capital development. (3-1)

continued

BOX 9-1 Continued

U.S. Department of Education

- Provide competitive grants and technical assistance to support state efforts to experiment with and evaluate interventions designed to improve graduation rates at high schools and colleges, as well as the rates at which high school dropouts receive their General Educational Development (GED) credential and enroll in college or job training. (4-1)
- Provide competitive grants and technical assistance to support state efforts to implement at a medium or large scale and evaluate education and workforce development approaches that are more closely tied to high-demand economic sectors. (4-2)
- Provide competitive grants and technical assistance to support state efforts to experiment with and evaluate providing performance-based subsidies to their public colleges and universities. (4-3)

U.S. Department of Labor

- Provide competitive grants and technical assistance to support state efforts to implement at a medium or large scale and evaluate education and workforce development approaches that are more closely tied to high-demand economic sectors. (4-2)
- Provide competitive grants and technical assistance to support state efforts to experiment with and evaluate providing performance-based subsidies for public colleges and universities. (4-3)
- Expand and improve opportunities for service for all young adults, and emphasize the short- and long-term effects of service on participants' health and well-being (in addition to community impact) in program evaluations. (5-1)

Corporation for National and Community Service

- Expand and improve opportunities for service for all young adults, and emphasize the short- and long-term effects of service on participants' health and well-being (in addition to community impact) in program evaluations. (5-1)

U.S. Preventive Services Task Force

- Develop a consolidated set of standardized evidence-based recommendations for clinical preventive services such as screenings, counseling services, and preventive medications specifically for young adults. Behavioral and oral health should be included in these recommendations. (7-2)

U.S. Department of Health and Human Services

Agency for Healthcare Research and Quality

- Develop quality performance metrics on the transition-of-care process to ensure continuity of care for young adults making the transition from pediatric to adult behavioral and medical health care. (7-1)

Centers for Medicare & Medicaid Services

- Encourage greater attention to the pediatric-to-adult transition-of-care process within the innovation models that it solicits and funds, such as those from the Center for Medicare & Medicaid Innovation. (7-1)
- Incorporate young adult transition-of-care metrics into pay-for-performance schemes, contracting, and other provider assessments. (7-1)
- Adopt the clinical preventive services recommended by the U.S. Preventive Services Task Force, include the delivery of those services in quality performance metrics used for pay-for-performance and other health care provider assessments, and require public reporting of compliance. (7-3)

Office of the National Coordinator for Health Information Technology

- Ensure that meaningful use criteria enable the capture of data on the pediatric-to-adult transition-of-care process. (7-1)

Health Resources and Services Administration, Maternal and Child Health Bureau

- Expand work on transition-of-care metrics for youth with special health care needs to include all youth and young adults, incorporate such metrics in Title V program requirements, and support related capacity development and training in states. (7-1)
- Adopt the clinical preventive services recommended by the U.S. Preventive Services Task Force, include the delivery of those services in quality performance metrics used for pay-for-performance and other health care provider assessments, and require public reporting of compliance. (7-3)

Other Agencies That Fund or Provide Physical or Behavioral Health Services—Including the Substance Abuse and Mental Health Services Administration and the Indian Health Service

- Adopt the clinical preventive services recommended by the U.S. Preventive Services Task Force, include the delivery of those services in quality performance metrics used for pay-for-performance and other health care provider assessments, and require public reporting of compliance. (7-3)

National Institutes of Health

- Support research aimed at developing a set of evidence-based practices for medical and behavioral health care, including prevention, for young adults. (7-4)

U.S. Departments of Defense and Veterans Affairs

- Adopt the clinical preventive services recommended by the U.S. Preventive Services Task Force, include the delivery of those services in quality performance metrics used for pay-for-performance and other health care provider assessments, and require public reporting of compliance. (7-3)

BOX 9-2
Recommendations for State and Local Governments

In addition to Recommendation 9-1 above, the committee provides the following recommendations to assist state legislatures and state and local agencies in developing policies, programs, and services designed to improve the health, safety, and well-being of young adults.

State Legislatures and Governors

- Amend laws and regulations to create accountability for achieving improvement on a limited set of key outcomes for marginalized young adults. (8-4)

State Agencies in the Areas of Education, Health and Human Services, Housing, Justice, and Labor, and Other Agencies Serving Large Numbers of Young Adults

- Incorporate a greater focus on marginalized young adults in ongoing and new population-based cross-sectional and longitudinal studies of young adults. (8-1)
- Expand on existing state and local efforts to integrate and use administrative data to better understand and serve marginalized young adults. (8-2)

State Education and Employment Agencies

- Experiment with and evaluate a range of interventions designed to improve graduation rates at high schools and colleges, as well as the rates at which high school dropouts receive their GED credential and enroll in college or job training. (4-1)

RESEARCH NEEDS

Given that the transition to adulthood encompasses a wide range of concerns (and thus research disciplines and policy targets), different disciplines will have to collaborate to ensure that the many relevant levels of explanation and intervention (from biological to cultural) are integrated in research designed to support efforts to improve the health, safety, and well-being of young adults. It would be sensible for philanthropic organizations interested in young adults, the National Institutes of Health, and other federal research agencies to collaborate in convening a forum or some other activity for the purpose of identifying priorities and formulating a national

- Experiment with and evaluate programs designed to reduce the enormous disparities in high school and college completion that now exist by race, family income, and geographic location (urban versus rural). (4-1)
- Implement at a medium or large scale and evaluate education and workforce development approaches that are more closely tied to high-demand economic sectors. (4-2)
- Experiment with and evaluate providing performance-based subsidies for public colleges and universities. (4-3)

State and Local Public Health Agencies

- Establish an office to coordinate programs and services bearing on the health, safety, and well-being of young adults. If a separate office is not established for young adults, these responsibilities should be assigned to the adolescent health coordinator. (6-1)
- Take the lead in convening a multistakeholder public-private coalition on "Healthy Transitions to Adulthood." (6-2)
- Include specific targets for young adults in plans to reach the 5-year measurable performance goals of Community Transformation Grants. (6-3)

State and Local Agencies That Fund or Provide Physical or Behavioral Health Services

- Adopt the clinical preventive services recommended by the U.S. Preventive Services Task Force, include the delivery of those services in quality performance metrics used for pay-for-performance and other health care provider assessments, and require public reporting of compliance. (7-3)

research agenda that can meet this need. As a starting point, Table 9-1 presents a listing of key research topics identified by the committee.

CONCLUDING REMARKS

Focusing on the health, safety, and well-being of the current cohort of young adults (those becoming adults in the first third of the 21st century) is especially important because of the powerful (and perhaps transformative) economic and social forces now at work—the restructuring of the economy, widening inequality, a rapidly increasing "elder dependency ratio" (i.e., the

BOX 9-3
Recommendations for Private Entities

The committee provides the following recommendations to assist private entities in developing and supporting policies, programs, and services designed to improve the health, safety, and well-being of young adults.

Philanthropic Funders and Other Entities That Fund Service Programs

- Expand and improve opportunities for service for all young adults, and emphasize the short- and long-term effects of service on participants' health and well-being (in addition to community impact) in program evaluations. (5-1)

Philanthropic Funders That Fund Programs for Marginalized Young Adults

- Actively monitor the outcomes of the young parent participants in addition to early childhood outcomes in the development, implementation, and evaluation of two-generation programs. Doing so would be valuable for programs that target primarily health and well-being (such as home visiting programs), as well as those that target primarily human capital development. (3-1)
- Emphasize evaluation of programs aimed at improving outcomes across multiple vulnerable populations while remaining sensitive to differences across subpopulations. (8-5)

ratio of the population aged 65 and older to the working-age population), a substantial increase in immigration, and the increasing diversity of the population. The future well-being of the nation rests on the investments made in all young adults today—particularly those whose background and characteristics put them at risk of experiencing the greatest struggles. Providing more of the educational, economic, social, and health supports they need will help ensure equal opportunity, erase disparities, and enable more young adults to embrace adult roles successfully as healthy workers, parents, and citizens.

Colleges and Universities, Employers, Youth Organizations; Nonprofit Organizations; Medical Specialties Providing Primary Care to Young Adults; and Other Community Organizations Serving, Supporting, or Investing in Young Adults

- Participate in a multistakeholder public-private coalition on "Healthy Transitions to Adulthood." (6-2)

Recipients of Community Transformation Grants

- Include specific targets for young adults in plans to reach the 5-year measurable performance goals of Community Transformation Grants. (6-3)

National Committee for Quality Assurance, National Quality Forum, and Other Quality Measurement Entities

- Incorporate pediatric-to-adult transition-of-care performance metrics into quality measurement and reporting frameworks. (7-1)

Health Care Delivery Systems and Provider Organizations Serving Young Adults

- Develop a coordinated pediatric-to-adult transition-of-care process within their organizations. (7-1)

Health Insurers and Purchasing Entities Such as Employer Coalitions

- Incorporate pediatric-to-adult transition-of-care performance metrics, to be developed by the Agency for Healthcare Research and Quality, into pay-for-performance initiatives, contracting, and other health care provider assessments. (7-1)

TABLE 9-1 Research Needed to Inform Policies and Programs Designed to Improve Young Adults' Health, Safety, and Well-Being

General Category	Specific Research Needs
Cross-Cutting	• Identify processes that underlie heterogeneity in trajectories in the health, safety, and well-being of young adults, including romantic relationships, family formation, childbearing and parenting, effective parenting of young adults, intergenerational patterns, peer relations, access to and utilization of behavioral and medical health care, involvement with social service and justice systems, and neurobiological processes. • Understand how social media and mobile technology influence young adults' social relations, health, safety, and well-being to inform the design of interventions.
Relationships	• Monitor evaluation results from ongoing two-generation programs, and extend successful programs to new implementation sites. • Examine the impact of the recent dramatic shift in union formation and childbearing on the health and well-being of young adults and their children. • Understand the ways in which social media can be used to impact young adults' social relations, health, safety and well-being.
Education and Employment	• Understand what works to improve success rates in higher education and the labor market for the most difficult-to-serve young adults who are already disconnected. • Identify effective practices for assisting high school students with disabilities in transitioning to postsecondary education or employment.
Civic Engagement and National Service	• Identify factors that contribute to and enhance civic engagement and involvement in national service among young adults. • Conduct more rigorous experimental studies to determine how civic engagement and involvement in national service impact the trajectories of health, safety, and well-being of young adult participants. • Examine institutional supports and individual characteristics that facilitate successful transitions into education, employment, social relationships, and citizenship following national service.

TABLE 9-1 Continued

General Category	Specific Research Needs
Public Health	• Assess the effectiveness of multilevel interventions with respect to health outcomes, including how to connect with difficult-to-reach young adults. • Better understand the influence of social media on health outcomes. • Better understand how social determinants, mechanisms, and trajectories contribute to health inequalities among young adults, including within different groups. • Better understand the impact of advertising and promotion of alcohol, tobacco, and marijuana on the health, safety, and well-being of young adults.
Health Care Systems	• Develop preventive care guidelines for young adults (see Recommendation 7-2). • Develop a set of evidence-based practices for medical and behavioral health care for young adults, including prevention and effective processes for the transition from pediatric to adult care (see Recommendations 7-1, 7-2, 7-3, and 7-4). • Examine the efficacy of integrating behavioral and physical health care in improving health outcomes for young adults. • Develop a comprehensive behavioral health screen.
Government Investments in Marginalized Young Adults	• Gain better knowledge of how marginalized young adults fare during young adulthood (see Recommendation 8-1). • Integrate information across the systems serving marginalized young adults and over time to provide a more complex, longitudinal perspective on their health and well-being (see Recommendation 8-2).

A

Open Session Agendas

The committee held data gathering sessions that were open to the public in Washington, DC, on December 5, 2013; January 30, 2014; and in Irvine, California, April 2, 2014. The open session agendas are presented below.

COMMITTEE ON IMPROVING THE HEALTH, SAFETY, AND WELL-BEING OF YOUNG ADULTS: OPEN SESSION

Thursday, December 5, 2013
National Academies' Keck Center
500 Fifth Street, NW, Room 208
Washington, DC

Open Session Goals:

1. Hold open session with representatives from the Health Resources and Services Administration and the Robert Wood Johnson Foundation to understand the sponsor perspectives on the study task.
2. Hold open session to provide an overview of federal policies and programs relevant to the health, safety, and well-being of young adults.

SPONSOR BRIEFING

Session Objective: To obtain a better understanding of the study background and the sponsors' charge to the committee.

1:00 PM	**Welcome and Introductions** Richard Bonnie, *Committee Chair* Harrison Foundation Professor of Medicine and Law University of Virginia
1:15 PM	**Background and Charge to the Committee** Trina Anglin Director, Adolescent Health Maternal and Child Health Bureau Health Resources and Services Administration Kristin Schubert *(by phone)* Team Director and Senior Program Officer Vulnerable Populations Program Robert Wood Johnson Foundation
1:45 PM	**Committee Discussion with Sponsors** Richard Bonnie
2:30 PM	Break

FEDERAL POLICIES AND PROGRAMS

Session Objective: To provide an overview of selected federal policies and programs relevant to young adults' health, safety, and well-being. Specific questions to be discussed include

- What existing federal policies and programs are targeted specifically at young adults?
- How are young adults impacted by current federal policies and programs, considering those specifically targeted at young adults as well as those applicable to the general population?
- What are the greatest gaps, challenges, and opportunities?
- How do the policies and programs for young adults contrast with policies and programs for children and adolescents?

2:45 PM **Welcoming Remarks**
Richard Bonnie

2:50 PM **Presentations by Representatives of Federal Agencies**
Martha Moorehouse
Chair, Interagency Working Group on Youth Programs
Office of the Assistant Secretary for Planning and Evaluation
U.S. Department of Health and Human Services
and Senior Advisor for the Social Innovation Fund
Corporation for National and Community Service

Stephen Cha
Chief Medical Officer
Center for Medicaid and CHIP Services
Centers for Medicare & Medicaid Services
U.S. Department of Health and Human Services

Rebecca Flatow
Public Health Analyst
Substance Abuse and Mental Health Services Administration
U.S. Department of Health and Human Services

Erica Zielewski
Social Science Research Analyst
Administration for Children and Families
U.S. Department of Health and Human Services

Aria Crump
Health Scientist Administrator
Prevention Research Branch
National Institute on Drug Abuse
U.S. Department of Health and Human Services

Jennifer Kemp
Unit Chief, Youth Policy and Performance
Employment and Training Administration
U.S. Department of Labor

Christopher Arendt
Deputy Director, Accessions Policy
Office of the Under Secretary of Defense for Personnel and Readiness
U.S. Department of Defense

4:15 PM **Committee Discussion with Representatives of Federal Agencies**
Richard Bonnie

4:45 PM Adjourn open session

IMPROVING THE HEALTH, SAFETY, AND WELL-BEING OF YOUNG ADULTS: A WORKSHOP ON STATE POLICIES AND PROGRAMS AND SOCIAL MEDIA AND INFORMATION TECHNOLOGY

January 30, 2014
National Academy of Sciences Building, Room 120
2101 Constitution Avenue, NW
Washington, DC

9:00-9:15 AM **Welcome**
Richard Bonnie, *Committee Chair*
Harrison Foundation Professor of Medicine and Law
University of Virginia

PART 1: STATE POLICIES AND PROGRAMS

9:15-10:30 AM **Session 1: Innovative State and Local Approaches**
Objective: Explore examples of innovative models for supporting young adults' health, safety, and well-being. Specific questions include

- How have the models been integrated/coordinated across the various agencies and services that are relevant to young adults' well-being?
- How have public-private partnerships been integrated into these models?
- What are the most promising approaches, and what lessons can be learned about what has not worked well?

- What evidence is available to support the approach?
- What methods have worked well to engage adult agencies that have not traditionally focused on young adults?
- What steps have been taken to develop a workforce to work with young adults?

Moderator:
Gladys Carrión, *Committee Member*
Commissioner, Administration for Children's Services
New York City

Speakers:
Steven A. Reeder
Director, Office of Adult Services
Mental Hygiene Administration
Maryland Department of Health and Mental Hygiene

David S. Berman
Director, Program Management and Policy
NYC Center for Economic Opportunity

Sam Wood
Special Projects Coordinator for Youth Engagement Programs
Kaiser Permanente Educational Theatre Programs
and Semira Abdu Kassahun and Paul Rastrelli
Former members of the youth advisory group for CO9to25

Kim McGaughey
Three Branch Project Manager
Virginia Department of Social Services

10:30-10:45 AM Break

10:45 AM-12:15 PM **Session 2: Overview of State Policies and Programs That Impact Young Adults' Health, Safety, and Well-Being**
Objective: Provide an overview of state policies and programs in various domains that are relevant to

young adults' health, safety, and well-being (e.g., access to and use of health services, substance abuse services, employment support, support for those aging out of foster care, income support), including the general population of young adults and those from at-risk groups. Specific questions include

- To what extent are states focusing on this age group?
- What state policies and programs are specifically targeted at young adults? And what state policies and programs are applicable to the general population but have an important impact on young adults?
- How do states organize services for this age group?
- What are the greatest gaps and most important opportunities to enhance young adults' health, safety, and well-being through changes to state policies and programs?

Moderator:
Mark Courtney, *Committee Member*
Professor, School of Social Service Administration
University of Chicago

Speakers:
Joy Johnson Wilson
Director, Health and Human Services Policy
National Conference of State Legislatures

Alexandra Cawthorne
Senior Policy Analyst
and Meghan Wills
Policy Analyst
Economic, Workforce, and Human Services Division
National Governors Association

Christina M. Crayton
Senior Policy Associate
American Public Human Services Association
and Staff Liaison
National Association of Public Child Welfare Administrators

Susan E. Foster
Vice President and Director of Policy Research and Analysis CASAColumbia®

12:15-1:15 PM Lunch

1:15-2:15 PM **Session 3: Implications of Federalism**

Objectives: Discuss state and federal roles in young adult services and systems; explore implications of the state-federal relationship; and examine the impact on young adults of variation across states in key policy decisions, such as states' decision about whether to expand Medicaid or whether to extend foster care to age 21. Specific questions include

- What data are available, including data collected by the federal government, to assess how these variations impact young adults' well-being?
- What is the range of actions (e.g., funding, technical assistance) that the federal government takes or could take for the impacted populations in the different policy contexts created by these decisions? What are the associated implications?

Moderator:
Mark Courtney

Speakers:
JooYeun Chang
Associate Commissioner, Children's Bureau
U.S. Department of Health and Human Services

Kathleen Nolan
Director of State Policy and Programs
National Association of Medicaid Directors

2:15-2:30 PM Break

PART 2: SOCIAL MEDIA AND INFORMATION TECHNOLOGY

2:30-4:00 PM Session Objectives:

- Explore how young adults use information technology and social media to influence their health and well-being.
- Identify and discuss opportunities and challenges in using information technology and social media to enhance young adults' health, safety, and well-being, with a particular focus on practices that could have a very important impact and those that are "low-hanging fruit."
- Explore the trajectory of social media in the near future and possible implications for health.

Moderator:
Kasisomayajula "Vish" Viswanath
Harvard School of Public Health

Speakers:
Gwenn Schurgin O'Keeffe
CEO and Editor-in-Chief, *Pediatrics Now*

Thomas Goetz
Co-founder, Iodine *and* Entrepreneur in Residence
Robert Wood Johnson Foundation

Chris Wegrzyn
Co-founder, BlueLabs

Amy Lin
Deputy Policy and Organizing Director, Young Invincibles

4:00 PM Adjourn public workshop

COMMITTEE ON IMPROVING THE HEALTH, SAFETY, AND WELL-BEING OF YOUNG ADULTS: MEETING 3 OPEN SESSION

April 2, 2014
The Beckman Center, Balboa Room
100 Academy Drive, Irvine, CA

Open Session Objectives:

1. Discuss young adults and the justice system with Vincent Schiraldi, Senior Advisor, New York City Mayor's Office of Criminal Justice.
2. Receive briefing from Patrice Cromwell of the Annie E. Casey Foundation, a new sponsor of this consensus study, on the foundation's areas of interest.

OPEN SESSION

8:30-8:35 AM PST	**Welcome** Richard Bonnie, *Committee Chair* Harrison Foundation Professor of Medicine and Law University of Virginia
8:35-8:50 AM PST	**Young Adults and the Justice System** Vincent Schiraldi *(by teleconference)*
8:50-9:15 AM PST	**Committee Discussion with Vincent Schiraldi**
9:15-9:25 AM PST	**Sponsor Briefing** Patrice Cromwell *(by teleconference)*
9:25-9:45 AM PST	**Committee Discussion with Sponsor**
9:45 AM PST	Adjourn open session

B

Diversity and the Effects of Bias and Discrimination on Young Adults' Health and Well-Being

This appendix focuses in greater detail on the adverse effects of continuing patterns of prejudice and discrimination[1] on the health and well-being of young adults summarized in Chapter 2. We take note of variations across racial and ethnic groups, and summarize what is known about factors that protect or buffer young people against these effects.

EXPERIENCE OF BIAS AND DISCRIMINATION

As noted in Chapter 2, the experience of being exposed to biased and discriminatory behavior has been characterized as a pervasive and normative stressor in the lives of people of color (García Coll et al., 1996) and can take a toll on adolescents and young adults, negatively affecting their future well-being. Importantly, during adolescence and young adulthood, many minority youth start to make meaning of their ethnic and racial group membership as a core component of their identity and may become increasingly aware of negative societal views of and prejudices toward their group, which can heighten sensitivity to perceived bias and discrimination (Cross and Cross, 2008). Thus, normative processes of identity development can

[1] *Prejudice* and *bias* are used synonymously to refer to attitudes even if unaccompanied by discriminatory behavior. Although surveys of minorities ascertain their perceptions of biased or discriminatory behavior rather than the intentions of the persons exhibiting the behavior, we have not inserted the word "perceived" in every instance. Finally, when used generally (and not being used to report on a specific study), the term *discrimination* is meant to encompass bias or prejudice. We generally do not use the term *racism* because we typically are referring to bias and discrimination based on either ethnicity or race.

potentially increase vulnerabilities; at the same time, these processes can play a protective role in attenuating the negative effects of bias and discrimination, which we address in more detail later in this appendix.

As reported in Chapter 2, results of a 2013 national survey of adults by the Pew Research Center (2013b) indicate that 88 percent of non-Hispanic blacks and 57 percent of non-Hispanic whites believe that African Americans are subject to "some"/"a lot" of discrimination in the United States, while another report found that among all adults, 73 percent and 65 percent, respectively, hold that view of Muslim Americans and Hispanics (Pew Research Center, 2013a). Interestingly, the perception that racial or ethnic minorities face discrimination is more widespread among young adults (aged 18-29) of all racial/ethnic backgrounds than among older age groups of all backgrounds (Pew Research Center, 2013a).

Until recently, research on racial/ethnic bias and discrimination in the United States focused primarily on African Americans. A substantial majority of blacks report that they have personally been exposed to race-related stimuli perceived as biased or discriminatory (Clark, 2000; Seaton et al., 2008; Simons et al., 2002; Williams et al., 2003). In the National Survey of African Life, the majority of black young adults (in this instance, African American and Caribbean blacks) reported experiencing at least one discriminatory event in the previous year, with increased episodes occurring as they transitioned into young adulthood (Seaton et al., 2008). A higher incidence of discrimination was reported among females from both ethnic groups. African Americans and Caribbean Americans reported equal numbers of discriminatory incidents; however, one interesting finding was that exposure to discrimination was associated with greater vulnerability and more negative outcomes for Caribbean American young adults compared with their African American counterparts. The authors speculate that lack of preparation for negative race-related stress among the recent Caribbean immigrants may explain the variability in the groups' responses. Importantly, these differences reveal that people from the same pan-racial group have diverse experiences with discrimination that are affected by differences in patterns of immigration and cultural norms. In addition to African Americans, evidence is growing that other immigrant groups, such as Asians and Hispanics, are reporting discrimination that is associated with physical and mental health issues, harmful health behaviors, and decreased access to quality health care (Viruell-Fuentes et al., 2012). Further, the longer immigrants reside in the United States, the more likely they are to have heightened exposure to bias and discrimination (Viruell-Fuentes et al., 2012), although bias and discrimination can be particularly salient for immigrants in the context of anti-immigration legal policies and social messages (Lopez et al., 2010).

According to the minority stress theory, minorities who are openly gay (e.g., gay African Americans, Asian Americans, or Hispanics) are at greater risk of experiencing discrimination at the structural and institutional levels (Krieger and Sidney, 1997; Kyung-Hee et al., 2013; Mays and Cochran, 2001; Schmitt et al., 2014), including in housing, employment, and health care, and are at increased risk of substance use, particularly when experiencing discrimination targeting multiple social group memberships (e.g., gender, race, sexual orientation) (McCabe et al., 2010). Of course, in the United States, *all* disadvantaged and marginalized groups, including people of color, individuals of low-income status, immigrants, religious minorities (e.g., Muslims), sexual minorities, individuals with disabilities, and those in low-resource settings (e.g., public housing) are at risk of experiencing some form of bias or discrimination. Results of a 2014 review of both correlational and experimental studies that manipulated perceptions of discrimination in laboratories offer support for the detrimental effects of perceived discrimination for groups stigmatized because of sexual orientation, race/ethnicity, gender, or disabilities (Schmitt et al., 2014).

EFFECTS OF DISCRIMINATION ON WELL-BEING

Impact on Educational Performance and Employment

As noted in Chapter 2, African Americans and Hispanics are overrepresented among high school dropouts. This problem, which has its roots in grade school, is widely perceived to have been magnified by harsh enforcement of "zero tolerance" school discipline policies, including suspension and expulsion, and by increased use of law enforcement officers in school settings, thereby creating the so-called schools-to-prisons pipeline (Alfaro et al., 2009; NRC, 2013; U.S. Department of Education and National Center for Education Statistics, 2014). The associations between early school leaving and young adults' future outcomes, including joblessness, have been well established (see Chapter 4 of this report). Future research is needed to determine the extent to which young adults' perceptions and experiences of racial discrimination at the interpersonal and structural levels limit their ability to succeed in education and employment.

Psychological and Physical Functioning

Several systematic reviews and recent studies (Lee et al., 2009; Priest et al., 2013; Williams and Williams-Morris, 2000; Williams et al., 2003) have found strong associations between racial discrimination and mental health outcomes among all racial/ethnic groups. According to the results of one review (Priest et al., 2013), 76 percent of 121 studies demonstrate a significant association between exposure to racial discrimination and mental health outcomes such as depression and anxiety. A recent meta-analytic review of experimental and correlational studies concludes that perceiving pervasive instances of discrimination negatively affects psychological well-being across a wide range of measures (Schmitt et al., 2014). Perceived discrimination by both peers and adults is significantly associated with decreased self-esteem and increased symptoms of depression among African American, Asian American, and Latino/a high school students (Greene et al., 2006). Exposure to race-related stress can evoke feelings of anger, hurt, frustration, bitterness, helplessness, and hopelessness and a desire to lash out (Wagner et al., 2011), which in turn can elevate depressive symptoms and anxiety. Individuals may attempt to manage their psychological state by relying on various self-soothers, such as overeating and use of alcohol and other substances, which over time can lead to chronic health problems (Karlamangla et al., 2006b; Ogden, 2012).

Negative emotions that may emanate from race-related stress also have been associated with the amplification of biological and physiological responses, including increased blood pressure, elevated fasting glucose, and increased plasma lipid levels, which forecast cardiovascular problems among African American young adults (Brody et al., 2014; Karlamangla et al., 2010); similar patterns are evinced among Asian Americans and Hispanics (Earnshaw et al., 2013; Lee et al., 2009). Living in a society where one's everyday life experiences are filtered through prejudice and racism triggers negative reactivity and the use of coping behaviors that may increase one's vulnerability to the onset and escalation of chronic diseases (Harrell et al., 2003; Williams and Williams-Morris, 2000). Further, exposure to racism, directly and indirectly, even during childhood, can have long-term consequences (Martin et al., 2011; Williams and Williams-Morris, 2000).

Persistent exposure to incidents of racism can negatively affect physical health by creating demands on individuals to respond to stress-inducing stimuli, requiring the activation of one's psychological and physiological systems to operate at high levels. This constant engagement of the "flight-fight" response, commonly referred to as "allostatic load," has been linked to increased inflammation and compromised autoimmune functioning, and is a significant predictor of the onset and escalation of major chronic diseases (Karlamangla et al., 2006a). Stress-response dysfunction increases blood pressure, which in turn increases vascular restriction and cardio output. Elevated blood pressure over time causes vascular resistance. The cycle of heightened physiological responses causes wear and tear on biological systems, including damage to the cardiovascular system. This cyclic link between race-related stress and cardiovascular risk vulnerabilities has been implicated as a major predictor of a range of developmental and health outcomes, including sleep disorders (Beatty et al., 2011), higher visceral fat, poor ambulatory blood pressure responses, and increases in vascular reactivity (Clark, 2000).

Childhood exposure to racism is associated with less healthy pregnancy outcomes among African American women of childbearing age (Hilmert et al., 2014). This finding reveals that one can be greatly affected by witnessing race-related events occurring to someone else, and that such experiences can be linked to blood pressure and depressive symptoms many years later (Caughy et al., 2004; Simons et al., 2002). Further, race-related stress has consistently been linked to preterm and low-birthweight infants among African American and Puerto Rican women (Earnshaw et al., 2013). Decline in psychological functioning and elevated blood pressure in response to race-related stress create a toxic maternal-fetal environment, causing reduced fetal growth and early delivery (Earnshaw et al., 2013; Hilmert et al., 2014). Additional research is needed to determine and explain how exposure to racism is transmuted from psychosocial experiences into physiological outcomes and to identify the etiological mechanisms by which experiences of racism and discrimination affect the health and well-being of adolescents and young adults of color.

Acculturation Stress

Acts of discrimination toward individuals because of immigrant status, legal status, skin tone, and language can contribute to acculturation stress. Immigrant status, skin tone, and phenotypic characteristics intersect through social interactions with members of the dominant culture among adolescents and young adults of color. They are faced with decisions that require negotiation of their "home culture" and internalization of the dominant culture, creating individual-level acculturation stress in determining the degree to which they should or can assimilate. Many, but not all, adolescents and young adults who abandon their home culture and fully assimilate in the dominant culture fare less well than those who maintain the home culture (Berry, 2005). Assimilation heightens family conflict that can reduce cultural support systems shown to buffer persons of color from negative outcomes often associated with stress-inducing events (Burnam et al., 1987; Cuéllar, 2000; Cuéllar et al., 1997; Heilemann et al., 2002).

Acculturation stress has been associated with increased depression in immigrants (Heilemann et al., 2002). It also has been associated with higher odds of a past suicide attempt among immigrants compared with individuals born in the United States (Gomez et al., 2011). Further, acculturative stress and perceived discrimination have been found to be strong predictors of hopelessness and depressive symptoms among Asian Americans, Latina/os, and Native Americans (Fritz et al., 2008; Kalibatseva and Leong, 2011; LaFromboise et al., 2010; Stein et al., 2012). On the other hand, the experience of bias or discrimination may foster stronger connections to one's own culture as young adults reject pressures to adapt and assimilate to the dominant society and instead maintain norms, attitudes, behaviors, and practices of their home culture (Padilla, 2002). Deeper understanding of this potentially protective process is needed.

PROTECTIVE PROCESSES

Current patterns of discrimination are associated with structural factors (e.g., economic and/or residential segregation, institutional racism) that restrict opportunity and well-being in pervasive ways. However, it is also important to recognize that disadvantaged cultural groups have developed productive, adaptive means of coping with their deprivations and that individual resilience and family strengths play important roles in supporting the healthy development of ethnic minority young adults even in the face of societal stressors (García Coll et al., 1996). Several studies have identified factors that buffer, protect against, or reduce the impact of racism and discriminatory experiences on individuals (Luthar, 2006).

Social Support, Connections, and Belongingness

Racial and ethnic identity, perceived to reflect closeness to members of one's own group, has been shown to serve a protective function for people of color. Across all racial/ethnic groups, high self-regard for one's ancestral heritage has been associated with the promotion of a sense of belongingness, supportiveness, and ethnic affirmation, which in turn bolsters self-esteem, self-control, and future orientation (Berkel et al., 2010; Seaton et al., 2011; Sellers et al., 2006; Wills et al., 2007). In addition, racial/ethnic group connections counteract potential adverse effects of perceived discrimination, protecting individuals from negative mental health outcomes, including internalizing behaviors, such as depression, shyness, and social isolation, and externalizing behaviors, such as aggression, violence, anger, and substance use (Neblett et al., 2012: Stock et al., 2013). Racial and ethnic identity, therefore, buffers the deleterious effects of discrimination on mental health functioning through parental/family adaptive cultural socialization (discussed in the following section) that prepares individuals to reject the internalization of bias and discriminatory messages (Berkel et al., 2010; Hughes et al., 2009). In addition, racial identity reduces the negative effects of discrimination on individual well-being through the protection of psychosocial resources, specifically social relationships and social support (Ida and Christie-Mizell, 2012).

Cultural Socialization

All individuals experience socialization processes that prepare them to be functional members of a society (Farver et al., 2007). Parents of racial and ethnic minorities also socialize their children into their own ethnic or natal culture and into the dominant culture, processes that include being aware of, understanding, and developing skills to resolve inconsistencies and conflicting views across cultures (Boykin, 1986; Farver et al., 2007). These parenting socialization processes, which encompass racial socialization (Harris-Britt et al., 2007; Hughes et al., 2006) and acculturation socialization (Dumka et al., 2009; Hill, 2011; Kim et al., 2013), may foster culturally specific forms of resilience and self-regulation, which can contribute to the development of adaptive coping mechanisms throughout childhood and lessen the likelihood of maladaptive behavior in adolescence and young adulthood (Yasui and Dishion, 2007).

Conclusion

A highly salient feature of growing up in America today is the increasingly multicultural character of the society, marked by significant increases in immigration from many different parts of the world. Today's young adults and their successors will be in their middle years when the country becomes majority minority. As the face of the nation changes, the social experiences of young people maturing in an increasingly diverse population will differ substantially from those of their elders. At the same time, this country still struggles to overcome its legacy of racial oppression and to ensure equal opportunity for all, regardless of race, ethnicity, sexual preference, and disability. By itself, the increasing diversity of the population provides no assurance that existing patterns of bias, stereotyping, and discrimination will be erased. However, young adults are the leading edge of the demographic change and can also become the most powerful force for equal rights in the 21st century.

REFERENCES

Alfaro, E. C., A. J. Umaña-Taylor, M. A. Gonzales-Backen, M. Y. Bámaca, and K. H. Zeiders. 2009. Latino adolescents' academic success: The role of discrimination, academic motivation, and gender. *Journal of Adolescence* 32(4):941-962.

Beatty, D. L., M. H. Hall, T. A. Kamarck, D. J. Buysse, J. F. Owens, S. E. Reis, E. J. Mezick, P. J. Strollo, and K. A. Matthews. 2011. Unfair treatment is associated with poor sleep in African American and Caucasian adults: Pittsburgh SleepSCORE project. *Health Psychology* 30(3):351.

Berkel, C., G. P. Knight, K. H. Zeiders, J. Y. Tein, M. W. Roosa, N. A. Gonzales, and D. Saenz. 2010. Discrimination and adjustment for Mexican American adolescents: A prospective examination of the benefits of culturally related values. *Journal of Research on Adolescence* 20(4):893-915.

Berry, J. W. 2005. Acculturation: Living successfully in two cultures. *International Journal of Intercultural Relations* 29:697-712.

Boykin, A. W. 1986. The triple quandary and the schooling of Afro-American children. *The School Achievement of Minority Children: New Perspectives* 57-92.

Brody, G. H., M. K. Lei, D. H. Chae, T. Yu, S. M. Kogan, and S. R. Beach. 2014. Perceived discrimination among African American adolescents and allostatic load: A longitudinal analysis with buffering effects. *Child Development* 85(3):989-1002.

Burnam, M. A., R. L. Hough, M. Karno, J. I. Escobar, and C. A. Telles. 1987. Acculturation and lifetime prevalence of psychiatric disorders among Mexican Americans in Los Angeles. *Journal of Health and Social Behavior* 28(1):89-102.

Caughy, M., P. J. O'Campo, and C. Muntaner. 2004. Experiences of racism among African American parents and the mental health of their preschool-aged children. *American Journal of Public Health* 94:2118-2124.

Clark, R. 2000. Perceptions of interethnic group racism predict increased vascular reactivity to a laboratory challenge in college women. *Annals of Behavioral Medicine* 22(3):214-222.

Cross, W. E., and T. B. Cross. 2008. Theory, research, and models. In *Handbook of race, racism, and the developing child*, edited by S. M. Quintana and C. McKown. Hoboken, NJ: Wiley. Pp. 154-181.

Cuéllar, I. 2000. Acculturation and mental health: Ecological transactional relations of adjustment. In *Handbook of multicultural mental health: Assessment and treatment of diverse populations*, edited by I. Cuéllar and F. A. Paniagua. San Diego, CA: Academic Press. Pp. 45-62.

Cuéllar, I., B. Nyberg, R. E. Maldonado, and R. E. Roberts. 1997. Ethnic identity and acculturation in a young adult Mexican-origin population. *Journal of Community Psychology* 25(6):535-549.

Dumka, L. E., N. A. Gonzales, D. D. Bonds, and R. E. Millsap. 2009. Academic success of Mexican origin adolescent boys and girls: The role of mothers' and fathers' parenting and cultural orientation. *Sex Roles* 60(7-8):588-599.

Earnshaw, V. A., L. Rosenthal, J. B. Lewis, E. C. Stasko, J. N. Tobin, T. T. Lewis, A. E. Reid, and J. R. Ickovics. 2013. Maternal experiences with everyday discrimination and infant birth weight: A test of mediators and moderators among young, urban women of color. *Annals of Behavioral Medicine* 45(1):13-23.

Farver, J. M., Y. Xu, B. R. Bhadha, S. Narang, and E. Lieber. 2007. Ethnic identity, acculturation, parenting beliefs, and adolescent adjustment: A comparison of Asian Indian and European American families. *Merrill-Palmer Quarterly* 53(2):184-215.

Fritz, M. V., D. Chin, and V. DeMarinis. 2008. Stressors, anxiety, acculturation, and North American students. *International Journal of Intercultural Relations* 32:244-259.

García Coll, C., G. Lamberty, R. Jenkins, H. P. McAdoo, K. Crnic, B. H. Wasik, and H. Vázquez García. 1996. An integrative model for the study of developmental competencies in minority children. *Child Development* 67(5):1891-1914.

Gomez, J., R. Miranda, and L. Polanco. 2011. Acculturative stress, perceived discrimination, and vulnerability to suicide attempts among emerging adults. *Journal of Youth and Adolescence* 40(11):1465-1476.

Greene, M. L., N. Way, and K. Pahl. 2006. Trajectories of perceived adult and peer discrimination among black, Latino, and Asian American adolescents: Patterns and psychological correlates. *Developmental Psychology* 42(2):218-236.

Harrell, J. P., S. Hall, and J. Taliaferro. 2003. Physiological responses to racism and discrimination: An assessment of the evidence. *American Journal of Public Health* 93(2):243-248.

Harris-Britt, A., C. R. Valrie, B. Kurtz-Costes, and S. J. Rowley. 2007. Perceived discrimination and self-esteem in African American youth: Racial socialization as a protective factor. *Journal of Research on Adolescence* 17:669-682.

Heilemann, M. V., K. A. Lee, and F. S. Kury. 2002. Strengths and vulnerabilities of women of Mexican descent in relation to depressive symptoms. *Nursing Research* 51(3):175-182.

Hill, N. E. 2011. Undermining partnerships between African-American families and schools: Legacies of discrimination and inequalities. In *African American children's mental health*, Vol. 1, edited by N. E. Hill, T. L. Mann, and H. E. Fitzgerald. Santa Barbara, CA: Praeger. Pp. 199-230.

Hilmert, C. J., T. P. Dominguez, C. D. Schetter, S. K. Srinivas, L. M. Glynn, C. J. Hobel, and C. A. Sandman. 2014. Lifetime racism and blood pressure changes during pregnancy: Implications for fetal growth. *Health Psychology* 33(1):43-51.

Hughes, D., J. Rodriguez, E. P. Smith, D. J. Johnson, H. C. Stevenson, and P. Spicer. 2006. Parents' ethnic-racial socialization practices: A review of research and directions for future study. *Developmental Psychology* 42(5):747-770.

Hughes, D., D. Witherspoon, D. Rivas-Drake, and N. West-Bey. 2009. Received ethnic-racial socialization messages and youths' academic and behavioral outcomes: Examining the mediating role of ethnic identity and self-esteem. *Cultural Diversity and Ethnic Minority Psychology* 15(2):112.

Hunter, B. 2009. Indigenous social exclusion: Insights and challenges for the concept of social inclusion. *Family Matters* 82:52-61.

Ida, A. K., and C. A. Christie-Mizell. 2012. Racial group identity, psychosocial resources, and depressive symptoms: Exploring ethnic heterogeneity among African Americans. *Sociological Focus* 45:41-62.

Kalibatseva, Z., and F. T. L. Leong. 2011. Depression among Asian Americans: Review and recommendations. *Depression Research and Treatment* 9.

Karlamangla, A. S., B. H. Singer, and T. E. Seeman. 2006a. Reduction in allostatic load in older adults is associated with lower all-cause mortality risk: Macarthur studies of successful aging. *Psychosomatic Medicine* 68(3):500-507.

Karlamangla, A., K. Zhou, D. Reuben, G. Greendale, and A. Moore. 2006b. Longitudinal trajectories of heavy drinking in adults in the United States of America. *Addiction* 101(1):91-99.

Karlamangla, A. S., S. S. Merkin, E. M. Crimmins, and T. E. Seeman. 2010. Socioeconomic and ethnic disparities in cardiovascular risk in the United States, 2001-2006. *Annals of Epidemiology* 20(8):617-628.

Krieger, N., and S. Sidney. 1997. Prevalence and health implications of anti-gay discrimination: A study of black and white women and men in the CARDIA cohort. *International Journal of Health Services* 27:157-176.

Kyung-Hee, C., J. Paul, G. Ayala, R. Boylan, and S. E. Rregorich. 2013. Experiences of discrimination and their impact on the mental health among African American, Asian and Pacific Islanders, and Latino men who have sex with men. *American Journal of Public Health* 103:868-874.

LaFromboise, T. D., K. Albright, and A. Harris. 2010. Patterns of hopelessness among American Indian adolescents: Relationships by levels of acculturation and residence. *Cultural Diversity and Ethnic Minority Psychology* 16(1):68-76.

Lee, S., H. S. Juon, G. Martinez, C. E. Hsu, E. S. Robinson, J. Bawa, and G. X. Ma. 2009. Model minority at risk: Expressed needs of mental health by Asian American young adults. *Journal of Community Health* 34(2):144-152.

Lopez, M. H., R. Morin, and P. Taylor. 2010. *Illegal immigration backlash worries, divides Latinos*. Washington, DC: Pew Hispanic Center. http://www.pewhispanic.org/files/reports/128.pdf (accessed October 1, 2014).

Luthar, S. S. 2006. Resilience in development: A synthesis of research across five decades. In *Developmental psychopathology*, Vol. 3, 2nd ed., edited by D. Cicchetti and D. J. Cohen. Hoboken, NJ: Wiley. Pp. 739-795.

Martin, M. J., B. McCarthy, R. D. Conger, F. X. Gibbons, R. L. Simons, C. E. Cutrona, and G. H. Brody. 2011. The enduring significance of racism: Discrimination and delinquency among black American youth. *Journal of Research on Adolescence* 21(3):662-676.

Mays, V. M., and S. D. Cochran. 2001. Mental health correlated of perceived discrimination among lesbian, gay, and bisexual adults in the U.S. *American Journal of Public Health* 91:1869-1876.

McCabe, S. E., W. B. Bostwick, T. L. Hughes, B. T. West, and C. J. Boyd. 2010. The relationship between discrimination and substance use disorders among lesbian, gay, and bisexual adults in the United States. *American Journal of Public Health* 100:1946-1952.

Meyer, I. H. 1995. Minority stress and mental health in gay men. *Journal of Health and Social Behavior* 36:38-56.

Neblett, E. W., D. Rivas-Drake, and A. J. Umaña-Taylor. 2012. The promise of racial and ethnic protective factors in promoting ethnic minority youth development. *Child Development Perspectives* 6(3):295-303.

NRC (National Research Council). 2013. *Reforming juvenile justice: A developmental approach*. Washington, DC: The National Academies Press.

Ogden, J. 2012. *Health psychology: A textbook*. New York: McGraw-Hill International.

Padilla, A. M. 2002. Hispanic psychology: A 25-year retrospective look. In *Online readings in psychology and culture* (Unit 3, Ch. 3), edited by W. J. Lonner, D. L. Dinnel, S. A. Hayes, and D. N. Sattler. Bellingham: Western Washington University.

Pew Research Center. 2013a. *After Boston, little change in views of Islam and violence*. Washington, DC: Pew Research Center.

Pew Research Center. 2013b. *For African Americans, discrimination is not dead*. Washington, DC: Pew Research Center. http://www.pewresearch.org/fact-tank/2013/06/28/for-african-americans-discrimination-is-not-dead (accessed September 26, 2014).

Priest, N., Y. Paradies, B. Trenerry, M. Truong, S. Karlsen, and Y. Kelly. 2013. A systematic review of studies examining the relationship between reported racism and health and wellbeing for children and young people. *Social Science & Medicine* 95:115-127.

Schmitt, M. S., N. R. Branscombe, T. Postmes, and A. Barcia. 2014. The consequences of perceived discrimination for psychological well-being: A meta-analytic review. *Psychological Bulletin* 140:921-948.

Seaton, E. K., C. H. Caldwell, R. M. Sellers, and J. S. Jackson. 2008. The prevalence of perceived discrimination among African American and Caribbean black youth. *Developmental Psychology* 44:1288-1297.

Seaton, E. K., E. W. Neblett, R. D. Upton, W. P. Hammond, and R. M. Sellers. 2011. The moderating capacity of racial identity between perceived discrimination and psychological well-being over time among African American youth. *Child Development* 82(6):1850-1867.

Sellers, R. M., N. Copeland-Linder, P. P. Martin, and R. H. Lewis. 2006. Racial identity matters: The relationship between racial discrimination and psychological functioning in African American adolescents. *Journal of Research on Adolescence* 16(2):187-216.

Simons, R. L., V. Murry, V. McLoyd, K. H. Lin, C. Cutrona, and R. D. Conger. 2002. Discrimination, crime, ethnic identity, and parenting as correlates of depressive symptoms among African American children: A multilevel analysis. *Development and Psychology* 14:371-393.

Stein, G. L., L. M. Gonzalez, and N. Huq. 2012. Cultural stressors and the hopelessness model of depressive symptoms in Latino adolescents. *Journal of Youth and Adolescence* 41(10):1339-1349.

Stock, M. L., F. X. Gibbons, M. Gerrard, A. E. Houlihan, C. Y. Weng, F. O. Lorenz, and R. L. Simons. 2013. Racial identification, racial composition, and substance use vulnerability among African American adolescents and young adults. *Health Psychology* 32(3):237.

U.S. Department of Education and National Center for Education Statistics. 2014. *The condition of education 2014* (NCES 2014-083). http://nces.ed.gov/pubs2014/2014083.pdf (accessed October 1, 2014).

Viruell-Fuentes, E. A., P. Y. Miranda, and S. Abdulrahim. 2012. More than culture: Structural racism, intersectionality theory, and immigrant health. *Social Science & Medicine* 75(12):2099-2106.

Wagner, J. A., C. Y. Osborn, E. A. Mendenhall, L. M. Budris, S. Belay, and H. A. Tennen. 2011. Beliefs about racism and health among African American women with diabetes: A qualitative study. *Journal of the National Medical Association* 103(3):224.

Williams, D., and R. Williams-Morris. 2000. Racism and mental health: The African American experience. *Ethnicity and Health* 5(3-4):243-268.

Williams, D. R., H. W. Neighbors, and J. S. Jackson. 2003. Racial/ethnic discrimination and health: Findings from community studies. *American Journal of Public Health* 93(2): 200-208.

Wills, T. A., V. M. Murry, G. H. Brody, F. X. Gibbons, M. Gerrard, C. Walker, and M. G. Ainette. 2007. Ethnic pride and self-control related to protective and risk factors: Test of the theoretical model for the strong African American families program. *Health Psychology* 26(1):50-59.

Yasui, M., and T. J. Dishion. 2007. The ethnic context of child and adolescent problem behavior: Implications for child and family interventions. *Clinical Child and Family Psychology Review* 10(2):137-179.

C

Youth-Focused National Service Programs[1]

In 2014, the top 10 National Direct Grantees (national organizations receiving grants) were YouthBuild National, City Year National, Notre Dame Mission Volunteers, Washington Service Corps, Minnesota Reading Corps, Public Allies National, Health Corps, Teach for America, Habitat for Humanity, and Jumpstart. Five of these organizations focus on youth explicitly, while two (YouthBuild and Public Allies) hire almost exclusively "opportunity youth."[2] Some programs, such as YouthBuild, Public Allies, and PASCO (a regional service corps that engages all of its members in leadership development), intentionally recruit "opportunity youth" and give priority to member development. Other programs that involve youth from marginalized communities in service, such as Wisconsin's Fresh Start program, vary by state. While these programs receive funding from a diverse array of sources, they, often with supplemental support from AmeriCorps, make up the networked community of service programs that engage

---

[1] This appendix draws on a paper commissioned by the committee titled "Civic Engagement, Volunteerism, and Young Adult Well-Being: Volunteer Work and National Service as Developmental Opportunities for Social Incorporation," by Constance Flanagan and Victoria Faust. Available online at http://www.iom.edu/youngadults.

[2] A 2012 report by Belfield and colleagues coins the term "opportunity youth" to describe young people disconnected from all major institutions who present an opportunity for society to devise new ways to reengage them. Note that the Serve America Act defines disadvantaged youth as out-of-school youth, including those who are unemployed, aging out of foster care, with limited English proficiency, homeless or runaway, at risk to leave secondary school without a diploma, former juvenile offenders or at risk of delinquency, or individuals with a disability.

disadvantaged youth participants in civic opportunities. This appendix summarizes some of the more common youth-focused programs, along with relevant research.

YOUTHBUILD

YouthBuild was developed in 1978 in East Harlem (Godsay et al., 2012). It expanded in 1988 to engage low-income youth aged 16-24 across the country in service while delivering educational programming to assist with high school or completion of the General Educational Development (GED) credential (Godsay et al., 2012). The Housing and Urban Development Act of 1992 put YouthBuild in the same ranks as the Peace Corps and Head Start, receiving yearly allocations from Congress (Godsay et al., 2012). Currently, the U.S. Department of Labor provides approximately $73 million to support YouthBuild programs serving around 4,950 youth (DOL, 2014). Some YouthBuild sites, called YouthBuild AmeriCorps, also receive support through AmeriCorps, either through half-time member stipended positions with an education award or just an education award (Tomberg, 2013).

As of 2013, more than 110,000 individuals had participated in YouthBuild (Tomberg, 2013). All members are low income; 94 percent enter without a high school diploma (Godsay et al., 2012); 71 percent are men; 53 percent are African American, 22 percent white, 20 percent Latino/a, 3 percent Native American, and 2 percent Asian American; 32 percent are court involved; and 45 percent have received public assistance (YouthBuild USA, 2014). According to the program's own statistics, 78 percent of entering students complete the program; of those, 63 percent obtain a high school diploma or equivalent by the time they finish, and 60 percent of alumni are placed in jobs or pursue further education (YouthBuild USA, 2014). In the YouthBuild program model, youth alternate weeks between participating in educational coursework and building housing for low-income and homeless individuals (Godsay et al., 2012). Youth serve in their own communities in contrast with other models, such as City Year, in which "opportunity youth" serve in groups with recruits from other communities (Anderson and Fabiano, 2007).

Core elements of the YouthBuild model are adopted by every site. In contrast to a "youth at risk" paradigm, the program's theory of change is founded on a belief in the transformative power of love (Godsay et al., 2012). Accordingly, program elements include family-like support and appreciation of members from adults and peers; protection and patient caring for each young person's development; profound respect for each person's intelligence, coupled with high standards and expectations for his/her performance; inspiring and caring role models; opportunities for career and leadership; opportunities for civic engagement; and skill development (Godsay et al., 2012).

YouthBuild also employs a unique approach to civic engagement with many opportunities for leadership and public action. Standard practices in the 12- to 16-month program include advocating for funding, shared governance established through an elected policy committee, team decision making about building projects, and community problem solving (Godsay et al., 2012). At the local program level, investments include staff training in youth and leadership development, staff time incorporating leadership into all aspects of the program, the director's time and involvement in the program policy committee, creation of leadership skills training, and funds to support leadership opportunities such as Statehouse Days and leadership learning trips (Godsay et al., 2012). In addition, several levels of leadership opportunities exist for program alumni (nationally, the organization devotes more than half a million dollars annually to these leadership pipeline programs). They include the National Young Leaders Council (elected by peers at an annual conference), the National Alumni Council, VOICES (Views on Improving Credential and Education Success) for alumni in postsecondary education, the National Speakers Bureau, and others (Godsay et al., 2012). Finally, in the last few years, YouthBuild has funded staff to mentor and provide support to alumni as they transition out of the program and into the next phase of their lives (Godsay et al., 2012). The U.S. Department of Labor also is funding 1 year of follow-up of alumni (Godsay et al., 2012).

Several studies of YouthBuild have documented its impact from baseline to program completion. Hahn and colleagues (2004) compared YouthBuild participants with high school dropouts who were not in the program. They found increases in youths' expected life span between the start and end of involvement in the program (Hahn et al., 2004). They also documented an 87 percent employment rate among graduates and a high correlation between how quickly youth found jobs and how much assistance their YouthBuild mentors provided in the search (Hahn et al., 2004). Finally, 7 years after graduating from the program, 75 percent of the graduates participating in this study were either working, in school, or in a job training program; 70 percent had registered to vote, and nearly half had voted in one or more elections (Hahn et al., 2004).

Tomberg (2013) found significant increases in civic outcomes between pre- and postprogram assessments. Specifically, regardless of age, race, or number of hours served, youths' reports of social trust and community orientations increased, and among 16- to 18-year-olds, there also were significant gains in commitments to service (Tomberg, 2013). Tomberg included 494 staff in her study as well and found that the staff were well versed in the implementation of the YouthBuild model and engaged youth in wraparound support services, in civic leadership development, and in ways to negotiate service opportunities (Tomberg, 2013).

Others have studied particular elements of the YouthBuild model or groups targeted by specific programs. Concerning the latter, Cohen and Piquero (2010) evaluated the YouthBuild Offenders project and documented reduced recidivism for young offenders who stayed with the program relative to a similar group not enrolled in the program. One retrospective study surveyed 344 alumni and conducted intensive interviews with a subset of 54, all of whom had engaged in one or more of YouthBuild's alumni leadership pipeline programs (Godsay et al., 2012). Two pathways to becoming leaders were identified. For some it was the result of a steady, incremental feeling of mattering to and receiving social support from staff that enabled them to step up to new challenges. Others identified turning points or transformational experiences. For example, many mentioned the Mental Toughness training module offered early in a YouthBuild program that pushes participants to aim higher, while others cited the Conference of Young Leaders, an intensive, multiday event held in Washington, DC (Godsay et al., 2012).

CITY YEAR

Established in 1988, City Year was the model on which the current AmeriCorps Program was built (Anderson and Fabiano, 2007). An independent program, its central office and statewide entities combined receive by far the largest National Direct AmeriCorps grant funding from the Corporation for National and Community Service (CNCS) (more than $30 million) (City Year, 2013; CNCS, 2014). City Year members perform service in curricular support, youth leadership development, after-school programs and day camps, health services/outreach, and park renovation/housing restoration, although currently almost all the positions have a focus on educational achievement (Anderson and Fabiano, 2007). A primary goal of the program has always been to promote attitudes and behaviors that alter the civic path of City Year members themselves by engaging 17- to 24-year-olds in social and civic institutions (Anderson and Fabiano, 2007).

In contrast to YouthBuild, which recruits only youth from low-income backgrounds, City Year seeks to establish integrated teams of members from different socioeconomic, racial, ethnic, and geographic backgrounds. In 2011, City Year developed a member diversity plan, which included forming strategic recruitment partnerships with African American and Latino/a fraternities and sororities to increase diversity among its members (Dickerson Wynder, 2014). City Year also has joined with the Peace Corps, Teach for America, and the Breakthrough Collaborative (a program focused on connecting low-income middle school students with college) in developing a Diversity Recruitment Collaborative (Dickerson Wynder, 2014).

In 2007, Policy Studies Associates (PSA) concluded a 5-year, three-part study of the impact of City Year on alumni, which consisted of a mail survey completed by more than 2,189 participants, focus groups with 37 participants, and 20 open-ended interviews with alumni, as well as a telephone survey of the parents and families of alumni (Anderson and Fabiano, 2007). Alumni were categorized into three cohorts—from 1988 to 1993, 1994 to 1998, and 1999 to 2003 (Anderson and Fabiano, 2007).

PSA gathered retrospective accounts of how alumni perceived City Year's impact on outcomes including their employment, education, civic attitudes, political engagement, leadership, and social capital development (Anderson and Fabiano, 2007). Some of the alumni responses were compared with those of a matched group from the National Election Studies and CIRCLE's National Civic Engagement Survey (Anderson and Fabiano, 2007).

Two trends in the demographics of program participants were noteworthy. First, between 1988 and 2003 across all sites, the percentage of youth entering with some college remained the same, while the percentage of youth entering with a GED or less decreased, and the percentage of those with a bachelor's degree doubled (Anderson and Fabiano, 2007). Second, from the first cohort to the last, the percentage of African American participants increased from 25 percent to 35 percent, while the percentage of white participants decreased from 51 percent to 41 percent (Anderson and Fabiano, 2007). Over the entire period of 1988 to 2003, the City Year programs in Boston, Rhode Island, and San Antonio had enrolled the highest number of members with no college experience—each just over 60 percent (Anderson and Fabiano, 2007).

Concerning outcomes reported by the alumni, those who entered the program without a GED were the most likely to report that their experience with City Year impacted their career. In addition, the greater the educational attainment of a participant upon entering the program, the less additional education he/she pursued upon completing the program (Anderson and Fabiano, 2007). In addition, alumni consistently reported that their City Year program had a positive impact on their self-efficacy and sense of egalitarianism. Compared with the national sample of 18- to 40-year-olds, City Year alumni in all racial, ethnic, and educational attainment groups were more likely to participate in organizations, to vote, and to volunteer (Anderson and Fabiano, 2007). The social capital (a combined measure of social trust, political efficacy, egalitarianism, and social and political expression) reported by City Year alumni also was higher than that reported by the national comparison group.

PUBLIC ALLIES

First established in Washington, DC, Public Allies was named a demonstration site for National Public Service in 1992 by President George H. W. Bush and was one of the first programs to receive AmeriCorps funding (Public Allies, 2013a). Public Allies now operates in 21 sites and recruits diverse participants from the communities for a service and leadership development apprenticeship program (Public Allies, 2013a). The program has evolved to a franchise-like model, with central offices providing training and technical assistance on program design to sites around the country and a member leadership development curriculum that includes units on asset-based community development, diversity and privilege, critical thinking, nonprofit management, and teamwork. Among program participants, two-thirds are people of color; 60 percent are female; 50 percent are college graduates; and 15 percent are lesbian, gay, bisexual, or transgender. Numbers vary for specific sites, with New York hiring approximately 90 percent people of color (Public Allies, 2013c).

Public Allies is relatively unique among national service programs in its focus on alumni engagement and continuing development (although, as noted above, YouthBuild involves some of its alumni in continuing leadership programs). Public Allies hosts a National Leadership Institute conference to share best practices in service and community building, particularly as regards engaging young diverse leadership (Public Allies, 2013b). Alumni are a key feature of Public Allies' overall recruitment strategy. The organization also has a commitment to diversity in leadership among its own staff.

One mechanism by which Public Allies is able to engage alumni is through its Personal Impact and Service Documentation portal (Goggins-Gregory, 2004). This online portal for data collection and management, developed with technology fellows and an advisory board, has been touted as a model for service programs. It also enables the program to share up-to-date outcomes (Goggins-Gregory, 2004). However, public reporting on member outcomes is not widely studied outside of the organization.

TEACH FOR AMERICA (TFA)

TFA participants commit to teaching for 2 years in a rural or urban school in a low-income community (TFA, 2010). The program, which recruits only those who have completed 4 years of college, aims to reduce educational inequality by placing teachers in these low-income schools. During these 2 years, teachers receive a salary ($24,000-$51,000, depending on the region); health benefits; and other benefits, such as an education award (TFA, 2014).

A retrospective study of TFA was conducted in 2001-2002. Three groups were compared: matriculants (who completed their 2 years of service), dropouts (who dropped out before completing their 2 years), and nonmatriculants (who completed all of the TFA paperwork but never joined the program) (McAdam and Brandt, 2009). The final sample comprised 1,583 graduates, 324 dropouts, and 634 nonmatriculants (McAdam and Brandt, 2009). Because TFA has never asked applicants for social class information, no such comparisons could be made. However, there were no differences in race/ethnicity and gender among the groups.

The main goal of the study was to test the "transformational" claims of the TFA organization. However, McAdam and Brandt (2009) found that TFA graduates lagged significantly behind the two comparison groups on seven dimensions of civic life—service, civic activity, institutional politics, social movements, voting, charitable giving, and prosocial employment (teaching, working in nonprofits). Note, however, that this finding must be put in perspective as this was a highly civically engaged sample. For example, 92 percent of the respondents across all three groups said they had voted in the last presidential election (almost twice what their peers in the general population reported), so the 89 percent of TFA graduates who reported voting needs to be interpreted in the context of this very high overall rate (McAdam and Brandt, 2009).

McAdam and Brandt offer some plausible explanations for their counterintuitive finding, including temporary exhaustion on the part of recent graduates (and dropouts); negative reactions to TFA; and for many, the isolating nature of the teaching experience (McAdam and Brandt, 2009). Analyses of the dropouts' experience are especially revealing: not only did their experience leave them disillusioned with TFA, but it also left them with negative views of educational service in general (McAdam and Brandt, 2009). Based on pretest interviews and other information, McAdam and Brandt conclude that five features of TFA placements contribute to a negative experience: urban school placement, lack of support within the school, lack of support from TFA, low sense of efficacy on the part of the volunteer, and disillusionment with TFA (McAdam and Brandt, 2009).

THE CIVIC JUSTICE CORPS

The Civic Justice Corps was a model initially developed through collaborations involving the U.S. Department of Labor, CNCS, the Open Society Institute, The Bill & Melinda Gates Foundation, the Cascade Center for Community Governance, and The Corps Network (The Corps Network, 2014). At the time, the incorporation of ex-offenders and disadvantaged youth through multisectoral partnerships was an explicit component of the CNCS strategic plan. The program engaged formerly incarcerated or court-involved youth aged 18-24 in community service projects and work experience, vocational training and academic interventions for skill improvement, and career development (DOL, 2011). Its pilot, implemented by the Corps Network and including wraparound support services and civic leadership development, demonstrated significant reductions in recidivism and increased educational and employment attainment. The U.S. Department of Labor subsequently began administering $20 million for the Civic Justice Corps in 2011 (DOL, 2011). Since then, $30 million in additional funding has been granted to programs that have adopted a similar model, although it is no longer administered under the auspices of the Civic Justice Corps program (DOL, 2012).

AMERICORPS-NCCC

AmeriCorps-NCCC is a 10-month, full-time, residential service program for men and women aged 18-24 (CNCS, 2014). Inspired by the Depression-era Civilian Conservation Corps, the program combines the best practices of civilian and military service (CNCS, 2014). AmeriCorps-NCCC members live and train in teams at five regional campuses and serve nonprofit organizations and government entities in communities across the country (CNCS, 2014). During their service period, members spend considerable time off campus providing services throughout the region, living temporarily in schools or other facilities provided by the community. Some NCCC members also participate in disaster relief efforts, such as flood relief or fighting wildfires. While the Serve America Act authorized the opportunity for NCCC programs to be developed in communities away from campus, these programs have yet to be enacted. However, one of the major new federal interagency partnerships built by CNCS is housed in NCCC. This collaboration places 18- to 24-year-olds with the Federal Emergency Management Agency to assist with disaster relief initiatives around the country (CNCS, 2014).

The Serve America Act also reinforced an existing goal of NCCC to hire 50 percent of its members from disadvantaged backgrounds (CNCS, 2009). Currently, CNCS and the Congress hold NCCC to a higher burden of proof of such participation relative to any other AmeriCorps program. Of the 2010-2011 class, about 50 percent of youth who served in NCCC had a college degree, and about 70 percent were Caucasian (CNCS, 2011a). In response to the Serve America Act, NCCC developed targeted recruitment strategies to engage youth from disadvantaged backgrounds, including outreach to specific institutions and programs around the country that serve at-risk youth (CNCS, 2011b).

YOUTH CORPS

Conservation and Service Corps, or Youth Corps, are a diverse set of programs (really a network) united in their common mission of engaging members, primarily young adults, in a combination of community service, workforce development, and education. Like AmeriCorps-NCCC, Youth Corps builds on the legacy of the Civilian Conservation Corps (Price et al., 2011). Today, Youth Corps are operated by local community-based organizations and local and state government agencies (Price et al., 2011). While they typically engage in educational, employment and training, and community service activities, there is no single program model. Youth Corps vary a good deal in their organizational structure, type of members targeted, and duration and intensity of participation. They receive support from CNCS, other federal agencies (including the U.S. Departments of Labor, Interior, and Housing and Urban Development), and local and state government and foundations (Price et al., 2011). Some programs receive additional support from fee-for-service projects, in which project sponsors, typically local or state government agencies, provide Youth Corps with direct funding for services.

REFERENCES

Anderson, L. M., and L. Fabiano. 2007. *The city year experience: Putting alumni on the path to lifelong civic engagement*. Boston, MA: City Year, Inc.

Belfield, C. R., H. M. Levin, and R. Rosen. 2012. *The economic value of opportunity youth*. Washington, DC: CNCS.

City Year. 2013. *Annual report 2013*. http://www.cityyear.org/sites/default/files/PDF/City%20Year%20-%202013%20Annual%20Report.pdf (accessed September 25, 2014).

CNCS (Corporation for National and Community Service). 2009. *Current law vs. Serve America Act: Side by side comparison*. http://www.nationalservice.gov/sites/default/files/documents/09_0519_serveact_sidebyside.pdf (accessed September 23, 2014).

CNCS. 2011a. *AmeriCorps National Civilian Community Corps*. http://www.serviceandinclusion.org/symp2011/electronic/NCCCLeaveYourMark (accessed September 23, 2014).

CNCS. 2011b. *The Corporation for National and Community Service strategic plan 2011-2015*. http://www.nationalservice.gov/pdf/strategic_plan_web.pdf (accessed September 23, 2014).

CNCS. 2014. *AmeriCorps NCCC*. http://www.nationalservice.gov/programs/americorps/americorps-nccc (accessed August 27, 2014).

Cohen, M. A., and A. R. Piquero. 2010. An outcome evaluation of the YouthBuild USA Offender Project. *Youth Violence and Juvenile Justice* 8(4):373-385.

The Corps Network. 2014. *Civic Justice Corps*. http://www.nascc.org/impact/workforce-development/civic-justice (accessed September 2, 2014).

Dickerson Wynder, B. 2014. *Celebrating black history month: City Year Corps' living witness to diversity and inclusion*. http://www.cityyear.org/blog/celebrating-black-history-month-city-year-corps%E2%80%99-living-witness-diversity-and-inclusion (accessed September 22, 2014).

DOL (U.S. Department of Labor). 2011. *U.S. Department of Labor announces $20 million in grants to support young people transitioning from justice facilities to the workforce.* http://www.dol.gov/opa/media/press/eta/eta20110944.htm (accessed September 2, 2014).

DOL. 2012. *Notice of availability of funds and solicitation for grant applications for serving young adult ex-offenders through training and service-learning.* http://www.doleta.gov/grants/pdf/training_and_service_learning_sga.pdf (accessed September 2, 2014).

DOL. 2014. *Approximately $73M in YouthBuild grants to help disadvantaged youth develop job and leadership skills made available by U.S. Labor Department.* http://www.dol.gov/opa/media/press/eta/ETA20140257.htm (accessed September 22, 2014).

Godsay, S., A. Kiesa, K. Kawashima-Ginsberg, W. Henderson, and P. Levine. 2012. *Pathways into leadership: A study of YouthBuild graduates.* Medford, MA: Center for Information and Research on Civic Learning and Engagement.

Goggins-Gregory, A. 2004. *Organizational transformation through technology at public allies.* Milwaukee, WI: Public Allies, Inc.

Hahn, A., T. Leavitt, E. M. Hovart, and J. E. Davis. 2004. *Life after YouthBuild: 900 YouthBuild graduates reflect on their lives, dreams, and experiences.* Somerville, MA: YouthBuild USA.

McAdam, D., and C. Brandt. 2009. Assessing the effects of voluntary youth service: The case of Teach For America. *Social Forces* 88(2):945-969.

Price, C., J. Williams, L. Simpson, J. Jastrzab, and C. Markovitz. 2011. *National evaluation of youth corps: Findings at follow-up.* Prepared for the Corporation for National and Community Service. Cambridge, MA: Abt Associates Inc.

Public Allies. 2013a. *Our story.* http://www.publicallies.org/site/c.liKUL3PNLvF/b.3117293/k.9D/Our_Story.htm (accessed August 28, 2014).

Public Allies. 2013b. *National Leadership Institute.* http://www.publicallies.org/site/c.liKUL3PNLvF/b.8103257/k.22F2/National_Leadership_Institute.htm (accessed August 28, 2014).

Public Allies. 2013c. *New York.* http://www.publicallies.org/site/c.liKUL3PNLvF/b.3158921/k.D04A/New_York.htm (accessed September 23, 2014).

TFA (Teach for America). 2010. *Teach For America fields largest teacher corps in its 20-year history.* http://www.teachforamerica.org/newsroom/documents/20100524_Teach.For.America.Fields.Largest.Teacher.Corps.In.Its.20.Year.History.htm (accessed July 17, 2014).

TFA. 2014. *Compensation and benefits.* http://www.teachforamerica.org/why-teach-for-america/compensation-and-benefits (accessed September 22, 2014).

Tomberg, K. A. 2013. *Youth development through service: A quality assessment of the YouthBuild AmeriCorps Program.* New York: Research and Evaluation Center, John Jay College of Criminal Justice, City University of New York.

YouthBuild USA. 2014. *YouthBuild demographics and outcomes.* https://youthbuild.org/youthbuild-demographics-and-outcomes (accessed April 25, 2014).

D

Biographical Sketches of Committee Members

Richard Bonnie, LL.B. (*Chair*), teaches and writes about criminal law, bioethics, and public policies relating to mental health, substance abuse, and public health. Professor Bonnie has been actively involved in public service throughout his career. Among other positions, he has been associate director of the National Commission on Marihuana and Drug Abuse (1971-1973); secretary of the first National Advisory Council on Drug Abuse (1975-1980); chair of Virginia's State Human Rights Committee, responsible for protecting the rights of persons with mental disabilities (1979-1985); and chief advisor for the American Bar Association's Criminal Justice Mental Health Standards Project (1981-1988). He recently chaired a Commission on Mental Health Law Reform at the request of the chief justice of Virginia (2006-2011). Professor Bonnie has served as an advisor to the American Psychiatric Association's (APA's) Council on Psychiatry and Law since 1979, received the APA's Isaac Ray Award in 1998 for contributions to the field of forensic psychiatry, and was awarded a special presidential commendation in 2003 for his contributions to American psychiatry. He also has served on three MacArthur Foundation research networks—on Mental Health and the Law (1988-1996), Mandated Community Treatment (2000-2010), and Law and Neuroscience (since 2008). In 1991, Professor Bonnie was elected to the Institute of Medicine (IOM) of the National Academies. He has chaired numerous National Academies studies on subjects ranging from elder mistreatment to underage drinking, including the landmark report *Ending the Tobacco Problem: A Blueprint for the Nation* (2007). Most recently, he chaired a major National Research Council study on juvenile justice reform. He received the Yarmolinsky

Medal in 2002 for his contributions to the IOM and the National Academies. In 2007, Professor Bonnie received the University of Virginia's highest honor, the Thomas Jefferson Award.

Claire D. Brindis, Dr.P.H., is director of the Philip R. Lee Institute for Health Policy Studies and professor of pediatrics and health policy in the Department of Pediatrics, Division of Adolescent Medicine, and the Department of Obstetrics, Gynecology and Reproductive Health Sciences at the University of California, San Francisco (UCSF). She is also a director of the Bixby Center for Global Reproductive Health and executive director of the National Adolescent and Young Adult Health Information Center at UCSF. Incorporating a variety of quantitative and qualitative methodologies, as well as community participatory research, Dr. Brindis's research focuses on program evaluation and the translation of research into policy at the local, state, and national levels. Dr. Brindis's specific content expertise is in the areas of young adult, adolescent, and child health policy and analyses of a wide array of health policies, including those related to improving health care access for underserved communities and pursuing strategies for closing the gap between the emergence of evidence-based innovation and its application to policy and programs. Her research portfolio includes policy analyses and evaluations of the state of California's comprehensive teenage pregnancy prevention programs; evaluation of California's Family Planning, Access, Care, and Treatment (Family PACT) program; the impact of health care reform on adolescents' and young adults' access to health care, including the incorporation of clinical preventive guidelines aimed at improving the health of young adults; and the University of Southern California Annenberg School of Journalism's Health Disparities Media Fellowship Program. Dr. Brindis recently served as a member of the Planning Committee on Improving the Health, Safety, and Well-Being of Young Adults. She is the recipient of numerous awards, including the California Department of Health Services' 2000 Beverlee A. Myers Award for Excellence in Public Health, the Federal Maternal and Child Health Bureau Director's Award, the Association of Maternal and Child Health Programs' John C. MacQueen Lecture Award, UCSF's Chancellor's Award for the Advancement of Women, and the University of California, Los Angeles' (UCLA's) 2012 Alumni Hall of Fame Award. She was elected to the IOM in 2010.

Gladys Carrión, J.D., was appointed commissioner of New York City's Administration for Children's Services in December 2013. Previously, she served as commissioner of the New York State Office of Children & Family Services (OCFS), starting in January 2007. The numerous responsibilities she oversaw at OCFS included foster care, adoption and adoption assistance, child protective services, preventive services for children and families, child care services, and protective programs for vulnerable adults. Commissioner Carrión was also responsible for directing the oversight, administration, and management of specialized programs for juvenile delinquents and juvenile offenders and residential facilities for youth placed in the custody of OCFS by the family and criminal courts. She also was responsible for directing the functions performed by the Commission for the Blind and state government responses to the needs of Native Americans on reservations and in communities. Previously, Commissioner Carrión was senior vice president for community investment with the United Way of New York City and executive director of Inwood House, one of the oldest youth-serving organizations in the city. She also served for 3 years as commissioner of the New York City Community Development Agency, where she developed citywide policy and programs designed to address the human services needs of the city's most vulnerable citizens and ensured the quality performance of more than 300 city-funded community-based organizations. Until her appointment, Commissioner Carrión was chair of the board of the New York Foundation and served on the advisory board of Child Welfare Watch. She has served on numerous boards, including the Executive Committee of Legal Services of New York, the Puerto Rican Policy Institute, and Youth Ministries for Peace and Justice. She served as chair of the Latino Child Welfare Collaborative, a project of the Committee for Hispanic Children and Families, and was a member of the Children's Defense Fund's New York Advisory Board and a co-chair of Agenda for Children Tomorrow (ACT). Commissioner Carrión is a graduate of Fordham University and New York University School of Law.

Mark E. Courtney, Ph.D., M.S.W., is a professor in the School of Social Service Administration at the University of Chicago. He also has served on the faculties of the University of Wisconsin (1992-2000) and University of Washington (2007-2010). His fields of special interest are child welfare policy and services, the connection between child welfare services and other institutions serving families living in poverty, and the transition to adulthood for vulnerable populations. He is a faculty affiliate of Chapin Hall at the University of Chicago, for which he served as director from 2001 to 2006. He was a member of the MacArthur Foundation Research Network on Transitions to Adulthood and Public Policy from 2003 to 2010. Dr. Courtney received the 2010 Peter W. Forsythe Award for leadership in public child welfare from the National Association of Public Child Welfare Administrators and in 2012 was elected as a fellow of the American Academy of Social Work and Social Welfare. He obtained his M.S.W. and Ph.D. degrees from the School of Social Welfare at the University of California, Berkeley.

Robert Crosnoe, Ph.D., is Elsie and Stanley E. (Skinny) Adams, Sr. centennial professor in liberal arts at The University of Texas at Austin, where he is a faculty member in the Department of Sociology, Department of Psychology (by courtesy), and Population Research Center. Prior to coming to the university, he received his Ph.D. in sociology from Stanford University and completed a postdoctoral fellowship at the University of North Carolina at Chapel Hill. Dr. Crosnoe's main field of interest is the connections among health, human development, and education and the contributions of these connections to socioeconomic and immigration-related inequalities in American society. This work has been published in *Child Development*, *Developmental Psychology*, *American Sociological Review*, *Social Forces*, *American Educational Research Journal*, and *Journal of Marriage and Family* and supported by grants from the National Institute of Child Health and Human Development (NICHD), the William T. Grant Foundation, and the Foundation for Child Development. His books include *Mexican Roots, American Schools: Helping Mexican Immigrant Children Succeed* (Stanford University Press), *Fitting In, Standing Out: Navigating the Social Challenges of High School to Get an Education* (Cambridge University Press); and *Physical Attractiveness and the Accumulation of Social and Human Capital from Adolescence into Adulthood* (forthcoming at SRCD Monographs, with Rachel Gordon). Dr. Crosnoe also is a member of the NICHD Early Child Care Network, the Governing Council of the Society for Research in Child Development, the Governing Council of the Society for Research on Adolescence, and the Advisory Board of the Council of Contemporary Families, and serves as deputy editor of the *Journal of Marriage and Family*.

Maryann Davis, Ph.D., is a research associate professor with the Center for Mental Health Services Research in the University of Massachusetts Medical School's Department of Psychiatry. She is also director of the Learning and Working During the Transition to Adulthood Rehabilitation Research and Training Center (Transitions RTC). Dr. Davis is an internationally recognized expert on services for transition-age youth and young adults with serious mental health conditions. Her focus is on improving treatments and services for this population that help support the development of adult role functioning during the transition from adolescence to mature adulthood. She has examined the ways in which policies and practices support or impede the healthy development of this unique age group. Dr. Davis's work also emphasizes the development of evidence-based interventions that can improve this population's transition to adulthood, including facilitation of mental health and related treatment, as well as interventions that reduce criminal behavior and substance abuse while supporting the successful completion of education and training and movement into mature work life.

Kathleen Mullan Harris, Ph.D., is James E. Haar distinguished professor of sociology, adjunct professor of public policy, and faculty fellow at the Carolina Population Center at the University of North Carolina at Chapel Hill. Her research addresses social inequality and health, with particular focus on family demography, the transition to adulthood, health disparities, and family formation. Dr. Harris is director and principal investigator of the National Longitudinal Study of Adolescent Health (Add Health), a longitudinal study of more than 20,000 teens who are being followed into adulthood. Under her leadership, the study has pioneered innovative study designs and integrative multidisciplinary research to understand social, environmental, behavioral, biological, and genetic linkages in developmental and health trajectories from adolescence into adulthood. Dr. Harris has been an advocate within the social science and population disciplines for bridging the social and biomedical sciences to advance knowledge of the development of health disparities from both an inter- and intragenerational perspective to inform public health and social policy. She is currently building Add Health into a nationally representative intergenerational study with parallel social, behavioral, biological, and genetic data across three generations. Her publications appear in journals in a wide range of disciplines, including demography, genetics, family, epidemiology, biology, public policy, survey methodology, medicine, and social and health behavior. Dr. Harris serves on several national advisory boards for leading National Institutes of Health (NIH) studies, as well as on the National Advisory Committee on Racial, Ethnic, and Other Populations of the Census Bureau and the Committee on Population of the National Academy of Sciences. She received her doctorate in demography from the University of Pennsylvania. She was awarded the 2004 Clogg Award for Early Career Achievement from the Population Association of America and was president of the Population Association of America in 2009. Dr. Harris was elected to the National Academy of Sciences in 2014.

Harry J. Holzer, Ph.D., is a professor of public policy at Georgetown University and an institute fellow at the American Institutes for Research. Since receiving his Ph.D. in economics from Harvard, he also has served as a professor of economics at Michigan State University, chief economist of the U.S. Department of Labor (in the Clinton Administration), and an institute fellow at the Urban Institute. Dr. Holzer was co-founder and co-director of the Georgetown Center on Poverty, Inequality and Public Policy. He serves on the board of directors of the National Skills Coalition and the Economic Mobility Corporation, as well as several other advisory or editorial boards. Dr. Holzer has authored or edited 11 books and published several dozen articles in peer-reviewed journals, focusing heavily on employer behavior and job quality but also on particular groups of low-income workers, such as current/former welfare recipients, less-educated young men, ex-offenders, and noncustodial fathers in the job market. His policy interests include workforce development, equal employment opportunity and affirmative action, the Earned Income Tax Credit, Pell Grant reform, immigration reform, and removing barriers to work for ex-offenders.

Charles E. Irwin, Jr., M.D., is distinguished professor of pediatrics, director of the Division of Adolescent & Young Adult Medicine, and director of health policy in the Department of Pediatrics at UCSF School of Medicine and UCSF Benioff Children's Hospital. Dr. Irwin is a graduate of Hobart College, Dartmouth Medical School, and UCSF. He heads two national policy centers focused on adolescents and young adults: the National Adolescent Health Information and Innovation Center and the Public Policy Analysis and Education Center for Adolescent and Young Adult Health. His current health services research focuses on improving preventive screening practices in clinical settings and the financial and structural issues altering adolescents' and young adults' ability to access health care in the United States. Dr. Irwin has received numerous awards, including the Society for Adolescent Medicine's Outstanding Achievement Award, the American Academy of Pediatrics' Adele D. Hofmann Lifetime Achievement Award in Adolescent Medicine, the Swedish Medical Society's Lectureship Award, the National Center for Youth Law's Annual Award for Improving the Lives of At Risk Youth, and the Society for Adolescent Medicine's Hillary E. C. Millar Award for innovative Approaches to Adolescent Health Care. He has published more than 150 peer-reviewed articles and several chapters in medical textbooks. He served as the first chairman of the Subspecialty Board in Adolescent Medicine of the American Board of Pediatrics, a member of the Executive Council of the Section of Adolescent Health of the American Academy of Pediatrics, and president of the Society for Adolescent Medicine. Currently, he is editor-in-chief of the *Journal of Adolescent Health*, the official journal of the Society for Adolescent Health and Medicine. He has just completed service as co-chair of the National Advisory Council on Healthcare Research and Quality's Subcommittee on Quality Measures for Children's Healthcare. Dr. Irwin has played an active role in the three reports issued by the IOM/National Academies on adolescent and young adult health: *Losing Generations: Adolescents in High Risk Settings* (1993); *Adolescent Health Services: Missing Opportunities* (2008); and *Improving the Health, Safety, and Well-Being of Young Adults: Workshop Summary* (2013).

Beatriz Luna, Ph.D., is Staunton Professor of Psychiatry and Pediatrics and professor of psychology at the University of Pittsburgh. Her research focuses on the brain basis underlying the transition from adolescent- to adult-level cognitive control of behavior. She uses neuroimaging methods to characterize changes in brain function underlying developmental improvements in core cognitive and reward processing tasks. In 2005 Dr. Luna received the Presidential Early Career Award in Science and Engineering for her pioneering work on the brain basis of development. Her work has informed three Supreme Court decisions related to extended sentences for juveniles, pediatric practice (National Alliance to Advance Adolescent Health), and education. Dr. Luna received her B.A. in psychology at American University, her M.A. in clinical psychology at Duquesne University, and her Ph.D. in developmental psychology at the University of Pittsburgh.

Velma McBride Murry, Ph.D., is Betts Chair of Education and Human Development in the Peabody School at Vanderbilt University. Her work has focused on the significance of context in studies of African American families and youth, particularly the impact of racism on family functioning. This research has elucidated the dynamics of this contextual stressor in the everyday life of African Americans and the ways in which family members buffer each other from the impact of the external stressors that cascade through African American lives. Prior to joining the Vanderbilt faculty in 2008, Dr. Murry was professor of child and family development and co-director of the Center of Family Research in the Institute for Behavioral Research at the University of Georgia. She received a Ph.D. in human development and family studies from the University of Missouri, Columbia.

Zizi Papacharissi, Ph.D., is professor and head of the Communication Department at the University of Illinois, Chicago. Her work focuses on the social and political consequences of online media. Her book *A Private Sphere: Democracy in a Digital Age* (Polity Press, 2010) examines how online media redefine understanding of public and private in late-modern democracies. She also recently edited a volume on online social networks titled *A Networked Self: Identity, Community, and Culture on Social Network Sites* (Routledge, 2010). Dr. Papacharissi is the author of 4 books and more than 40 journal articles, book chapters, and reviews, and she serves on the editorial boards of 11 journals, including the *Journal of Communication*, *Human Communication Research*, and *New Media and Society*. She is editor of the *Journal of Broadcasting and Electronic Media* and the new open-access and free Sage journal *Social Media and Society*. Her latest book, titled *Affective Publics: Sentiment, Technology and Politics*, will be published in late 2014 by Oxford University Press.

John Schulenberg, Ph.D., is professor of developmental psychology, research professor at the Institute for Social Research and Center for Human Growth and Development, and associate director of the Survey Research

Center, all at the University of Michigan. He has published widely on several topics concerning adolescence and the transition to adulthood, focusing on how developmental tasks and transitions relate to health risks and adjustment difficulties. His current research is on the etiology and epidemiology of substance use and psychopathology, focusing on risk factors, course, comorbidity, and consequences during adolescence and the transition to adulthood. Dr. Schulenberg is co-principal investigator of the national Monitoring the Future study, funded by the National Institute on Drug Abuse (NIDA), concerning substance use and psychosocial development across adolescence and adulthood. He collaborates on two international interdisciplinary projects involving several long-term studies addressing key questions about life-course pathways. His work has been funded by NIDA, the National Institute on Alcohol Abuse and Alcoholism (NIAAA), NICHD, the National Institute of Mental Health (NIMH), the National Science Foundation (NSF), and the Robert Wood Johnson Foundation. For these and other institutes and foundations, he has served on numerous advisory and review committees, including as chair of the NIH Psychosocial Development and Risk Prevention Study Section. He also serves on several editorial boards and for guest-edited special issues of *Addiction*, *Applied Developmental Science*, *Development and Psychopathology*, and the *Journal of Longitudinal and Life-course Studies*. He is a fellow of the APA and president-elect of the Society for Research on Adolescence.

Martin Sepúlveda, M.D., FACP, is an IBM fellow and vice president of health systems and policy research in the Research Division of IBM Corporation. He collaborates in research with a diverse global team of computational, informatics, and other IBM scientists to advance population health improvement through health systems and health care innovation. Previously, he served as IBM vice president for integrated health services and led in the areas of health policy and strategy, health benefits and clinical care program design, occupational and behavioral health, wellness, safety, and productivity for IBM globally. He is a fellow of the American College of Physicians, the American College of Preventive Medicine, and the American College of Occupational and Environmental Medicine. He was elected an honorary member of the American Academy of Family Medicine and serves on the IOM's Board on Population Health and Public Health Practice, the American Board of Internal Medicine Foundation, and the Council on Health Research for Economic Development. Dr. Sepúlveda received his M.D. and M.P.H. degrees from Harvard University. He completed residencies in internal medicine at the UCSF Hospitals and occupational/environmental medicine at the National Institute for Occupational Safety and Health; trained in the Epidemic Intelligence Service of the U.S. Centers for Disease Control and Prevention (CDC); and completed a fellowship in internal medicine at the University of Iowa Hospitals and Clinics.

Kasisomayajula "Vish" Viswanath, Ph.D., is an associate professor in the Department of Social and Behavioral Sciences at the Harvard School of Public Health (HSPH), a faculty member with the Center for Community-Based Research at the Dana-Farber Cancer Institute, and faculty director of the Health Communication Core of the Dana-Farber/Harvard Cancer Center (DF/HCC). Dr. Viswanath is also the leader of DF/HCC's Cancer Risk and Disparities Program. He is the founding director of DF/HCC's Enhancing Communications for Health Outcomes Laboratory. He also chairs the steering committee for the health communication concentration at HSPH and teaches health communication courses within this concentration. Before coming to Harvard, Dr. Viswanath was acting associate director of the Behavioral Research Program, Division of Cancer Control and Population Sciences at the National Cancer Institute. His work draws on literature in communication science, social epidemiology, and social and health behavior sciences and focuses on the use of translational communication science to influence public health policy and practice. He focuses in particular on elucidating the relationship between communication inequalities and disparities in public and individual health in diverse populations and the implications for the use of knowledge translation to influence public health practice and policy. His research is supported by funding from private and public agencies, including NIH and CDC.

Leslie R. Walker, M.D., is chief of the Division of Adolescent Medicine at Seattle Children's Hospital and professor of pediatrics at the University of Washington School of Medicine. She also directs the University of Washington's Leadership Education in Adolescent Health training program. Dr. Walker was the 2011-2012 president of the Society for Adolescent Health and Medicine, and has served on many national committees and boards dedicated to the health and well-being of adolescents. She has been a member of previous committees of the National Academies/IOM, including Adolescent Health Care Services and Models of Care for Treatment, Prevention and Healthy Development, and the Standing Committee on Family Planning. Dr. Walker is currently involved in national and local efforts to address workforce diversity in the field of pediatrics. Her research interests and publications are in the areas of attention-deficit hyperactivity disorder and substance abuse, adolescent health care transition, and teenage pregnancy prevention.

Index

A

D

E

F

H

I

N

T

Y